Respiratory System

Series editor
Daniel Horton-Szar
BSc (Hons)
United Medical and Dental Schools of Guy's and St Thomas's Hospitals (UMDS), London

Faculty advisors
Simon Cross
BSc, MD, MRCPath
Senior Lecturer and Honorary Consultant, Department of Pathology, University of Sheffield Royal Hallamshire Hospital

Jacqueline Hardcastle
BSc, PhD
Senior Lecturer, Department of Biomedical Science, University of Sheffield

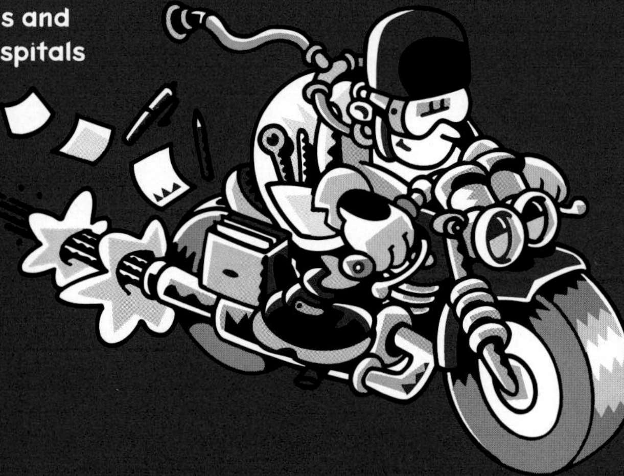

Respiratory System

Angus Jefferies
BEng (Hons)
United Medical and Dental Schools of Guy's and St Thomas's Hospitals (UMDS), London

Andrew Turley
BMedSci (Hons)
University of Sheffield Royal Hallamshire Hospital Sheffield

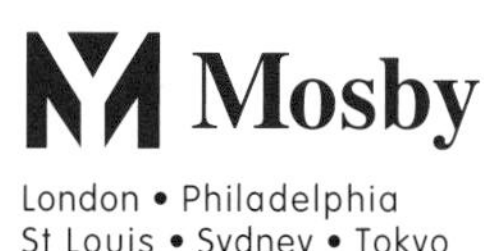

London • Philadelphia
St Louis • Sydney • Tokyo

Editor Louise Crowe
Development Editor Filipa Maia
Project Manager Dave Burin
Designer Greg Smith
Layout Gisli Thor
Illustration Management Mike Saiz
Illustrators Sandie Hill
Jenni Miller
Marion Tasker
David Graham
Robin Dean
Amanda Williams
Debra Woodward
Kevin Faerber
Cover Design Greg Smith
Production Andrea Ford
Index Jan Ross

ISBN 0 7234 2991 X

Published by Harcourt Publishers Limited, Robert Stevenson House,
1-3 Baxter´s Place, Leith Walk, Edinburgh EH1 3AF.

Printed by GraphyCems, Navarrra, Spain.
Text set in Crash Course-VAG Light; captions in Crash Course-VAG Thin.

Published 1999.
Reprinted 2001.

The publisher, authors and faculty advisors have undertaken reasonable endeavours to check drugs, dosages, adverse effects and contraindications in this book. We recommend that the reader should always check the manufacturer's instructions and information in the British National Formulary (BNF) or similar publication before administering any drug.

Cataloguing in Publication Data
A catalogue record for this book is available from the British Library.

Preface

Whether you aspire to be a hospital-based physician, a surgeon or a general practitioner, respiratory medicine will play a pivotal part in your daily workload. However, first things first and to pass the medical finals, which is every student's immediate aim, you are going to need to have a good grasp of respiratory medicine both factually and clinically.

As students, we are partly assessed on how much factual information we can remember from a wide diversity of specialities. Bearing this in mind, we have written *Crash Course: Respiratory Medicine* with the aim of combining the core information of basic clinical skills with the preclinical factual base, providing a fully integrated basic review. Numerous illustrations, hints and tips boxes, and comprehension check boxes at the end of each section, will hopefully make things a little easier around exam time.

We hope that *Crash Course: Respiratory Medicine* proves to be most useful in the pre-exam cramming period!

Angus Jefferies
Andrew Turley

Physiology and pathology of the respiratory system enter into all aspects of medicine. Lung disease accounts for a large proportion of morbidity and mortality - asthma, emphysema, chronic bronchitis and lung cancer all being common diseases. A patient cannot be safely anaesthetised or ventilated without a good working knowledge of respiratory physiology, and this knowledge can also be applied in other areas including sports medicine.

Crash Course: Respiratory System offers a succinct, yet comprehensive, coverage of respiratory physiology and pathophysiology that is essential information for all medical students. It contains many useful distillations of knowledge in the form of clinical algorithms, tables and hints and tips boxes. There are also multiple-choice, short-answer and essay questions for you to test your knowledge.

Diligent study of *Crash Course: Respiratory Medicine* will provide a core knowledge of respiratory medicine that will be useful for a professional lifetime as well as ensuring success in relevant examinations.

Simon Cross
Jacqueline Hardcastle
Faculty Advisors

OK, no-one ever said medicine was going to be easy, but the thing is, there are very few parts of this enormous subject that are actually difficult to understand. The problem for most of us is the sheer volume of information that must be absorbed before each round of exams. It's not fun when time is getting short and you realize that: a) you really should have done a bit more work by now; and b) there are large gaps in your lecture notes that you meant to copy up but never quite got round to.

This series has been designed and written by senior medical students and doctors with recent experience of basic medical science exams. We've brought together all the information you need into compact, manageable volumes that integrate basic science with clinical skills. There is a consistent structure and layout across the series, and every title is checked for accuracy by senior faculty members from medical schools across the UK.

I hope this book makes things a little easier!

Danny Horton-Szar
Series Editor (Basic Medical Sciences)

Acknowledgements

Andrew Turley would like to gratefully acknowledge the help, advice, criticism and encouragement of Professor Alyn H. Morice who has nurtured his interest in respiratory medicine from an early stage in his medical career.

Figure Credits

Figures 9.13, 9.14, 9.16, 9.23, 9.24, 11.1 and 11.34 are taken from *A Concise Textbook of Clinical Imaging 2e,* David Sutton and Jeremy W R Young, Mosby, 1995.

Figures 9.18, 9.19, 9.20 and 11.36 are taken from *Color Atlas and Text of Clinical Medicine 2nd edition,* Charles D Forbes and William F Jackson, Mosby–Wolfe, 1997.

Figures 1.1, 1.2 and 2.2 are taken from *Human Histology 2nd edition,* A Stevens and J Lowe, Mosby, 1997.

Figures 11.5 and 11.8A–E are taken from *Pathology,* A Stevens and J Lowe, Mosby, 1995.

Figures 6.27, 6.31 and 6.39 are taken from *Clinical Examination 2nd edition,* O Epstein, GD Perkin, DP de Bono and J Cookson, Mosby, 1997.

Contents

To Naomi (AJ)

To Charlotte and our families (AT)

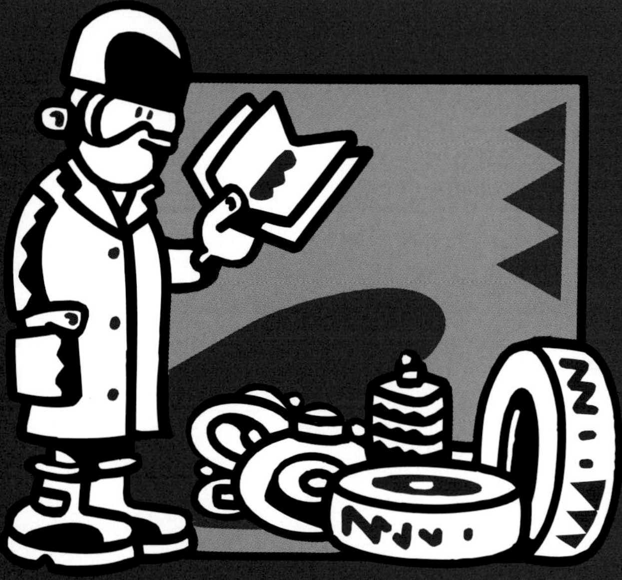

DEVELOPMENT, STRUCTURE, AND FUNCTION

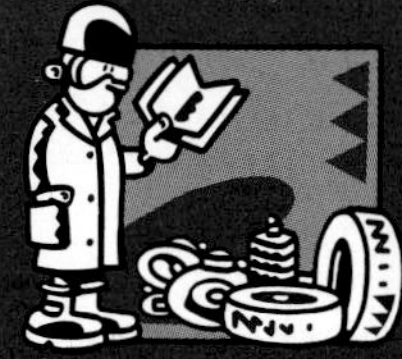

1. Overview of the Respiratory System

OVERALL STRUCTURE AND FUNCTION

Respiration

Respiration is considered to be the processes involved in oxygen transport from the atmosphere to the body tissues and the release and transportation of carbon dioxide produced in the tissues to the atmosphere.

This book will not discuss the oxygen-requiring biochemical reactions of tissue respiration, so for further information see *Crash Course, Metabolism and Nutrition.*

In addition, respiration is also concerned with:

- Regulation of the pH of body fluids.
- Regulation of body temperature.

Microorganisms rely on diffusion to and from their environment for the supply of oxygen and removal of carbon dioxide. Humans, however, are unable to rely on diffusion because:

- Their surface area : volume ratio is too small.
- The diffusion distance from the surface of the body to the cells is too large and the process would be far too slow to be compatible with life.

Remember that diffusion time increases with the square of the distance and as a result, the human body has had to develop a specialized respiratory system to overcome these problems. This system has two components:

- A gas-exchange system that provides a large surface area for the uptake of oxygen from, and the release of carbon dioxide to, the environment. This function is performed by the lungs.
- A transport system that delivers oxygen to the tissues from the lungs and carbon dioxide to the lungs from the tissues. This function is carried out by the cardiovascular system.

Structure

The respiratory system can be neatly divided into upper respiratory tract (nasal and oral cavities, pharynx, larynx, and trachea) and lower respiratory tract (main bronchi and lungs) (Fig. 1.1).

Upper respiratory tract

The upper respiratory tract has a large surface area, a rich blood supply, and its epithelium (respiratory epithelium) is covered by a mucous secretion. Within the nose, hairs are present, which act as a filter. The function of the upper respiratory tract is to warm, moisten, and filter the air so that it is in a suitable condition for gaseous exchange in the distal part of the lower respiratory tract.

Lower respiratory tract

The lower respiratory tract consists of the lower part of the trachea, the two primary bronchi, and the lungs. These structures are contained within the thoracic cavity.

Lungs

The lungs are the organs of gas exchange and act as both a conduit for air flow (the airway) and a surface for movement of oxygen into the blood and carbon dioxide out of the blood (the alveola capillary membrane).

The lungs consist of airways, blood vessels, nerves, and lymphatics, supported by parenchymal tissue. Inside the lungs, the two main bronchi divide into smaller and smaller airways until the end respiratory unit (acinus) is reached (Fig. 1.2).

Acinus

The acinus is that part of the airway that is involved in gaseous exchange (i.e. the passage of oxygen from the lungs to the blood and carbon dioxide from the blood to the lungs). The structure of the acinus is considered in detail in Chapter 2.

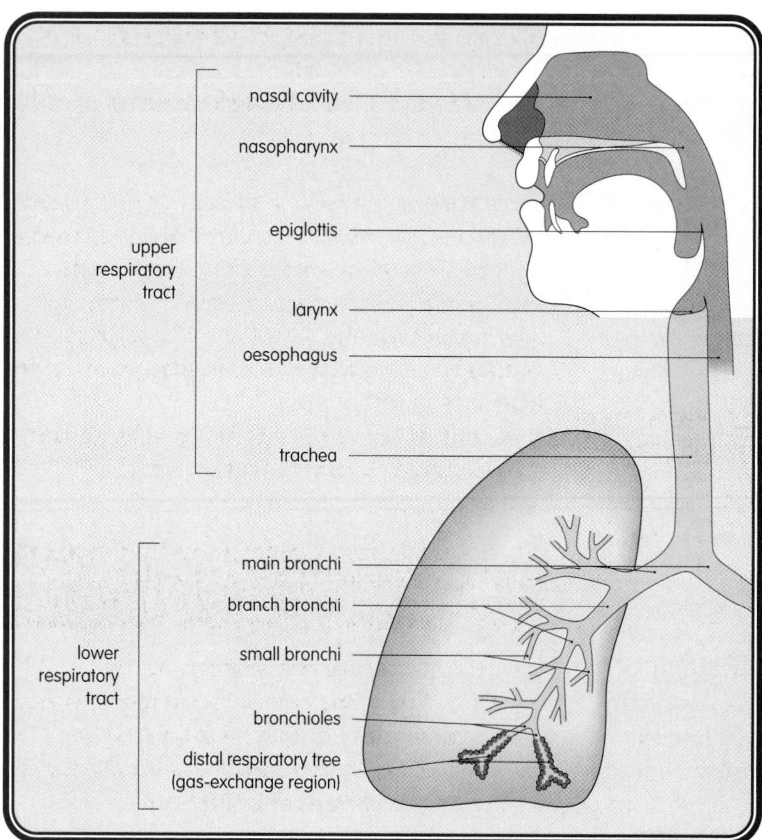

Fig. 1.1 A schematic diagram of the respiratory tract.

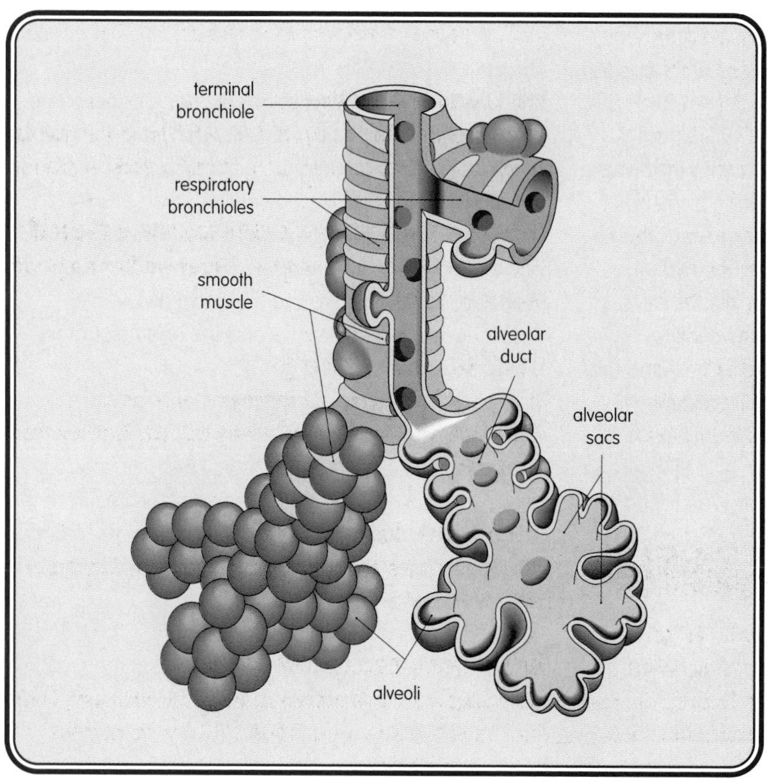

Fig. 1.2 The acinus, or respiratory unit. This part of the airway is involved in gas exchange.

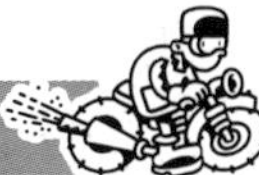

Pleurae

The lung, chest wall, and mediastinum are covered by two continous layers of epithelium known as the pleurae. The inner pleura covering the lung is the visceral pleura and the outer pleura covering the chest wall and mediastinum is the parietal pleura. These two pleurae are closely opposed and are separated by only a thin layer of liquid. The liquid acts as a lubricant and allows the two surface to slip over each other during breathing.

THE DYNAMICS OF BREATHING

The aim of breathing is to increase air flow into the lungs so that gaseous exchange can occur between the alveoli and the blood.

Air flows from a high-pressure area to a low-pressure area. We cannot change the local atmospheric pressure around us to a level higher than that inside our lungs; the only obvious alternative is to lower the pressure within the lungs. We achieve this pressure reduction by expanding the size of the chest.

The main muscle of respiration is the diaphragm, upon which the two lungs sit. The diaphragm is dome shaped; contraction flattens the dome, increasing intrathoracic volume. This is aided by the external intercostal muscles, which raise the rib cage; this results in a lowered pressure within the thoracic cavity and hence the lungs, supplying the driving force for air flow into the lungs.

Expiration is largely a result of elastic recoil of the lung tissue. However, in forced expiration (e.g. during coughing), the abdominal muscles increase intra-abdominal pressure, forcing the contents of the abdomen against the diaphragm. In addition, the internal intercostal muscles lower the rib cage. These actions greatly increase intrathoracic pressure and enhance expiration.

CONTROL OF BREATHING

Respiration must respond to the metabolic demands of the body. This is achieved by a control system within the brainstem (the respiratory centres—see Chapter 5, pp 83) which receives information from various sources in the body where sensors monitor:

- Partial pressures of oxygen and carbon dioxide (PO_2 and PCO_2) in the blood.
- pH of the extracellular fluid within the brain.
- Mechanical changes in the chest wall

On the basis of information they receive, the respiratory centres modify ventilation to ensure that oxygen supply and carbon dioxide removal from the tissues matches their metabolic requirements. The actual mechanical change to ventilation is carried out by the respiratory muscles: these are known as the effectors of the control system.

Respiration can also be modified by higher centres (e.g. during speech, anxiety, emotion, etc.).

SUMMARY OF RESPIRATORY FUNCTIONS

The functions of the respiratory system can be summarized as air flow, gaseous exchange, transport of oxygen and carbon dioxide, control of breathing, acid–base regulation, body temperature regulation, metabolism, excretion, and hormonal activity.

Air flow

Air flow causes ventilation of the lungs.

Gaseous exchange

Gaseous exchange of oxygen and carbon dioxide occurs between the alveolar gas and pulmonary capillary blood.

Transport of oxygen and carbon dioxide

Oxygen and carbon dioxide are carried within the blood stream to the tissues.

Control of breathing

Breathing is controlled to match perfusion and ventilation with the body's biochemical and behavioural requirements.

Acid–base regulation

By controlling the partial pressure of carbon dioxide, pH may be altered (see Chapter 4).

Body temperature regulation

Body temperature is achieved mainly by insensible heat loss. Thus, by altering ventilation, body temperature may be regulated.

Metabolism

The lungs have a huge vascular supply and thus a large number of endothelial cells. Hormones such as noradrenaline, prostaglandins, and 5-hydroxytryptamine are taken up by these cells and destroyed. Some exogenous compounds are also taken up by the lungs and destroyed (e.g. amphetamine and imipramine).

Excretion

Carbon dioxide and some drugs (notably those administered through the lungs; e.g. general anaesthetics) are excreted by the lungs.

Hormonal activity

Hormones (e.g. steroids) act on the lungs. Insulin enhances glucose utilization and protein synthesis. Angiotensin II is formed in the lungs from angiotensin I (by angiotensin-converting enzyme). Damage to the lung tissue causes the release of prostacyclin PG I_2, which prevents platelet aggregation.

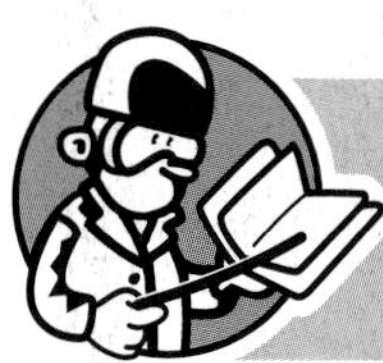

- **Why have humans developed a respiratory system?**
- **Describe how breathing is brought about.**
- **List the main functions of the respiratory system.**

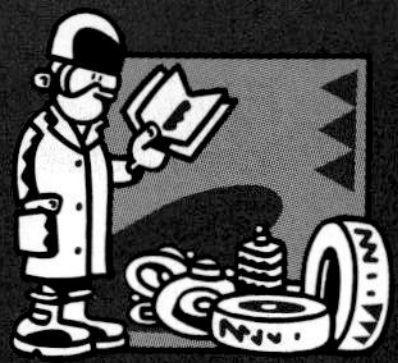

2. Organization of the Respiratory System

UPPER RESPIRATORY TRACT

Macroscopic structure of the upper respiratory tract

Nasal cavities

The nose consists of an external part (the external nose) and an internal part (the nasal cavities). The nose is used for smelling and breathing. This book will be concerned only with the internal nose (Figs 2.1 and 2.2) and its function in breathing.

Blood and nerve supply, and lymphatic drainage

The nose is richly supplied with blood and nerve fibres. Lymphatic vessels drain into the submandibular node, then drain into deep cervical nodes.

Pharynx

The tube of the respiratory tract becomes common with the alimentary tract in the middle part of the pharynx. The pharynx lies anteriorly to the cervical vertebra and is described as being divided into three parts: the nasopharynx, oropharynx, and the laryngopharynx, which open anteriorly into the nose, the mouth, and the larynx, respectively (Fig. 2.3).

- Superiorly, the pharynx is attached to the base of the skull, but opens anteriorly into the nasal cavities at the choanae (posterior nares).
- Inferiorly, the pharynx is continuous with the oesophagus at the level of the cricoid cartilage. At this level, the pharynx also opens anteriorly into the larynx below the epiglottis, which covers the opening to the larynx during swallowing.

Important openings into the nasal cavity (from top to bottom) are:

- **In the sphenoethmoidal recess—opening of the sphenoid sinus.**
- **In the superior meatus openings of the posterior ethmoidal air sinuses.**
- **In the middle meatus openings (anteriorly to posteriorly) of the frontal nasal duct, maxillary sinus, and anterior and middle ethmoid air sinus through the hiatus semilunaris.**
- **In the inferior meatus—the nasolacrimal duct, draining the conjunctival sac.**

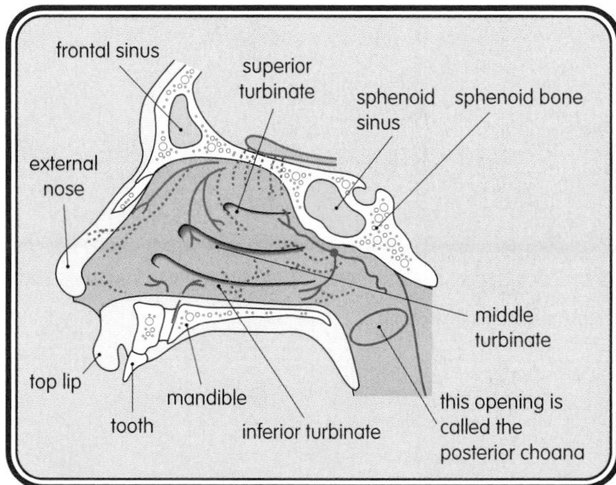

Fig. 2.1 Lateral view of the nasal cavity showing the rich blood and nerve supply

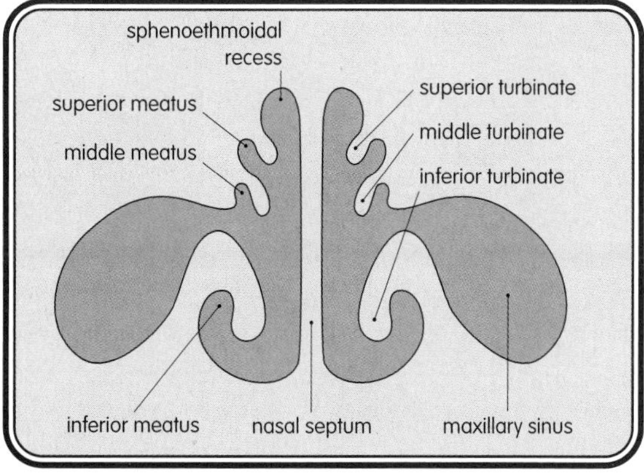

Fig. 2.2 Frontal view of the nasal cavity showing the superior, middle and inferior turbinates and the air spaces created by these: the superior, middle and inferior meatus.

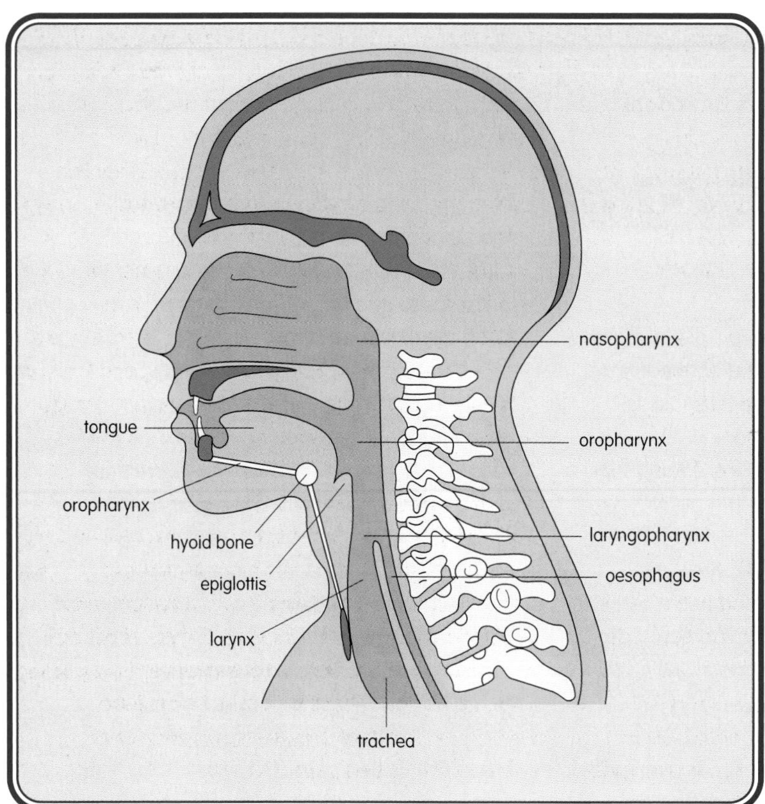

Fig. 2.3 Schematic diagram showing midline structures of the head and neck.

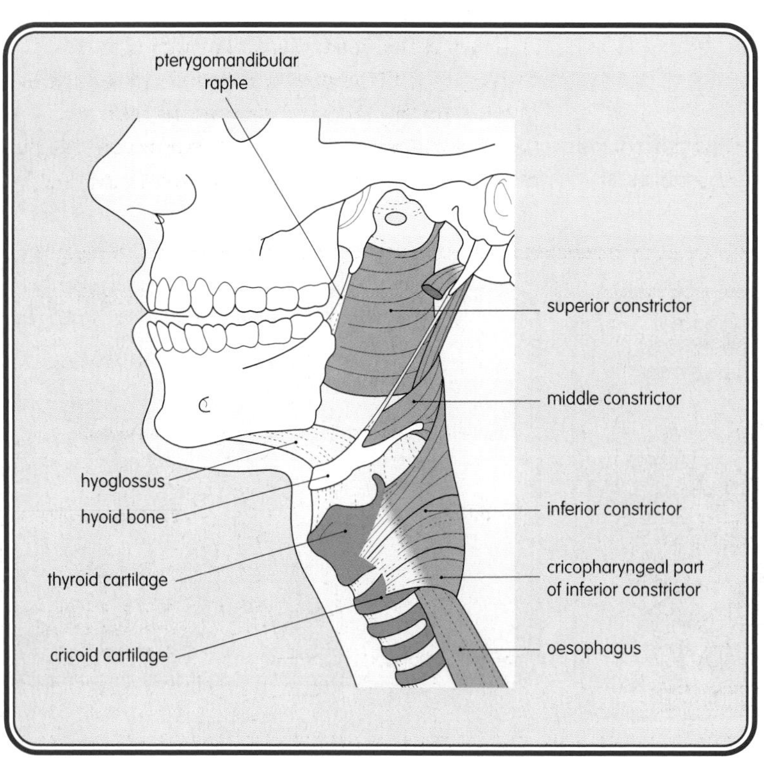

Fig. 2.4 The pharynx, showing the superior, middle and inferior constrictors.

Musculature, blood and nerve supply, and l ymphatic drainange

Three muscles surround the fascial tube of the pharynx: the superior, middle, and inferior constrictor muscles (Fig. 2.4).

The arterial blood supply of the pharynx is from the external carotid through the superior thyroid, ascending pharyngeal, facial, and lingual arteries. Venous drainage is by a plexus of veins on the outer surface of the pharynx to the internal jugular vein.

Both sensory and motor nerve supplies are from the pharyngeal plexus (cranial nerves IX and X); the maxillary nerve (cranial nerve V) supplies the nasopharynx with sensory fibres.

Lymphatic vessels drain directly into the deep cervical lymph nodes.

Nasopharynx

The nasopharynx is situated above the soft palate and opens anteriorly into the nasal cavities. During swallowing, the nasopharynx is cut off from the oropharynx by the soft palate. The nasopharynx contains the opening of the eustachian canal (pharyngotympanic or auditory tube) and the adenoids, which lie beneath the epithelium of its posterior wall.

The oropharynx and laryngopharynx are not discussed here in detail because this is beyond the scope of this book.

Larynx

At its inferior end, the larynx is continuous with the trachea. At its superior end, it is attached to the U-shaped hyoid bone and lies below the epiglottis of the tongue. The larynx is made up of a cartilaginous skeleton linked by a number of membranes. This cartilaginous skeleton consists of the epiglottis, thyroid, arytenoid, and cricoid cartilages. Fig. 2.5 shows an external view and a median section through the larynx.

The larynx has three main functions:

- As an open valve, to allow air to pass when breathing.
- Protection of the trachea and bronchi during swallowing. The vocal cords close, the epiglottis folds back covering the opening to the larynx, and the larynx is pulled upwards and forwards beneath the tongue.
- Speech production (phonation).

Other functions of the larynx are in:

- Coughing—on entering the larynx, mucus that has been brought up from the lungs by the ciliary action of respiratory epithelium triggers a cough reflex.
- Lifting—the larynx is closed so that the chest wall can act as a solid base for the muscles during lifting.
- Fixing the diaphragm to allow a rise in intra-abdominal pressure, pushing inferiorly as in defecation or micturition.

Musculature

The muscles of the larynx are split into external and internal muscles. There is only one external muscle of the larynx (cricothyroid), although many other muscles attach to the thyroid membrane and cartilage. Cricothyroid has its origin at the arch of the cricoid and attaches to the lower border of the thyroid cartilage. The

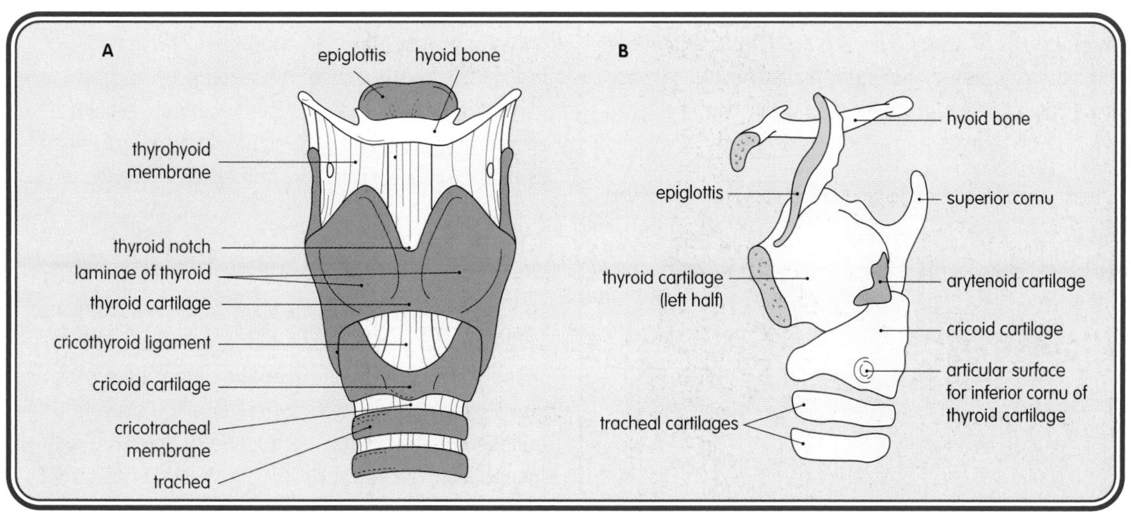

Fig. 2.5 The larynx. (A) External view—anterior aspect. (B) Median section through the larynx, hyoid bone, and trachea.

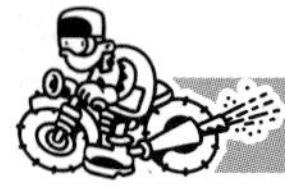

internal muscles may change the shape of the larynx: they protect the lungs by a sphincter action and adjust the vocal cords in phonation.

The internal laryngeal muscles consist of:

- Posterior and lateral cricoarytenoid muscles.
- Thyroarytenoid muscle.
- Thyroepiglottic muscle.
- Aryepiglottic muscle.
- Interarytenoid muscles.

Blood and nerve supply

The blood supply of the larynx is from superior and inferior laryngeal arteries, which are accompanied by the superior and recurrent laryngeal branches of the vagus nerve (cranial nerve X). The internal branch of the superior laryngeal nerve supplies the mucosa of the larynx above the vocal cords, the external branch supplies the cricothyroid muscle. The recurrent laryngeal nerve supplies the mucosa below the vocal cords and all the intrinsic muscles apart from the cricothyroid.

Lymphatic drainage

Lymph vessels above the vocal cords drain into the upper deep cervical lymph nodes; below the vocal cords lymphatic vessels drain into the lower cervical lymph nodes.

Trachea

The trachea is a membranous tube about 10 cm in length, running from the cricoid cartilage (at the level of the sixth cervical vertebra) to its bifurcation at the carina (at the level of the fourth or fifth thoracic vertebra). The trachea is approximately 2.5 cm in diameter and is supported by C- shaped rings of hyaline cartilage. The rings are completed posteriorly by the trachealis muscle. Important relations of the trachea within the neck are:

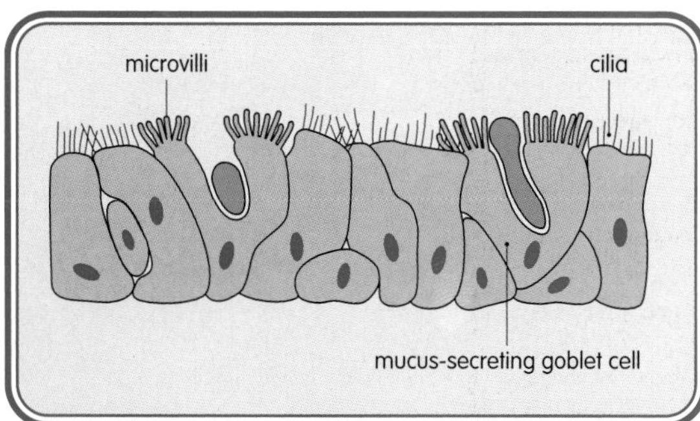

Fig. 2.6 Respiratory epithelium.

- The thyroid gland, which straddles the trachea, its two lobes sitting laterally and its isthmus anteriorly with the inferior thyroid veins.
- The common carotid arteries, which lie lateral to the trachea.
- The oesophagus, which lies directly behind the trachea, and the recurrent laryngeal nerve, which lies between these two structures.

Microscopic structure of the upper respiratory tract

Nasal sinuses and nasopharynx

The upper one-third of the nasal cavity is covered in yellowish olfactory epithelium.

The lower two-thirds of the nasal cavity, the nasal sinuses, and the nasopharynx are lined with pseudostratified columnar epithelium (Fig. 2.6). Throughout these cells are mucus-secreting goblet cells with microvilli on their luminal surface. This pattern of epithelium is known as respiratory-type epithelium which, with the exception of a few areas, lines the whole of the respiratory tract down to the terminal bronchioles.

Adenoids

The nasopharyngeal tonsil is a collection of mucosa-associated lymphoid tissue (MALT) that lies behind epithelium of the roof and the posterior surface of the nasopharynx. Together with the palatine tonsils and the lymphoid tissue on the dorsum of the tongue these form Waldeyer's ring.

Oropharynx and laryngopharynx

The oropharynyx and laryngopharynx have two functions as parts of both the respiratory and alimentary tracts. They are lined with nonkeratinized stratified squamous (NKSS) epithelium several layers thick and are kept moist by numerous salivary glands.

Larynx and trachea

The epithelium of the larynx is made up of two types: NKSS epithelium covers the vocal folds, vestibular fold, and larynx above this level; below the level of the vestibular fold (with the exception of the vocal folds, which are lined with keratinized stratified squamous epithelium), the larynx and trachea are covered with respiratory-type epithelium.

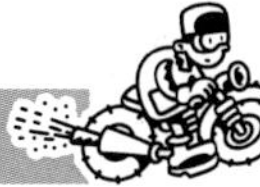

Development of the upper respiratory tract

Branchial arches and pharyngeal pouches

During week 4 of development, the branchial arches are formed; these are gill-like pairs of folds at the cranial (head) end of the embryo. Eventually, six pairs of branchial arches are formed, which are numbered craniocaudally (head to tail) from first to sixth arches. Not all arches are present at once; the first two branchial arches degenerate before the sixth arch is formed. The branchial arches form the major part of the branchial apparatus, which consists of:

- Branchial arches.
- Pharyngeal pouches: evaginations of endodermal tissue, situated inside the primitive pharynx.
- Branchial grooves: located between the branchial arches.
- Branchial membrane: bilaminar layer of ectodermal and endodermal tissue between the branchial arches.

The branchial arches form the skeletal and muscular components of the head and neck. Mesenchymal cells group together within the arches to form clusters called branchial arch cartilages, which form skeletal structures. Mesenchymal cells also form myoblasts (primitive muscle cells), which migrate to form the musculature of the head and neck.

Fig. 2.7 shows the formation of structures from the branchial arches and branchial pouches.

The nerve supply of the branchial arches is derived from the cranial nerves. The first and second branchial arches receive sensory fibres from cranial nerve V and motor fibres from cranial nerve VII. The nerve supply to

A	Branchial arch derivatives			
Arch No.	**Bones and cartilage**	**Muscles**	**Nerves**	**Ligaments**
1	incus and malleus	tensor tympani tensor veli palatini muscles of mastication mylohyoid anterior belly of digastric	cranial nerve V (trigeminal nerve)	anterior ligament of malleus sphenomandibular ligament
2	stapes styloid process lesser coruna of the hyoid bone superior part of hyoid	stapedius stylohyoid posterior belly of digastric muscles of facial expression	cranial nerve VII (facial nerve)	stylohyoid ligament
3	inferior part of body of hyoid greater coruna of hyoid	stylopharyngeus	cranial nerve IX (glossopharyngeal nerve)	
4/6	thyroid cartilage cricoid cartilage arytenoid cartilage corniculate and cuneiform cartilage	cricothyroid levator veli palatini pharyngeal constrictors intrinsic laryngeal muscles striated oesophageal muscle	cranial nerve X recurrent laryngeal nerve superior laryngeal nerve branches of the vagus nerve	

B	Pharyngeal pouch derivatives
Pouch No.	**Development**
1	tubotympanic recess → auditory tube and tympanic cavity
2	mostly obliterate → intratonsillar cleft endoderm → epithelium of tonsil and crypts
3	endoderm (dorsal) → inferior parathyroids endoderm (ventral) → thymus
4	endoderm (dorsal) → superior parathyroid endoderm (ventral) → ultimobranchial bodies, which fuse with the thyroid gland to form the parafollicular cells

Fig. 2.7 Derivatives of (A) branchial arches and (B) pharyngeal pouches.

the third branchial arch is from cranial nerve IX, which also supplies stylopharyngeus. The fourth and sixth branchial arches are supplied by two branches of the vagus nerve (cranial nerve X): the superior laryngeal and recurrent laryngeal nerves.

Primitive mouth, nasal and oral cavities, and nasopharynx and oropharynx

The primitive mouth is formed by a depression in the ectoderm at the cranial end of the embryo called the stomodeum, initially separated from the primitive pharynx by a bilaminar membrane called the oropharyngeal membrane. This membrane ruptures at about day 24–26, by which time the ectoderm of the cranial end of the embryo has already invaginated, forming the nasal and oral cavities.

Respiratory system (larynx and trachea)

The respiratory tract starts as a groove in the median plane of the primitive pharynx, the laryngotracheal groove. This groove deepens to form the laryngotracheal diverticulum and continues caudally (towards the tail) into the splanchnic mesenchyme, its distal end forming the lung bud. The cartilage and smooth muscle of the larynx are formed from the mesenchyme surrounding the diverticulum (Fig. 2.8). The foregut is separated from the diverticulum by the tracheoesophageal septum; when the diverticulum lengthens this is called the laryngotracheal tube. Defects in development may result in a tracheo-oesophageal fistula.

The connective tissue, cartilages, and smooth muscle of trachea develop from the splanchnic mesenchyme, the glandular tissue developing from the endoderm.

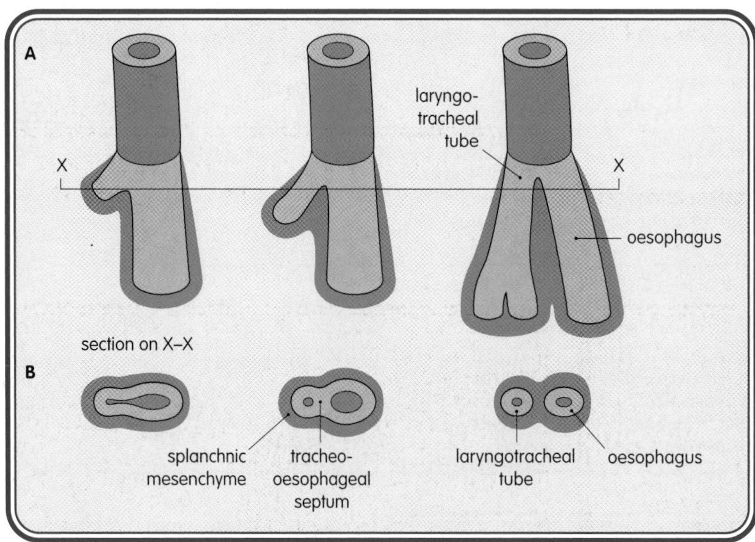

Fig. 2.8 Formation of the trachea and larynx: (A) lateral view; (B) cross-section on X–X.

- **Describe the anatomy of the upper respiratory tract, giving significant clinical details where appropriate.**
- **Draw and describe respiratory-type epithelium.**
- **Briefly describe the development of the upper respiratory tract.**
- **List the derivatives of the branchial arches and pharyngeal pouches.**

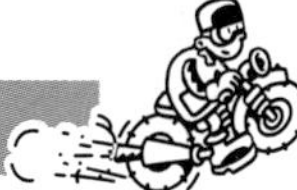

LOWER RESPIRATORY TRACT

Macroscopic structure of the lower respiratory tract

The lower respiratory tract consists of:

- The lower part of the trachea.
- The two main bronchi.
- Lobar bronchi, segmental bronchi, and smaller bronchi.
- Bronchioles and terminal bronchioles.
- The end respiratory unit.

These structures make up the tracheobronchial tree (Fig. 2.9). The structures distal to the two main bronchi are contained within a tissue known as the lung parenchyma.

Thorax

The cone-shaped thoracic cavity is bounded superiorly by the first rib and inferiorly by the diaphragm. The thorax is narrow at the top (thoracic inlet) and wide at its base (thoracic outlet).

The thoracic wall is supported and protected by the bony thoracic cage consisting of:

- Thoracic vertebrae.
- Manubrium.
- Sternum.
- Twelve pairs of ribs with associated costal cartilages (Fig. 2.10).

Each rib makes an acute angle with the spine and:

- Articulates with the body and transverse process of its equivalent thoracic vertebra.
- Articulates with the body of the vertebra above.

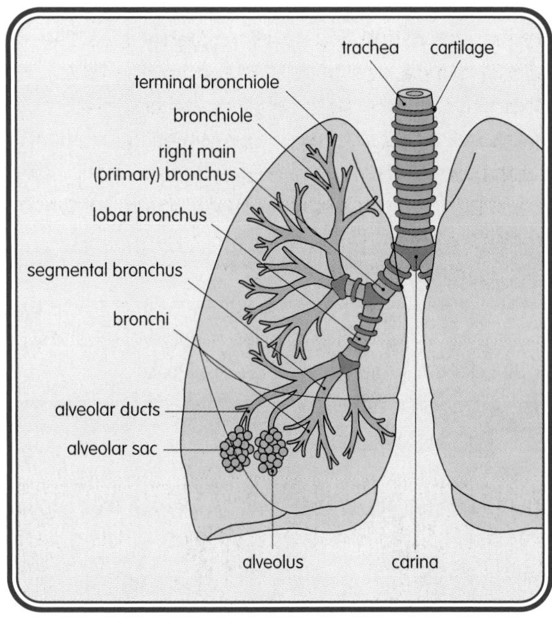

Fig. 2.9 Tracheobronchial tree. Schematic showing the divisions of the airway down to the end respiratory unit (acinus).

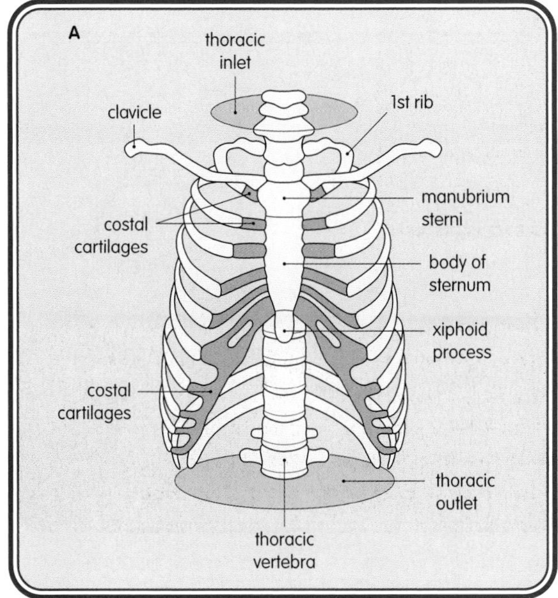

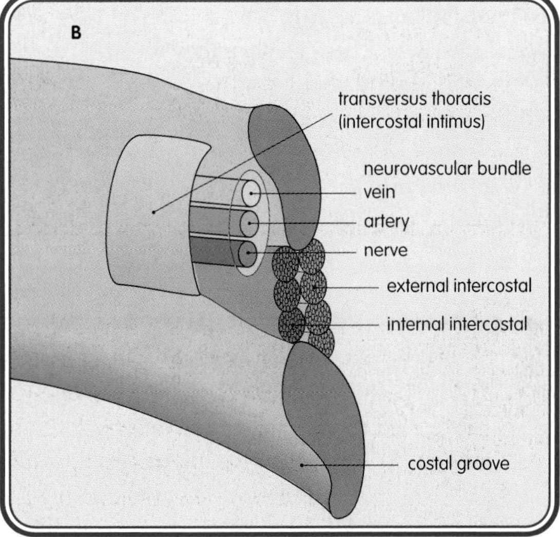

Fig. 2.10 The thoracic cage (A) and details of the subcostal neurovascular bundle (B).

The upper seven ribs (true ribs) articulate anteriorly through their costal cartilages with the sternum. The eighth, ninth, and tenth ribs (false ribs) articulate with the costal cartilages of the next rib above. The eleventh and twelfth ribs (floating ribs) are smaller and their tips are covered with a cap of cartilage.

The space between each rib is known as the intercostal space. Lying obliquely between adjacent ribs are the internal and external intercostal muscles. The intercostal muscles support the thoracic cage; their other functions include:

- External intercostal muscles—raise the rib cage and increase intrathoracic volume.
- Internal intercostal muscles—lower the rib cage and reduce intrathoracic volume.

The mechanics of ventilation breathing will be covered in detail in Chapter 3. Deep to the intercostal muscles and under cover of the costal groove lies a neurovascular bundle of vein, artery, and nerve (see Fig. 2.10). This anatomy is important during some procedures (e.g. when inserting a chest drain into a pneumothorax, the drain is inserted through the intercostal space just above the rib to avoid hitting the subcostal vessels).

The thorax contains:

- Lungs, heart, and major vessels.
- Oesophagus, lower part of the trachea, and main bronchi.

Mediastinum

The mediastinum is situated in the midline and lies between the two lungs. It contains the:

- Heart and great vessels.
- Trachea and oesophagus.
- Phrenic and vagus nerves.
- Lymph nodes.

To gain an understanding of the functions and relations of the lower respiratory tract, it is important to know the anatomy of the thorax.

Pleurae and pleural cavities

The pleurae consist of a continuous serous membrane, which covers the external surface of the lung and is then reflected to cover the inner surface of the thoracic cavity (Fig. 2.11).

The differences between the visceral and parietal pleurae are:

- The visceral pleura lines the surface of the lungs.
- The parietal pleura lines the thoracic wall and the diaphragm.

The pleurae form a double layer, creating a potential space known as the pleural cavity. The visceral and parietal pleurae are so closely apposed that only a thin film of fluid is contained within the pleural cavity. This allows the pleurae to slip over each other during breathing, thus reducing friction. Normally, no cavity is actually present, although in pathological states this potential space may expand.

Where the pleura is reflected off the diaphragm onto the thoracic wall, a small space is created which is not filled by the lung tissue; this space is known as the costodiaphragmatic recess. At root of the lung (the hilum), the pleurae become continuous and form a double layer known as the pulmonary ligament (see Fig. 2.14).

The parietal pleura has a blood supply from intercostal arteries and branches of the internal thoracic artery. Venous and lymph drainage follow a return course similar to the arterial supply. Nerve supply is from the phrenic nerve; thus, if the pleura becomes

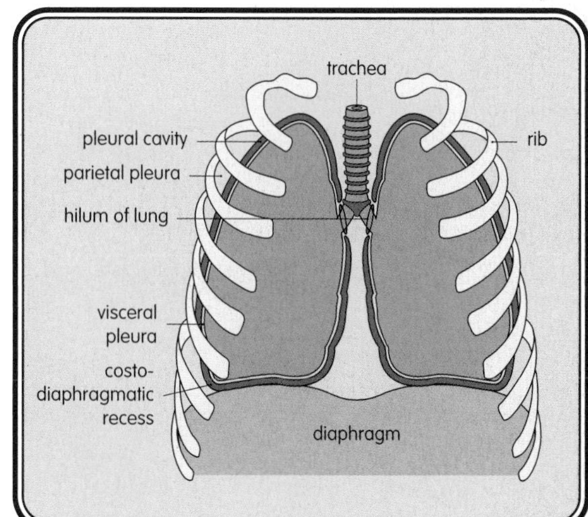

Fig. 2.11 The two pleurae form a potential space called the pleural cavity (shown in dark blue).

inflamed this may cause ipsilateral (on the same side of the body) shoulder-tip pain.

The visceral pleura has a blood supply from bronchial arteries. Venous drainage is through the bronchial veins to the azygous and hemiazygous veins. Lymph vessels drain through the superficial plexus over the surface of the lung to bronchopulmonary nodes at the hilum. The visceral pleura has an autonomic nerve supply and therefore does not give rise to the sensation of pain.

Inflammation of the pleurae can cause an increase in fluid between the parietal and visceral pleurae. This inflammation may give rise to a pleural rub on auscultation, which is said to mimic the sound of a foot crunching through fresh snow. Excess liquid or air may be present within the pleural cavity caused by:

- Pneumothorax.
- Haemothorax.
- Pleurisy and pneumonia.
- Malignancy.

Lungs

The two lungs are situated within the thoracic cavity and lie on either side of the mediastinum. During life, they appear pink and spongy, although carbon deposits give patchy discoloration. The lungs contain:

- Airways: bronchi, bronchioles, respiratory bronchioles, alveolar ducts, alveolar sacs, and alveoli.
- Vessels: pulmonary artery and vein and bronchial artery and vein.
- Lymphatics and lymph nodes.
- Nerves.
- Supportive connective tissue (lung parechyma), which has elastic qualities.

Figs 2.12 and 2.13 show the lateral and medial surfaces of the lung.

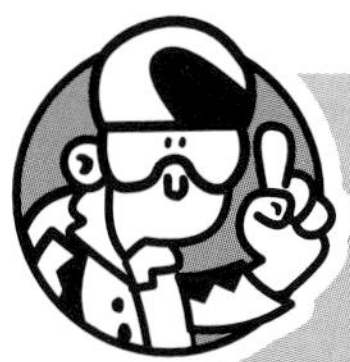

Lists are more difficult to remember than diagrams. Remember Fig. 2.13 and construct a list of medial relations from it.

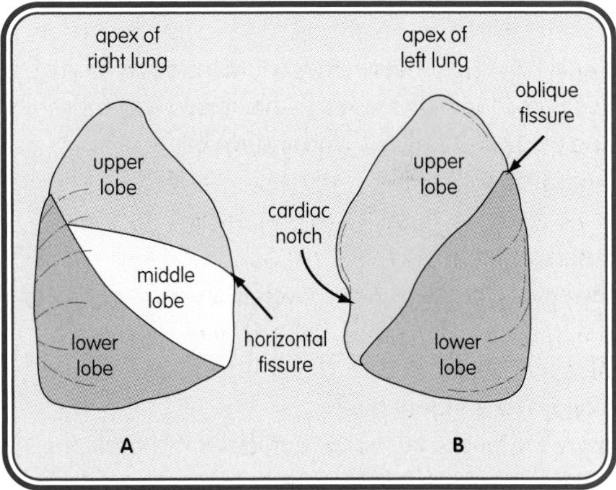

Fig. 2.12 Lateral aspect of the lungs. The outer surfaces show impression of the ribs. (A) left lung. (B) right lung.

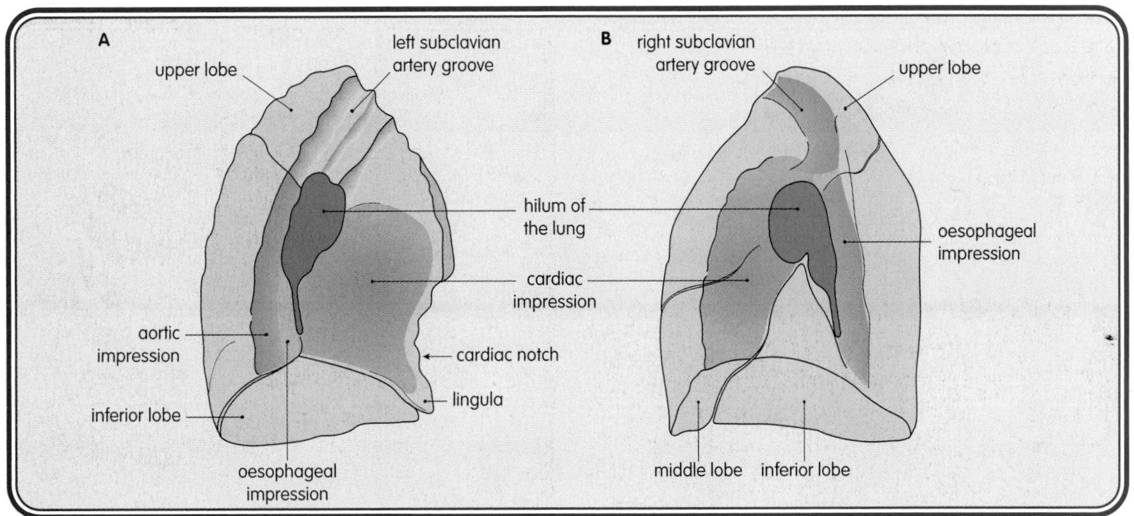

Fig. 2.13 Relations of the lung. (A) left lung. (B) right lung.

Hilum of the lung

The hilum or root of the lung (Fig. 2.14) consists of:

- Bronchi.
- Vessels: pulmonary artery and vein.
- Nerves.
- Lymph nodes and lymphatic vessels.
- Pulmonary ligament.

Bronchopulmonary segments

The trachea divides to form the left and right primary bronchi, which in turn divide to form lobar bronchi, supplying air to the lobes of each lung. The lobar bronchi divide again to give segmental bronchi, which supply air to regions of lung known as a bronchopulmonary segments. The bronchopulmonary segment is both anatomically and functionally distinct. This is important because it means that a segment of diseased lung can be removed surgically (e.g. in tuberculosis).

Surface anatomy

The surface anatomy of the lungs is shown in Fig. 2.15.

Airways and the blood–air interface

Airways (respiratory tree)

Inside the thorax, the trachea divides into the left and right primary bronchi. The right main bronchus is shorter and more vertical than the left; for this reason, inhaled foreign bodies are more likely to pass into the right lung.

The primary bronchi within each lung divide into secondary or lobar bronchi. The lobar bronchi divide again into tertiary or segmental bronchi. The airways continue to divide, always splitting into two daughter airways of progressively smaller calibre until eventually forming bronchioles.

Fig. 2.9 outlines the structure of the respiratory tree. Each branch of the tracheobronchial tree can be classified by its number of divisions (called the generation number); the trachea is generation number 0. The trachea and bronchi contain cartilage in their walls for support and to prevent collapse of the airway. At about generation 10 or 11, the airways contain no cartilage in their walls and are known as bronchioles. Airways distal to the bronchi that contain no cartilage rely on lung parenchymal tissue for their support and are kept open by subatmospheric intrapleural pressure (radial traction).

Bronchioles continue dividing for up to 20 or more generations before reaching the terminal bronchiole. Terminal bronchioles are those bronchioles which supply the end respiratory unit (the acinus).

The tracheobronchial tree can be classified into two zones:

- The conducting zone (airways proximal to the respiratory bronchiole), involved in air movement by bulk flow to the end respiratory units.
- The respiratory zone (airways distal to the terminal bronchiole), involved in gaseous exchange.

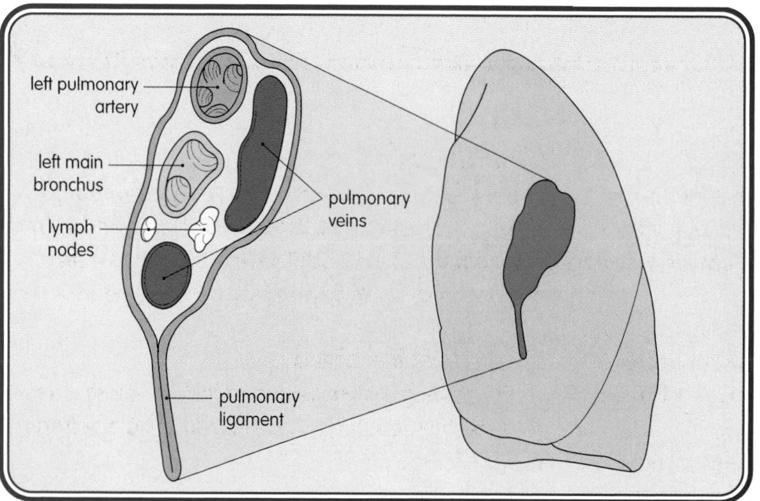

Fig. 2.14 Contents of the hilum.

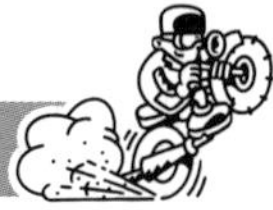

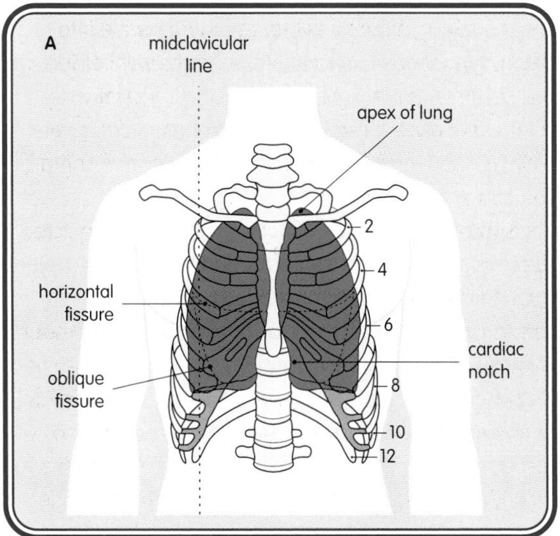

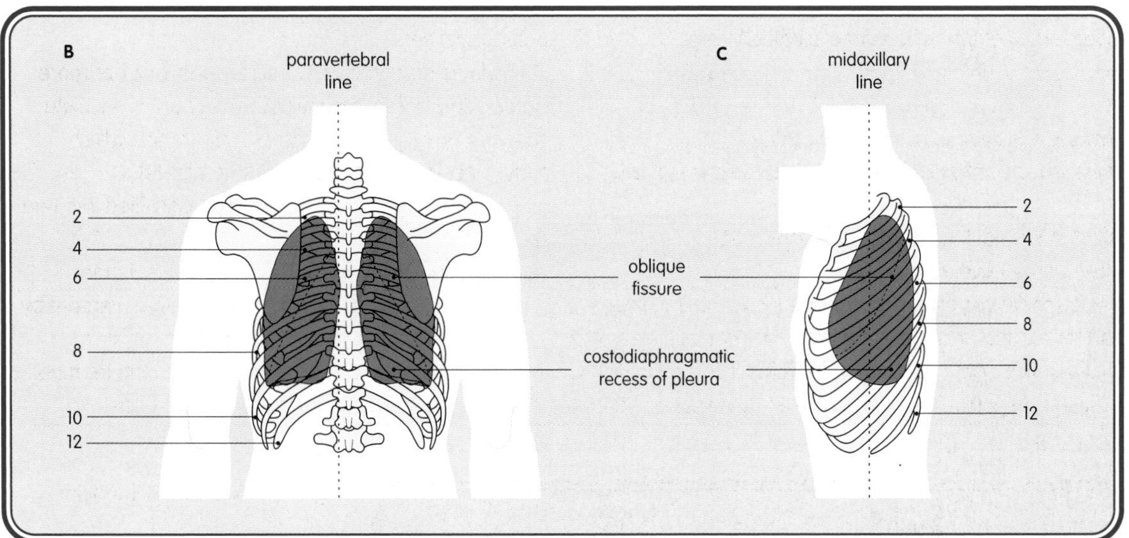

Fig. 2.15 Surface anatomy of the lungs and pleura (shaded area). (A) Anterior aspect; (B) posterior aspect; (C) lateral aspect.

Acinus

The acinus is that part of the airway that is involved in gaseous exchange (i.e. the passage of oxygen from the lungs to the blood and carbon dioxide from the blood to the lungs). The acinus consists of:

- Respiratory bronchioles, leading to the alveolar ducts.
- Alveolar ducts, opening into two or three alveolar sacs, which in turn open into several alveoli (see Fig. 1.2 on page 4).
- Alveoli also open directly into alveolar ducts and a few open directly into the respiratory bronchiole.

Lung lobules

Lung lobules (Fig. 2.16) are areas of lung containing groups of between three and five acini surrounded by parenchymal tissue. Each lobule is separated from a neighbouring lobule by an interlobular septum.

Structure of the airways

Descending the tracheobronchial tree, the structure of the airways changes; these differences are outlined in Fig. 2.17.

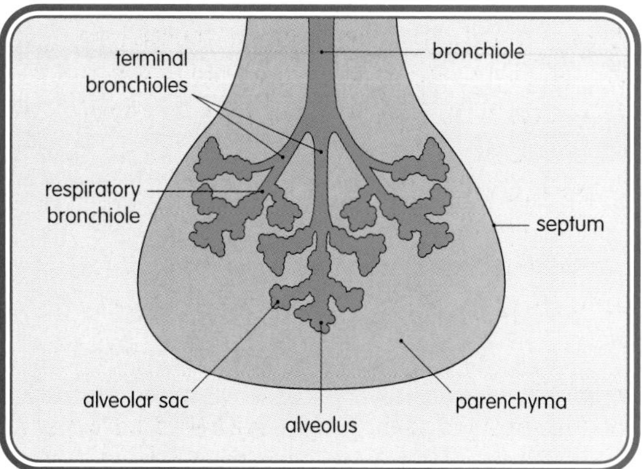

Fig. 2.16 The lung lobule.

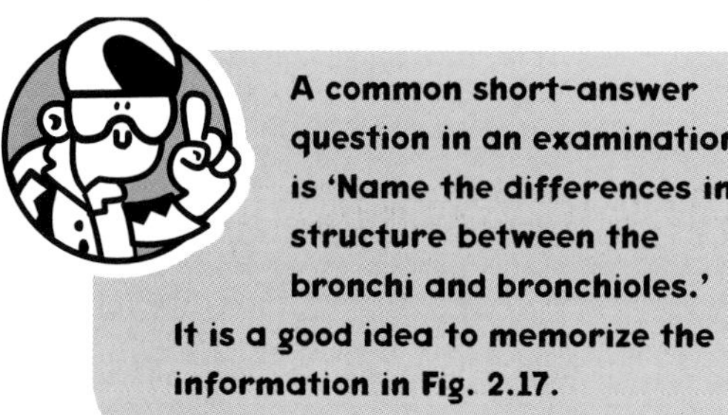

A common short-answer question in an examination is 'Name the differences in structure between the bronchi and bronchioles.' It is a good idea to memorize the information in Fig. 2.17.

The blood–air interface

The blood–air interface is a term that describes the site at which gaseous exchange takes place within the lung (Fig. 2.18).

The alveoli are microscopic blind-ending air pouches, of which there are 150–400 million in each normal lung. The alveoli open into alveolar sacs and then into alveolar ducts (see Fig. 1.2 on page 4). The walls of the alveoli are extremely thin and the alveoli are lined by a single layer of pneumocytes (types I and II) lying on a basement membrane. The alveolar surface is covered with alveolar lining fluid. The walls of the alveoli also contain capillaries.

It should be noted that:

- Average surface area of the alveolar–capillary membrane = 50–100 m^2 (about the same size as two tennis courts) .
- Average thickness of alveolar–capillary membrane = 0.4 μm.

This allows an enormous area for gaseous exchange and a very short diffusion distance.

Differences in structure of the airways						
Airway	**Generation No.**	**Lining**	**Wall structure**	**Diameter**	**Function**	**Contractile**
trachea	0	respiratory epithelium	membranous tube supported by C-shaped rings of cartilage loose submucosa and glands	25 mm	Con	No
bronchus	1–11	respiratory epithelium	fibromuscular tubes containing smooth muscle reinforced by β-receptors; incomplete rings of cartilage	1–10 mm	Con	Yes
bronchiole	12–16	simple ciliated cuboidal epithelium and Clara cells	membranous and smooth muscle in the wall; no submucosal glands and no cartilage	1.0 mm	Con	Yes
respiratory bronchiole	18+	simple ciliated cuboidal epithelium and Clara cells	merging of cuboidal epithelium with flattened epithelial lining of alveolar ducts; membranous wall	0.5 mm	Con/Gas	Yes
alveolar duct	20–23	flat nonciliated epithelium; no glands	outer lining of spiral smooth muscle; walls of ducts contain many openings laterally into alveolar sacs	0.5 mm	Gas	Yes
alveolus	24	pneumocytes types I and II	types I and II pneumocytes lie on an alveolar basement membrane; capillaries lie on the outer surface of the wall and form the blood–air interface	75–300 mm	Gas	No

Fig. 2.17 Differences in structure of the airways. Function: Con = conduction of air; Gas = gas exchange.

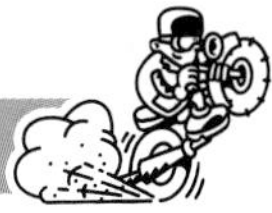

Microscopic structure of the lower respiratory tract

The basic structural components of the walls of the airways are shown in Fig. 2.19. The proportions of these components vary in different regions of the tracheobronchial tree. The absence of cartilage in the bronchioles and distal airways means that these airways must be kept open by radial traction (see Chapter 3). The walls of the airways are composed of:

- Respiratory epithelium (ciliated columnar type).
- Basement membrane.
- Lamina propria.
- Elastic fibres.
- Smooth muscle.
- Cartilage.

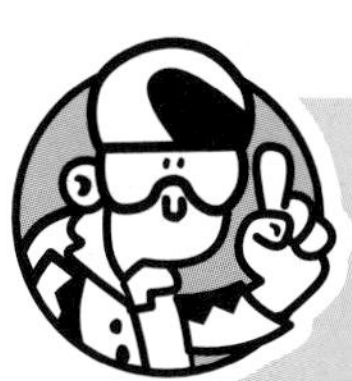

Layers through which gaseous exchange occurs are:

- **Alveolar lining fluid.**
- **Pneumocytes.**
- **Alveolar basement membrane.**
- **Capillary endothelium.**

Trachea

The respiratory epithelium of the trachea is tall and sits on a particularly thick basement membrane separating it from the lamina propria. The lamina propria of the trachea is loose and highly vascular, with a fibromuscular band of elastic tissue. Under the lamina propria lies a loose submucosa containing numerous

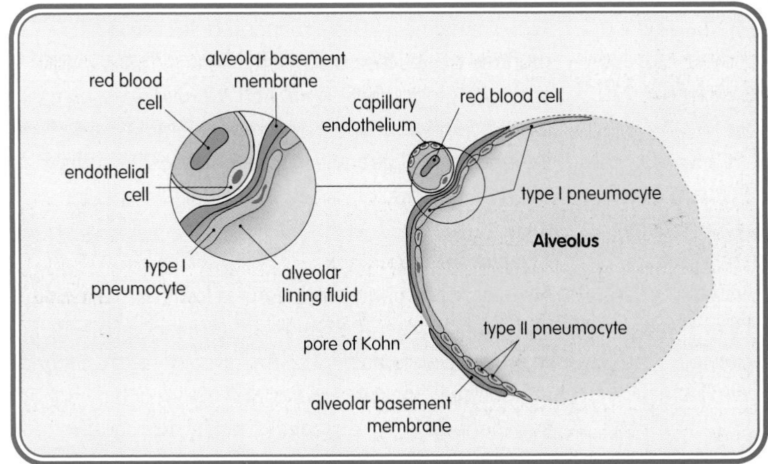

Fig. 2.18 Blood–air interface.

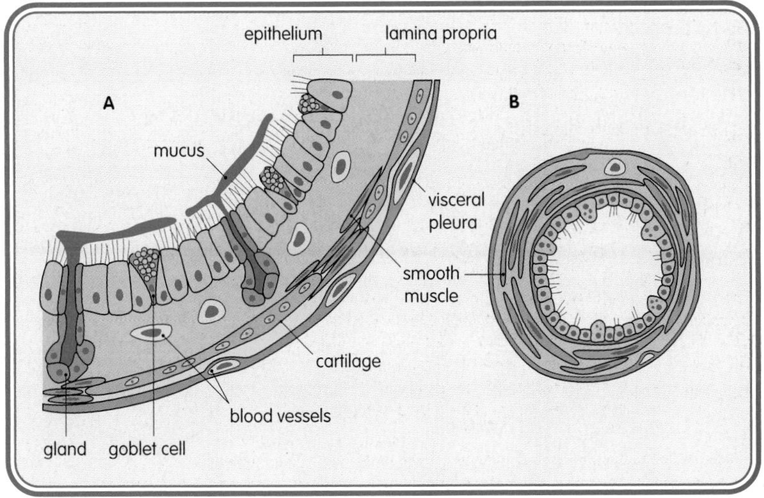

Fig. 2.19 Structure of the airways: (A) bronchial structure; (B) bronchiolar structure. (Redrawn with permission from Widdicombe and Davis.)

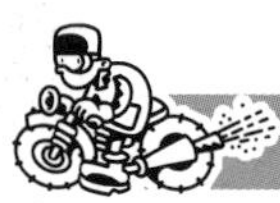

glands that secrete mucinous and serous fluid. The C-shaped cartilage found within the trachea is hyaline in type and merges with the submucosa.

Bronchi

Respiratory epithelium of the bronchi is shorter than the epithelium of the trachea and contains fewer goblet cells. The lamina propria is denser with more elastic fibres and it is separated from the submucosa by a discontinuous layer of smooth muscle. The lamina propria also contains mast cells.

The cartilage of the bronchi forms discontinuous flat plates and there are no C-shaped rings.

Tertiary bronchi

The epithelium in the tertiary bronchi is similar to that in the bronchi. The lamina propria of the tertiary bronchi is thin and elastic, being completely encompassed by smooth muscle. Submucosal glands are sparse and the submucosa merges with surrounding adventia. Mucosa-associated lymphoid tissue (MALT) is present (see p. 27).

Bronchioles

The epithelium of a bronchiole is ciliated cuboidal and contains clara cells, which are nonciliated and secrete proteinaceous fluid. Bronchioles contain no cartilage and no glands in the submucosa. The smooth muscle layer is prominent. Adjusting the tone of the smooth muscle layer alters airway diameter, enabling resistance to air flow to be effectively controlled.

Respiratory bronchioles

The respiratory bronchioles are lined by ciliated cuboidal epithelium, which is surrounded by smooth muscle. Clara cells are present within the walls of the respiratory bronchioles. Goblet cells are absent but there are a few alveoli in the walls; thus, the respiratory bronchiole is a site for gaseous exchange.

Alveolar ducts

Alveolar ducts consist of rings of smooth muscle, collagen, and elastic fibres. They open into two or three alveolar sacs, which in turn open into several alveoli. There are alveoli present in the walls and this is a site for gaseous exchange.

Alveoli

An alveolus is a blind-ending terminal sac of respiratory tract (Fig. 2.20). Most gaseous exchange occurs in the alveoli. Because alveoli are so numerous, they provide the majority of lung volume and surface area. The majority of alveoli open into the alveolar sacs. Communication between adjacent alveoli is possible through perforations in the alveolar wall called pores of Kohn. The alveoli are lined with type I and type II pneumocytes, which sit on a basement membrane. Type I pneumocytes are structural, whereas type II pneumocytes produce surfactant (see Chapter 3).

Type I pneumocytes

To aid gaseous diffusion, type I pneumocytes are very thin; they contain flattened nuclei and few mitochondria. Type I pneumocytes make up 40% of the alveolar cell population and 90% of the surface lining of the alveolar wall. Cells are joined by tight junctions.

Type II pneumocytes

Type II pneumocytes are rounded cells containing rounded nuclei; their cytoplasm is rich in mitochondria and endoplasmic reticulum, and microvilli exist on their exposed surface. Type II pneumocytes make up 60% of the alveolar cell population and 5–10% of the surface lining of the alveolar wall. They produce surfactant.

Alveolar macrophages

Alveolar macrophages are derived from circulating blood monocytes. They lie on an alveolar surface lining or on alveolar septal tissue. The alveolar macrophages phagocytose foreign material and bacteria; they are transported up the respiratory tract by mucociliary clearance.

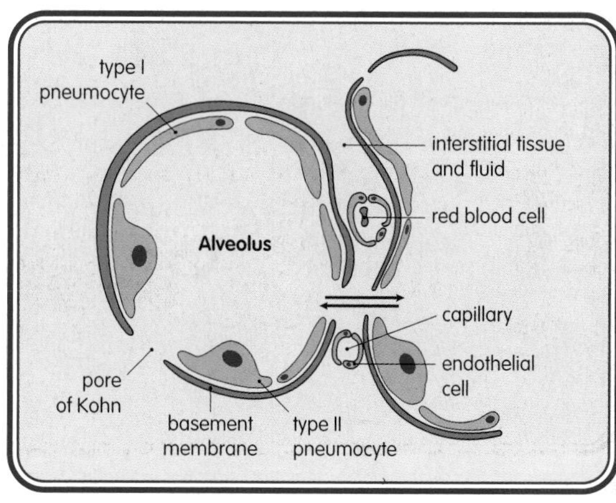

Fig. 2.20 The alveolus.

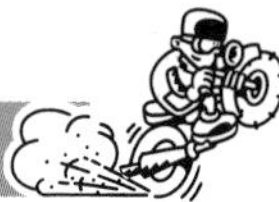

Development of the lower respiratory tract

Development of the bronchi

The laryngotracheal diverticulum develops into the lung bud, which divides into two bronchial buds by the end of week 4 (Fig. 2.21). As the bronchial bud enlarges, it forms two primary bronchi: the right and left primary bronchi (occurring in week 5). The right main bronchus is slightly larger and more vertical than the left. By the end of week 5, the secondary bronchi start to form.

By week 8, the segmental bronchi develop and together with the splanchnic mesenchyme form the bronchopulmonary segment. The splanchnic mesenchyme forms:

- Visceral pleura (mesoderm).
- Pulmonary capillaries and vasculature.
- Bronchial smooth muscle.
- Pulmonary connective tissue.

Development of the lungs

Lung development is divided into four stages: pseudoglandular, canalicular, terminal sac, and alveolar periods.

Stage 1—pseudoglandular period

During the pseudoglandular period, the major parts of the lung are formed; however, because there are no areas for gaseous exchange, respiration is not possible, and premature births at this stage do not survive.

Stage 2—canalicular period

During the canalicular period, there are increases in the diameter of airways, bronchi, and terminal bronchioles. The lung vasculature develops, and primitive end respiratory units are formed: respiratory bronchiole, alveolar duct, and terminal sac (primitive alveolus). Some gaseous exchange is possible, and there is a very small chance of survival if born after week 22 (although intensive care is required).

Stage 3—terminal sac period

During the terminal sac period, numerous terminal sacs develop; there is thinning of epithelial lining of terminal sacs. The squamous epithelium (type I pneumocytes) develops at about week 24, whereas secretory cells (type II pneumocytes) develop at around weeks 24–28. Type II pneumocytes produce surfactant, reducing surface tension within the liquid film within an alveolus and thus preventing alveolar collapse. After week 32, sufficient surfactant has been produced to allow the neonate to inflate its own lungs and allow the alveoli to continue to develop.

Stage 4—alveolar period

During the alveolar period, clusters of primitive alveoli are formed. Breathing occurs *in utero* by aspiration of amniotic fluid. The lungs are half full of liquid at birth; fluid is emptied through mouth and also absorbed into the blood and lymph. The alveoli mature after birth: for the first 3 years after birth, alveoli increase only in number, not size; between the ages of 3 and 8 years, alveoli increase in both size and number.

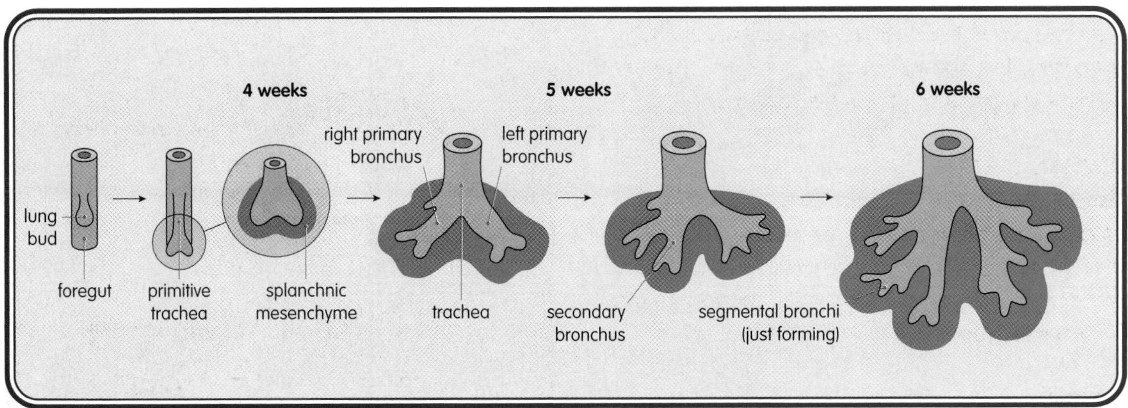

Fig. 2.21 Development of primary bronchi and the formation of the secondary and segmental bronchi.

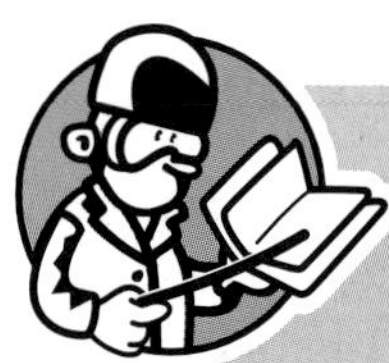

- Draw the anatomy of the thorax.
- Describe the anatomy and function of the pleurae.
- List the medial relations of the lungs and the contents of the hilum.
- Describe the structure of the tracheobronchial tree and define the differences between conducting and respiratory zones.
- Give an account of the blood–air interface.
- List the differences between bronchi and bronchioles.
- Describe the ultrastructure of the airways.
- Briefly describe the development of the lower respiratory tract.

ORGANIZATION OF THE PULMONARY CIRCULATION

Blood vessels

The lungs have a dual blood supply from the pulmonary and bronchial circulations. The bronchial circulation is part of the systemic circulation.

Pulmonary circulation

Function

The primary function of the pulmonary circulation is to allow the exchange of oxygen and carbon dioxide between the blood in the pulmonary capillaries and air in the alveoli. Oxygen is taken up into the blood while carbon dioxide is released from the blood into alveolar air.

Anatomy

Mixed venous blood is pumped from the right ventricle through the pulmonary arteries and thence through the pulmonary capillary network, which is in contact with the respiratory surface (Fig. 2.22). Gaseous exchange

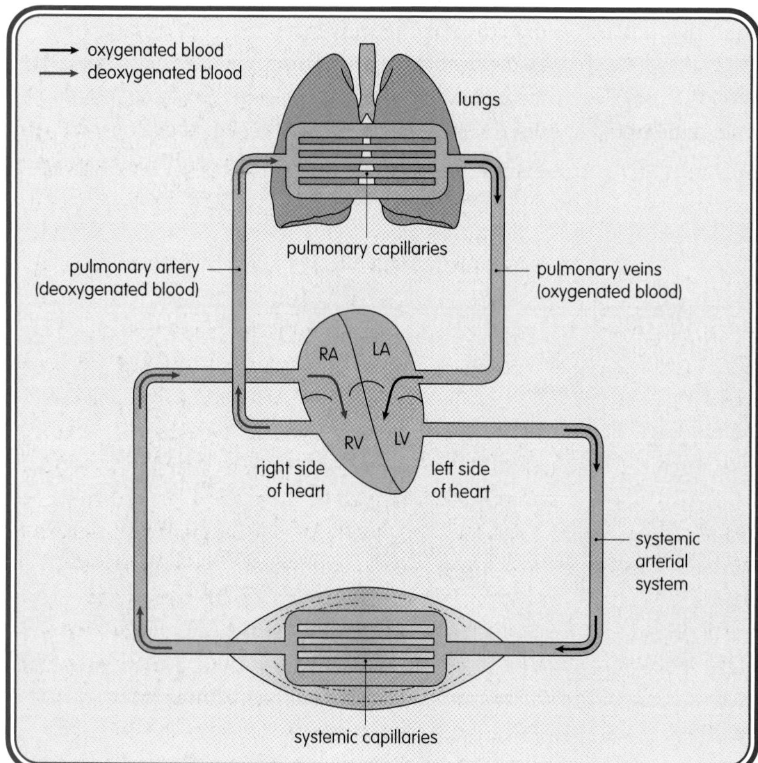

Fig. 2.22 Pulmonary circulation. Contained within the lungs are the pulmonary capillaries. These are situated in the alveolar walls. They are in contact with alveolar gas and this is the site where gaseous exchange takes place.

occurs (carbon dioxide given up by the blood, oxygen taken up by the blood) and the oxygenated blood returns through the pulmonary venules and veins to the left atrium. The pulmonary capillary network offers a huge gas exchange area of approximately 50–100 m^2.

Bronchial circulation

The bronchial circulation is part of the systemic circulation; bronchial arteries are branches of the descending aorta.

Function

The function of the bronchial circulation is to supply oxygen, water, and nutrients to:

- Lung parenchyma.
- Airways—smooth muscle, mucosal and glands.
- Pulmonary arteries and veins.
- Pleurae.

An additional function of the bronchial circulation is in the conditioning (warming) of inspired air. The airways distal to the terminal bronchiole are supplied only by alveolar wall capillaries. For this reason,a pulmonary embolus may result in infarction of the tissues supplied by the alveolar wall capillaries shown as a wedge-shaped opacity on the lung periphery of a chest X-ray.

Development of the pulmonary circulation

The primitive heart is divided into four chambers during weeks 4 and 5. This involves:

- Formation of endocardial cushions.
- Division of the primitive atrium.

During week 6, the six primitive aortic arches are transformed into the adult arterial layout. However, the ductus arteriosus is still patent. For further information on development of the heart see *Crash Course, Cardiovascular System*.

Fetal circulation

The main difference between adult and fetal circulation (Fig. 2.23) is that oxygenation of the fetal blood is by the maternal placental circulation. Consequently, the pulmonary circulation is largely bypassed through:

- The foramen ovale—which connects the right atrium to the left atrium.
- The ductus arteriosus—which connects the pulmonary artery to the aorta.

Deoxygenated fetal blood flows through the two umbilical arteries (branches of the common iliacs) to the placenta (Fig. 2.23). Oxygen and nutrients are taken up from the maternal blood by the fetal circulation. Waste products of metabolism and carbon dioxide are passed from fetal blood to the maternal circulation. Oxygenated blood returns back to the fetal heart through the umbilical vein, ductus venosus, and inferior vena cava. The oxygenated blood from the umbilical vein mixes with deoxygenated blood from the portal circulation and lower limbs and is returned to the right side of the heart. The majority of the fetal blood bypasses the pulmonary circulation, passing through the foramen ovale into the left atrium (see large arrow in Fig. 2.23).

In fetal life, the pressure in the pulmonary circulation is greater than systemic circulation and less than one-third of the right ventricular output passes through the lungs; the remainder flows from the pulmonary artery through the ductus arteriosus into the aorta.

Changes of circulation after birth

At birth, blood flow through the umbilical vessels stops. When blood flow through the umbilical vein ceases, the ductus venosus, a thick-walled vessel with a muscular sphincter, closes. As the neonate takes its first breath, the lungs fill with air and pulmonary vascular resistance falls to 10% of its value before lung expansion. Left atrial pressure is raised above that in the inferior vena cava by three methods:

- Decreased pulmonary vascular resistance leading to a large increase in blood flow through the lungs to the left atrium.
- Decreased blood flow to the right atrium caused by occlusion of the umbilical vein.
- Increased resistance to the left ventricular output produced by occlusion of the umbilical arteries.

The reversal of pressure gradient between the atria closes the valve over the foramen ovale. Fusion of the septal leaflets occurs over a period of several days.

The fall in pulmonary arterial pressure reverses the flow through the ducus arteriosus, but within a few moments of birth the ductus arteriosus begins to constrict, producing a turbulent flow heard as a murmur in the newborn child. The constriction is progressive and usually complete within 1–2 days after birth.

The exact mechanism for closure of the ductus arteriosus is not entirely clear, although it is thought to

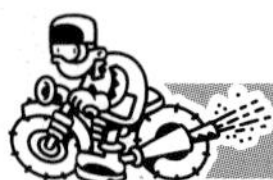

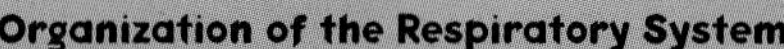

The following fetal vessels lose their function and become ligaments at birth:

- **Ductus arteriosus—becomes the ligamentum arteriosum**
- **Ductus venosus—becomes the ligamentum venosum**
- **Umbilical arteries—become the medial umbilical ligaments**
- **Umbilical veins—become the ligamentum teres**

involve bradykinin, prostaglandins (because indomethacin can delay closure), and adenosine.

The following factors have been suggested as causes of closure of the ductus arteriosus:

- Cutting of the umbilical cord.
- Exposure to cold air.
- Increase in arterial partial pressure of oxygen.
- Pressure difference between pulmonary and systemic circulations.

At birth, the walls of the left and right ventricles are the same thickness. After birth, the thickness of the right ventricular wall diminishes whereas that of the left ventricle increases.

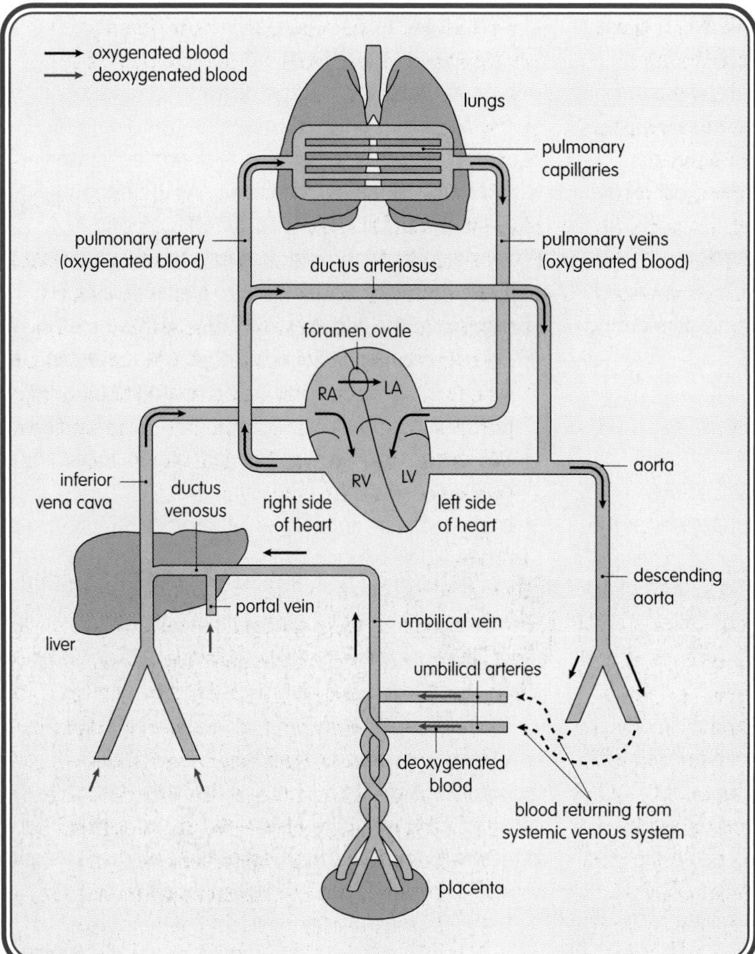

Fig. 2.23 Fetal circulation. A large proportion of blood entering the right atrium passes through the foramen ovale into the left atrium. A large proportion of blood entering the pulmonary artery passes along the ductus arteriosus directly to the aorta.

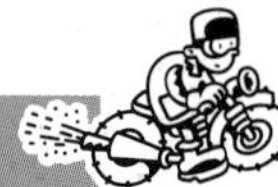

Patent ductus arteriosus

Patent ductus arteriosus (PDA) is a common congenital heart defect, especially in girls. It is associated with maternal rubella (togavirus infection) in early pregnancy. As discussed above, the ductus arteriosus normally closes within 24 hours of birth. If closure fails to occur, blood flows from the aorta through the patent ductus and into the pulmonary artery (a left-to-right shunt). This increases pulmonary artery pressure (hydrodynamic pulmonary hypertension). The defect is classified as either small ductus or large ductus. The murmur heard has a machine-like quality and extends throughout the cardiac cycle. The treatment of choice is surgical ligation of the ductus. If the defect is large, the infant may require medical treatment to alleviate heart failure.

Atrial septal defect

Atrial septal defect (ASD) is a defect in the atrial septum around the area of the fossa ovalis, caused by a defect in the ostium secundum. Blood flows from the left atrium to the right atrium and then into the right ventricle (a left-to-right shunt), increasing the pulmonary blood flow, causing hydrodynamic pulmonary hypertension. Symptoms do not usually occur until about 30–40 years of age, when patients present with heart failure; at presentation, a soft heart murmur is usually heard, and a fixed splitting of the second heart sound.

- **Describe the differences in function between the pulmonary and bronchial circulations.**
- **Outline the fetal circulation.**
- **How does the circulation change at birth?**
- **Name two congenital defects of the heart**

DEFENCE MECHANISMS OF THE LUNGS

Overview

The lungs have a very large surface area for gaseous exchange and present a small barrier to diffusion between air and the blood flowing through the lungs. In fact, they possess the largest surface area of the body in contact with the environment and, therefore, are extremely susceptible to damage by foreign material and provide an excellent gateway for infection. The lungs are exposed to many foreign materials:

- Dust particles.
- Pollen.
- Fungal spores.
- Bacteria.
- Viruses.
- Airborne pollutants.

Therefore, it is necessary for defence mechanisms to prevent infection and reduce the risk of damage by inhalation of foreign material. There are two main mechanisms of defence:

- Physical.
- Immunological.

Physical defences

Preventing entry to distal lower respiratory tract

Entry is restricted by the following three mechanisms:

- Filtering at the nasopharynx—hairs within the nose act as a coarse filter for inhaled particles; sticky mucus lying on the surface of the respiratory epithelium traps particles, which are then transported by the wafting of cilia to the nasopharynx; the particles are then swallowed into the gastrointestinal tract.

Smaller inhaled particles will travel further down the respiratory tract. The method that is used to deal with inhaled particles depends upon which area of the respiratory tract the particle finally reaches (e.g. large particles may be filtered out by the nasopharynx).

- Swallowing—during swallowing, the epiglottis folds back, the laryngeal muscles constrict the opening to the larynx, and the larynx itself is lifted; this prevents aspiration of food particles.
- Irritant C fibres—stimulation of receptors within the bronchi by inhalation of chemicals, particles, or infective material produces a reflex contraction of bronchial smooth muscle; this reduces the diameter of airways and increases mucus secretion, thus limiting the penetration of the offending material.

Removal of foreign material

Material is removed by four mechanisms:

- Cough reflex.
- Mucociliary clearance.
- Alveolar macrophages.
- α_1-Antitrypsin.

Cough reflex

Inhaled material and material brought up the bronchopulmonary tree to the trachea and larynx by mucociliary clearance can trigger a cough reflex (see Chapter 5). This is achieved by a reflex deep inspiration, increasing intrathoracic pressure while the larynx is closed. The larynx is suddenly opened, producing a high-velocity jet of air, which ejects unwanted material at high speed through the mouth.

Mucociliary clearance

Mucociliary clearance deals with a lot of the large particles trapped in the bronchi and bronchioles and debris brought up by alveolar macrophages. Respiratory epithelium is covered by a layer of mucus secreted by goblet cells and submucosal glands. Approximately 10–100 mL of mucus is secreted by the lung daily. The mucus film is divided into two layers:

- Periciliary fluid layer about 6 μm deep, immediately adjacent to the surface of the epithelium. The mucus here is hydrated by epithelial cells. This reduces its viscosity and allows movement of the cilia.
- Superficial gel layer about 5–10 μm deep. This is a relatively viscous layer forming a sticky blanket, which traps particles.

The cilia beat synchronously at 1000–1500 strokes per minute. Coordinated movement causes the superficial gel layer, together with trapped particles, to be continually transported towards the mouth at 1–3 cm/min. The mucus and particles reach the trachea and larynx where they are swallowed or expectorated (coughed up).

Mucociliary clearance is inhibited by:

- Tobacco smoke.
- Cold air.
- Many drugs (e.g. general anaesthetics).
- Sulphur oxides.
- Nitrogen oxides.

In cystic fibrosis, a defect in chloride channels throughout the body leads to hyperviscous secretions. In the lung, inadequate hydration causes excessive stickiness of the mucus lining the airways, preventing the action of the cilia in effecting mucociliary clearance. Failure to remove bacteria leads to repeated severe respiratory infections, which progressively damage the lungs. Impaired mucociliary clearance is the major cause of morbidity and mortality in cystic fibrosis.

Alveolar macrophages

Because the lining cells of the alveoli have no cilia, another mechanism is necessary to transport particles and debris from the alveoli. Alveolar macrophages are differentiated monocytes, and are both phagocytic and mobile. These cells ingest bacteria and debris, transporting it to the bronchioles where it can be removed from the lungs by mucociliary clearance.

α_1-Antitrypsin

α_1-Antitrypsin is an enzyme (an antiprotease) that breaks down the destructive proteases released from dead bacteria, macrophages and neutrophils.

Cigarette smoke increases the number of pulmonary macrophages; these release a chemical that attracts leucocytes to the lung. The leucocytes in turn release proteases, including elastase, that attack elastic tissue in the lungs. This process is usually inhibited by α_1-antitrypsin, but this itself is inhibited by oxygen radicals released by leucocytes. The result is a protease–antiprotease imbalance that leads to the destruction of lung tissue and the development of emphysema.

A deficiency in α_1-antitrypsin (inherited as an autosomal dominant condition) leads to a reduction in the breakdown of proteolytic enzymes released from neutrophils in acute inflammation. This results in increased destruction of the alveolar wall and lung parenchymal tissue. Thus, any insult to the lungs (e.g. smoking) will lead to increased destruction of tissue and emphysema. It should be noted, however, that only 2%

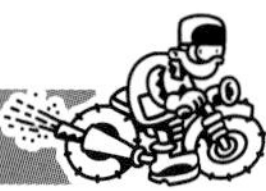

of individuals who have emphysema have α_1-antitrypsin deficiency; the vast majority of cases of emphysema are related to smoking.

Immune system defences

The immune system has a major role in the defence against pathogens (Fig. 2.24). Because of the nature of the blood–air interface, the importance of the immune system is paramount. To aid this key role of the immune system, lymphoid cells concentrate in the mucosal surfaces of the body to provide defence; thus, there is a specialized local system of lymphoid tissue, known as mucusa-associated lymphoid tissue (MALT).

MALT is noncapsulated lymphoid tissue located in the walls of the gastrointestinal, respiratory and urogenital tracts, providing immunological protection. These tissues are also a main site of lymphocyte activation and activated lymphocytes will specifically return to respiratory mucosa.

Examples of MALT were mentioned among the tissues of the upper respiratory tract (e.g. the adenoids and the tonsils). MALT in the lung is termed BALT (bronchus-associated lymphoid tissue). BALT is located beneath the mucosa of the bronchi and is covered by M cells, specialized epithelial cells that sample and transport antigen to the lymphoid tissue.

The lymphoid tissue of the respiratory tract is similar to that in the gut; aggregates are a diffuse distribution of mostly B lymphocytes within the lamina propria, covered by similar antigen-targeting and antigen-transporting cells (M cells). The lymphatic vessels associated with MALT are all efferent lymphatics, which drain to regional (hilar) lymph nodes. Large aggregations function in a similar manner to lymph nodes, containing T cell and B cell zones.

Protective proteins produced by the respiratory mucosa

Effector B lymphocytes (plasma cells) in the submucosa produce immunoglobulins. All classes of antibody are produced, but IgA production predominates. The immunoglobulins are contained within the mucous secretions in the respiratory tract and are directed against specific antigens. In addition, bacteriostatic and bactericidal proteins are produced by the respiratory epithelium and secreted in the mucous layer.

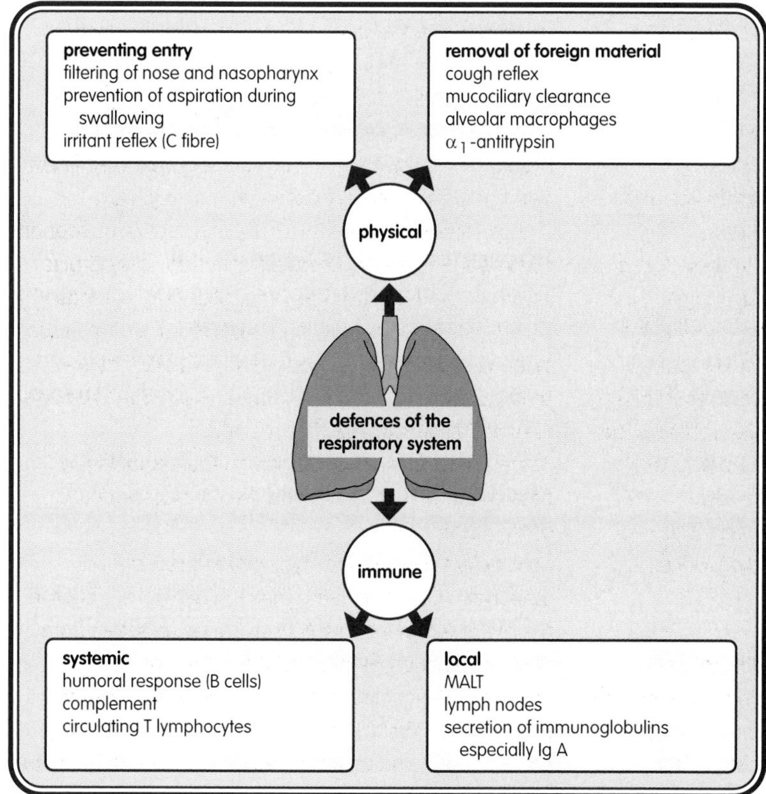

Fig. 2.24 Summary of defences of the respiratory system.

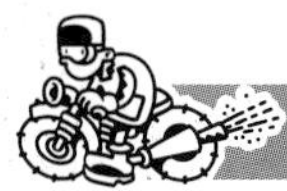

- Explain why the lungs are susceptible to damage.
- Describe the mechanisms available to the lung to prevent entry of particulate matter.
- Outline the mechanisms for removal of foreign material.
- Describe the local immune system, which protects the lung from infection.

METABOLIC FUNCTIONS OF THE LUNGS

Overview

The lungs, in addition to their role as gas exchange organs, have some important metabolic functions, notably:

- Conversion of angiotensin I to angiotensin II.
- Deactivation of vasoactive substances.
- Removal of serotonin, prostaglandins, and leukotrienes.
- Arachidonic acid metabolism.
- Phospholipid synthesis.
- Protein synthesis.

Conversion of angiotensin I

Renin released from the juxtaglomerular cells of the kidney enters the blood stream where it acts on a plasma protein, angiotensinogen, to produce angiotensin I (Fig. 2.25). Angiotensin I is further converted by angiotensin-converting enzyme (ACE) to angiotensin II, which stimulates aldosterone secretion and acts as a potent vasoconstrictor. ACE is produced by the vascular endothelial cells of the lungs.

Deactivation of vasoactive substances

An example of this is the degradation of bradykinin (a potent vasodilator) to inactive peptides by ACE (Fig. 2.26).

The administration of an ACE inhibitor (such as captopril) inhibits both the production of angiotensin II and the breakdown of bradykinin.

Arachidonic acid metabolism

The lungs are capable of both production and removal of arachidonic acid metabolites. The following metabolites are removed by the lung:

- Prostaglandin E_2.
- Prostaglandin $F_{2\alpha}$.
- Leukotrienes.

Arachidonic acid is released from membrane phospholipids by the action of phospholipase A_2 (Fig. 2.27). Arachidonic acid is converted into the endoperoxides (e.g. prostaglandins) by the action of cyclo-oxygenase or into leukotrienes by the action of lipoxygenase.

Arachidonic acid synthesis

Leukotrienes (LTB_4, LTC_4, LTD_4) are implicated as the cause of bronchoconstriction in asthma (Chapter 11). Thromboxane A_2 increases platelet aggregation and vasoconstriction, whereas prostacyclin has opposite effects. The prostaglandins produced have vasodilatory and vasoconstrictory effects.

Phospholipid synthesis

Type II pneumocytes produce surfactant which contains an important phospholipid (dipalmityol phosphotidylcholine, DPC). Surfactant has the property of reducing surface tension in proportion to its surface concentration (Chapter 3).

Phospholipids are produced from fatty acids in association with smooth endoplasmic reticular membrane. Synthesis occurs at the interface between cytosol and the endoplasmic reticular membrane. The synthesized phospholipids are transported to vesicles by 'membrane budding' (endoplasmic reticular membrane fuses with the vesicle).

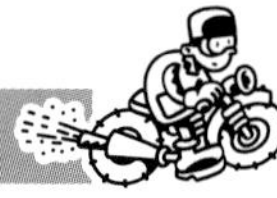

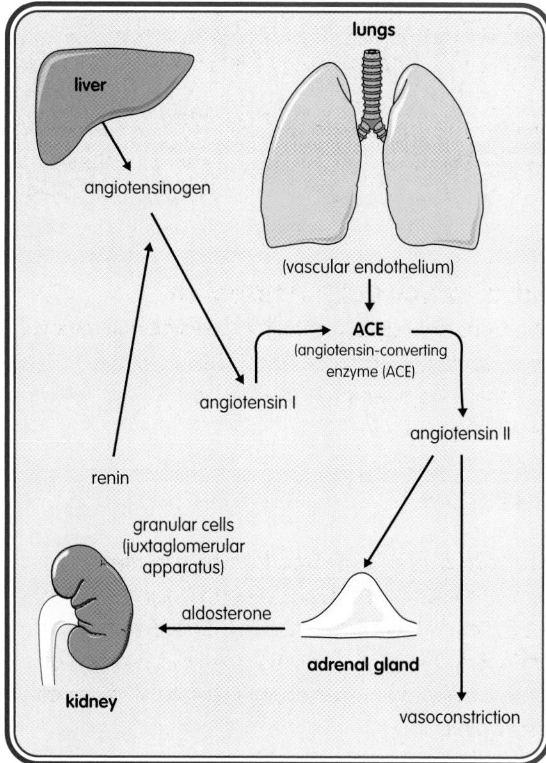

Fig. 2.25 The renin–angiotensin system. Conversion of angiotensin I to angiotensin II by angiotensin-converting enzyme (ACE) occurs mainly in the pulmonary vascular endothelium.

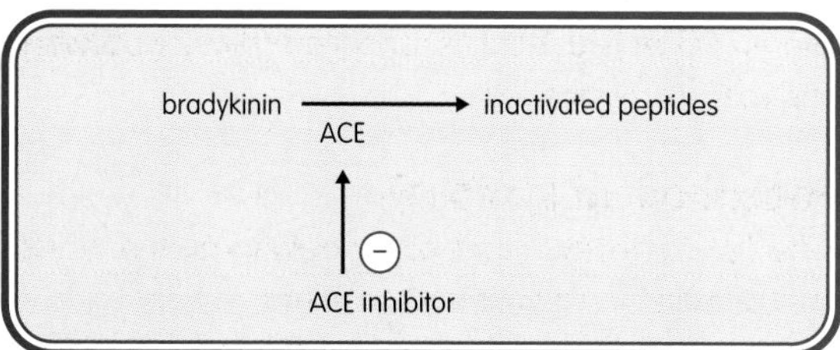

Fig. 2.26 Bradykinin degradation.

The surfactant mixture is extruded into the alveolus and lowers the surface tension. The synthesis is rapid and allows quick turnover of surfactant.

Protein synthesis

Structural proteins, collagen, and elastin form the parenchyma of the lung; their synthesis and breakdown are important to the normal functioning of the lung. An increase in their breakdown is associated with increased protease activity (as seen in α_1-antitrypsin deficiency) and leads to emphysema.

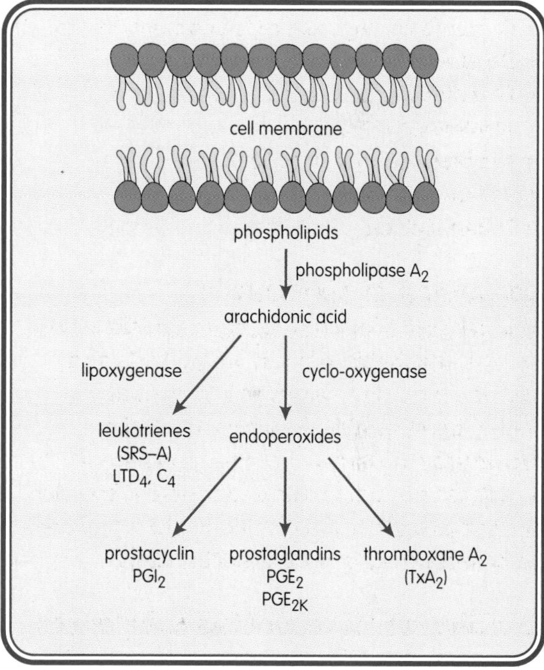

Fig. 2.27 Arachidonic acid metabolism. The production of endoperoxides and leukotrienes.

- **List the metabolic functions of the lung.**
- **Describe with the use of a diagram the conversion of angiotensin I.**
- **Outline with the aid of a diagram arachidonic acid metabolism.**

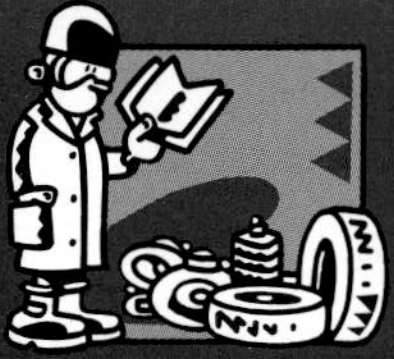

3. Ventilation and Gas Exchange

VENTILATION

Lung volumes

Lung volumes can be affected by disease; therefore, a knowledge of their normal values is important, for understanding both lung disease and function.

After breathing out, the lungs are not completely emptied of air. A completely deflated lung would require a much greater amount of energy to inflate it than one in which the alveoli have not collapsed (see Fig. 3.17). Even a maximum respiratory effort (forced expiration) fails to expel all the air from the lungs. When the expiratory muscles contract, all the structures in the lungs (not only the alveoli but also the airways) are compressed by the positive intrapleural pressure. During forced expiration, the smaller airways collapse before the alveoli empty completely. Thus, some air remains within the lungs; this is known as the residual volume (Fig. 3.1).

During normal breathing (quiet breathing), the lung volume oscillates between inhalation and exhalation. The total volume inhaled and exhaled is known as the tidal volume. In quiet breathing, after the tidal volume has been expired:

- Pressure outside the chest is equal to pressure inside the alveoli (i.e. atmospheric pressure).
- Elastic forces tending to collapse the lung are balanced by the elastic recoil trying to expand the chest (Fig. 3.2).
- This creates a subatmospheric (negative) pressure in the intrapleural space.

The lung volume at this condition is known as functional residual capacity. See Fig. 3.3 for definitions of lung volumes.

Measuring lung volumes

There are four main methods of measuring lung volumes:

- Spirometry.
- Nitrogen washout.
- Helium dilution.
- Plethysmography

Nitrogen washout and helium dilution work on the principle of conservation of mass (mass balance; i.e. what goes into a system must equal what comes out, otherwise there is accumulation). When a mass balance is applied to a particular component, this is known as a component balance.

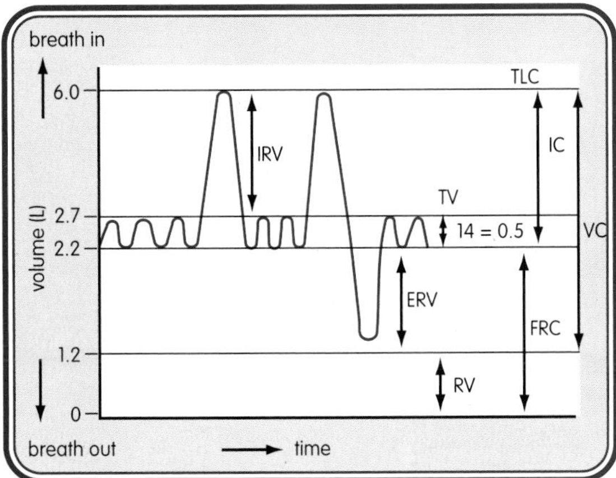

Fig. 3.1 Typical spirometer trace. Note that functional residual capacity (FRC) and residual volume (RV) cannot be measured using a spirometer; thus, neither can total lung capacity (TLC). ERV = expiratory reserve volume; IRV = inspiratory reserve volume;TV = tidal volume; IC = inspiratory capacity; VC = vital capacity.

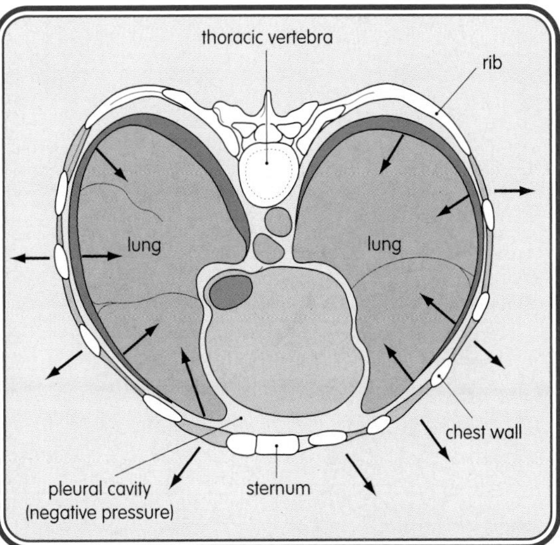

Fig. 3.2 Pressures within the thoracic cavity. The tendency for the lungs to collapse (elastic recoil) and the opposing forces tendency to expand the chest wall creates a subatmospheric (negative) pressure in the intrapleural space.

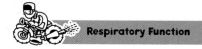

Descriptions of lung volumes and capacities	
Air in lungs is divided into 4 volumes	
tidal volume (TV)	volume of air breathed in and out in a single breath: 0.5 L
inspiratory reserve volume (IRV)	volume of air breathed in by a maximum inspiration at the end of a normal inspiration: 3.3 L
expiratory reserve volume (ERV)	volume of air that can be expelled by a maximum effort at the end of a normal expiration: 1.0 L
residual volume (RV)	volume of air remaining in lungs at end of a maximum expiration: 1.2 L
Pulmonary capacities are combinations of 2 or more volumes	
inspiratory capacity (IC) = TV + IRV	volume of air breathed in by a maximum inspiration at the end of a normal expiration: 3.8 L
functional residual capacity (FRC) = ERV + RV	volume of air remaining in lungs at the end of a normal expiration. Acts as buffer against extreme changes in alveolar gas levels with each breath: 2.2 L
vital capacity (VC) = IRV +TV + ERV	volume of air that can be breathed in by a maximum inspiration following a maximum expiration: 4.8 L
total lung capacity (TLC) = VC + RV	only a fraction of TLC is used in normal breathing: 6.0 L
Most of these volumes can be measures with a spirometer (see Figs 3.1 and 3.4)	

Fig. 3.3 Descriptions of lung volumes and capacities.

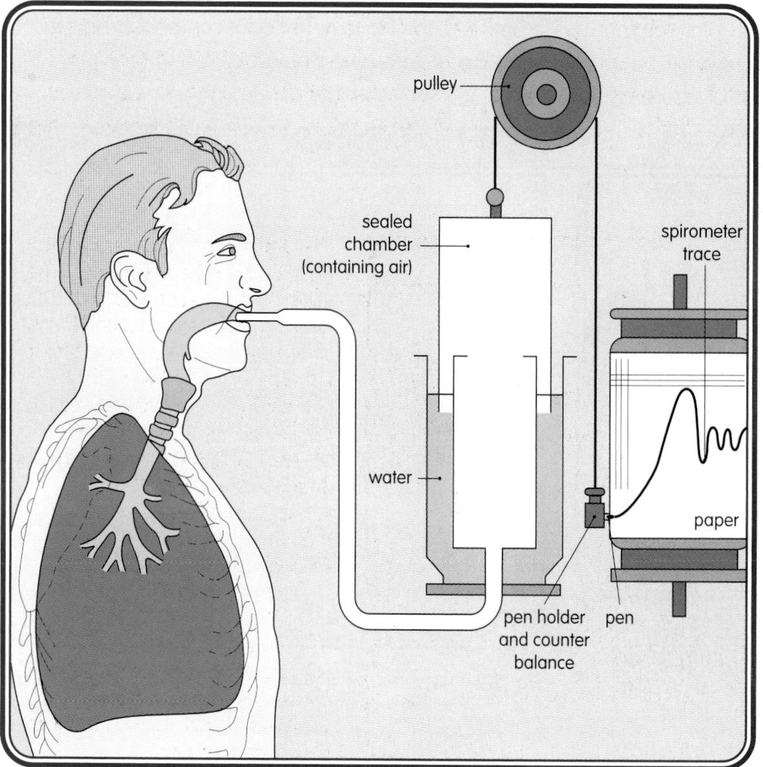

Fig. 3.4 Spirometry. The measurement of lung volume by displacement of a float within a sealed chamber is recorded on a paper roll by a pen.

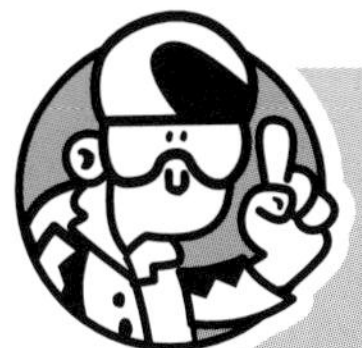

If there are two things in life that are certain, one is death, the other is that you will be asked to reproduce definitions and values for lung volumes in your exams.

Spirometry

Spirometry can measure all lung volumes except residual volume and functional residual capacity (thus neither can total lung capacity be measured). The spirometer converts volumes of inspiration and expiration into a single line trace. The subject is connected by a mouthpiece to a sealed chamber (Fig. 3.4). Each time the subject breathes, the volume inspired or expired is converted into the vertical position of a float. The position of the float is recorded on a rotating drum by means of a pen attachment. The residual volume remains trapped in the lungs and therefore requires an indirect method of measurement.

Nitrogen washout

Nitrogen washout measures the dilution of nitrogen in the lungs. After expiration of tidal volume, the subject breathes 100% O_2 and the exhaled gas is collected in a Douglas bag until approximately all the N_2 has been exhaled. The method can be used to determine functional residual capacity, total lung capacity, or residual volume.

Nitrogen washout is inaccurate; it is not considered useful as a method of determining lung volumes.

Helium dilution

Dilution techniques are commonly used to assess volumes that are not readily accessible for direct measurement. Helium dilution relies on helium being inert and not absorbed. Therefore, if helium is inhaled, it will be diluted by the volume of gas already within the lungs. The degree of dilution of a known amount of inert marker by an unknown lung volume is used to calculate that lung volume (Fig. 3.5). This technique can be used to calculate residual volume, total lung capacity, or functional residual capacity. Usually 10% He in a known amount of air is used as the marker.

Plethysmography

Plethysmography is the process of recording changes in pressure when a subject is placed within a sealed box to determine the change in lung volume. The idea behind plethysmography is Boyle's law: 'At a constant temperature the volume (*V*) of a perfect gas varies inversely with the pressure (*P*), and the pressure varies inversely with the volume.'

$P \cdot V = \text{constant}$, or $P_1V_1 = P_2V_2$

The subject sits in a sealed chamber (Fig. 3.6) that allows the subject to breathe through a mouthpiece. Initial volume of the box is known and pressures in both

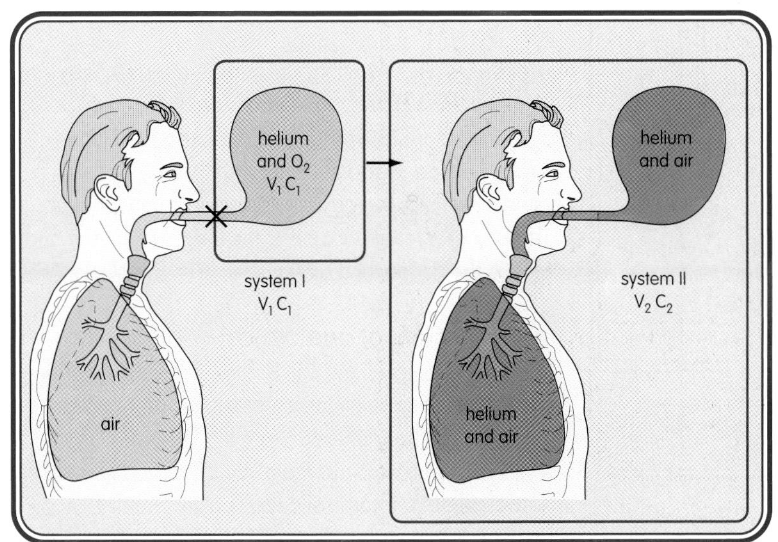

Fig. 3.5 Measurement of RV, FRC, and TLC using helium dilution. The subject inhales a specific volume of a helium–oxygen mixture of known concentration. The concentration of the exhaled gas allows calculation of the initial volume of the lungs (V_L). We know He in system I = He in system II ($V_1C_1 = V_2C_2$), therefore it is possible to calculate V_L.
$V_2 = V_L + V_1$, therefore $V_1C_1 = V_LC_2 + V_1C_2$.
$V_LC_2 = V_1C_1 - V_1C_2$.
Therefore, $V_L = \dfrac{V_1(C_1 - C_2)}{C_2}$.

V_1 = volume system I; C_1 = concentration of helium in system I (inhaled He concentrate); V_2 = volume system II; C_2 = concentration of helium in system II.

the lung and box can be measured. At the end of a normal breath:

- The shutter in the mouthpiece closes.
- The subject takes a breath in.
- This expands the chest, but no air flow into the lungs takes place.
- Lung volume (V_L) increases and lung pressure (P_L) decreases.
- Box volume (V_B) decreases and the box pressure (P_B) increases.

Thus applying Boyle's law:

$$P_1V_1 = P_2V_2$$

We know P_{B1}, V_{B1} and P_{B2}; therefore, we can calculate V_{B2}.

Assuming that $V_{B2} = V_{B1} + \Delta V$, where ΔV is the change in volume of the box, we can calculate the value of ΔV (which is negative). The lungs have expanded by an equal change in volume.

Applying Boyle's law to the change in lung volume, we get:

$$P_{L1}V_{L1} = P_{L2}V_{L2}$$

but $V_{L2} = V_{L1} + \Delta V$

Because we know P_{L1}, P_{L2}, and ΔV, we can calculate V_{L1}, which is functional residual capacity.

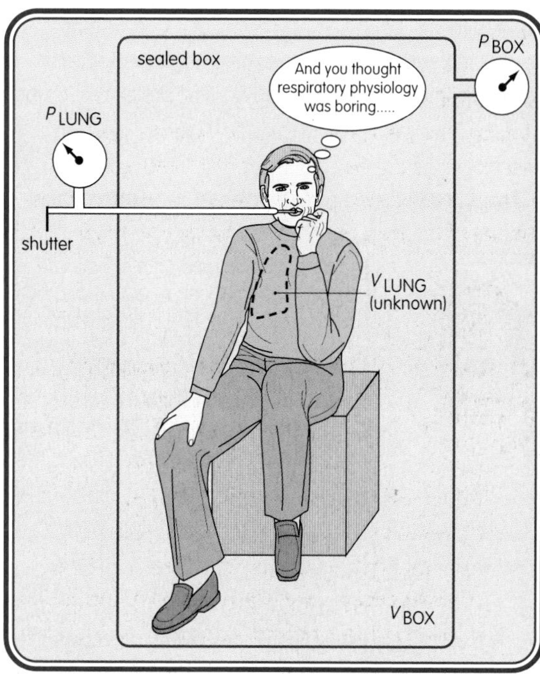

Fig. 3.6 Plethysmography. This assumes pressure at the mouth is the pressure within the lung.

Ventilation

Ventilation is the flow of air in and out of the respiratory system (breathing); it is defined physiologically as the amount of air breathed in and out in a given time. Not all the air inspired reaches the alveoli; some stays within the trachea or other conducting airways. Therefore, there are two values of ventilation to be considered:

- Minute ventilation ($\dot{V}_E$), which is the total amount of air entering the respiratory tract through the nose and mouth in 1 minute.
- Minute alveolar ventilation ($\dot{V}_A$), which is the amount of air that reaches the alveoli in 1 minute.

If a subject with a tidal volume of 500 mL took 12 breaths a minute, it would seem obvious that the volume exhaled per minute (minute ventilation) would be $500 \times 12 = 6000$ mL/min. Or, more generally:

$$\dot{V}_E = V_T f$$

where $\dot{V}_E$ = minute ventilation, V_T = the volume inhaled in one breath (approximately 500 mL in quiet breathing), and f = the respiratory rate (breaths/minute).

Anatomical dead space

Those areas of the airway not involved in gaseous exchange (i.e. the conducting zone) are known as the anatomical dead space; included in this space are:

- Nose and mouth.
- Pharynx.
- Larynx.
- Trachea.
- Bronchi and bronchioles, down to and including the terminal bronchioles.

Inspired air held within these areas is referred to as dead air. The volume of the anatomical dead space (V_D) is usually about 150 mL (or 2 mL/kg of bodyweight). Anatomical dead space varies with the size of the subject and also increases with increased inspiration because greater expansion of the lungs lengthens and widens the conducting airways.

Measurement of anatomical dead space

Anatomical dead space can be measured by recording the partial pressure of carbon dioxide in air leaving the mouth after a normal expiration; this assumes:

- There will be no carbon dioxide in expired gas from the area of anatomical dead space.
- No diffusion or turbulent mixing occurs between gas

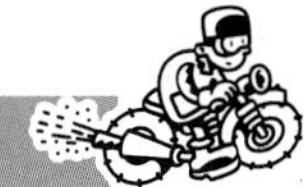

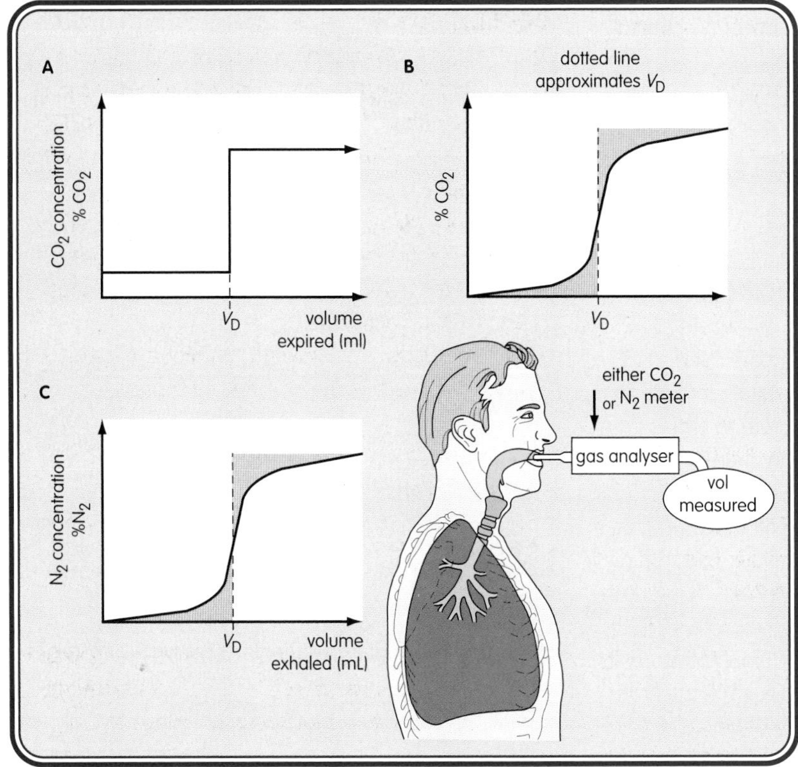

Fig. 3.7 Measurement of anatomical dead space. (A) Method 1—graphical method using carbon dioxide. It would be expected that the gas expired from those areas not undergoing gaseous exchange (anatomical dead space) would contain no carbon dioxide and thus a stepwise change would occur to the carbon dioxide concentration of expired gas; the volume at which this occurs would be equal to the anatomical dead space volume. (B) On a graph showing the real-world results, a dotted line has been drawn to approximate the step change in carbon dioxide concentration. (C) Method 2—Fowler's method. This works on the same principle as above, but 100% O_2 is inhaled. The expired nitrogen concentration is measured.

from the end respiratory unit and gas in the anatomical dead space.

If these conditions were met, there would be a stepwise increase in carbon dioxide concentration when alveolar gas was exhaled (Fig. 3.7A), showing the initially expired gas from the dead space containing little carbon dioxide, followed by gas from respiratory airways and alveoli containing high concentrations of carbon dioxide.

In the real situation, some mixing does occur. This means that initially the carbon dioxide concentration increases slowly, then sharply rises and reaches a plateau (the alveolar plateau, Fig. 3.7B). The alveolar plateau equates to the concentration of carbon dioxide in the alveoli (P_ACO_2). Mixing occurs because:

- There are unequal lengths between the respiratory surfaces and the mouth.
- Turbulence occurs at branches within the airways, causing mixing.
- The lungs are not uniformly ventilated

A vertical line approximates the errors caused by mixing and gives an estimated volume of anatomical dead space.

Fowler's method relies on the same principle but uses nitrogen concentration. The subject inhales 100% O_2; nitrogen concentration in expired gas is measured. (Fig. 3.7C)

Alveolar ventilation

Alveolar ventilation per minute ($\dot{V}_A$) is that amount of fresh air reaching the alveoli within 1 minute.

From our knowledge that alveolar ventilation is the amount of inspired air reaching the alveoli and from our

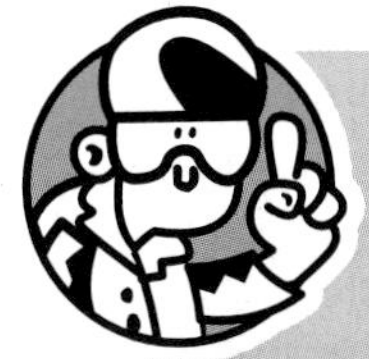

Examiners love equations. They are fooled into thinking that if you've learned them parrot-fashion, you understand them. Therefore, you will be tested on them. Try to understand the methodology behind them (e.g. mass balances, helium dilution, N_2 washout, etc.). If this fails, then learn them parrot-fashion.

understanding of anatomical dead space, we can say that for one breath:

$$V_A = V_T - V_D$$

where V_A = the volume reaching the alveolus in one breath, Hence, in 1 minute:

$$\dot{V}_A = (V_T - V_D)f$$

Physiological dead space

If each acinus (or end respiratory unit) were perfect, the amount of air received by each alveolus would be matched by the flow of blood through the pulmonary capillaries. Alas, the lung is not perfect:

- Some areas receive less ventilation than others.
- Some areas receive less blood flow than others.

In both these cases, ventilation does not match perfusion and efficient gaseous exchange will not take place. If an area of lung is not perfused, the ventilation is 'wasted'; the volume is known as alveolar dead space.

Physiological deadspace is a functional measure; it is the sum of the anatomical deadspace volume (from the conducting zone) and the volume of any nonfunctional areas of the respiratory zone (alveolar dead space). This is shown in Fig. 3.8.

In a normal, healthy person, anatomical and physiological dead space are almost equal, alveolar dead space being very small (<5 mL); however, alveolar dead space can increase in disease.

Measurement of physiological dead space

Knowing that carbon dioxide is not blown off from end respiratory units that are not perfused, it is possible to carry out a component balance for carbon dioxide to establish the volume of physiological dead space (Fig. 3.8).

Variation in ventilation within the lung

Not all regions of the lungs are ventilated equally. It has been shown that the lower zones of the lungs are ventilated better that the upper zones. The causes of regional differences in ventilation will be discussed in the next section. Ventilation per unit volume can be measured by inhalation of a radioactive isotope of xenon (^{133}Xe). If radiation counters are placed at different levels of the lungs, the volume of inhaled radioactive xenon in various areas of the lung can be measured.

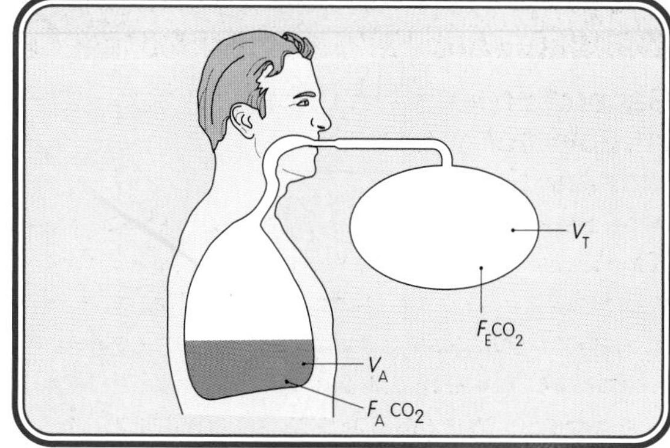

Fig. 3.8 The Bohr equation for physiological dead space. This method is another component balance using carbon dioxide. We assume:

- All carbon dioxide in alveolar gas is expired.
- Amount of carbon dioxide in alveolar gas = amount in mixed expired gas.
- Alveolar ventilation (V_A) = tidal volume (V_T) – physiological dead space (V_{pD}).
- (F_ECO_2) = mixed expired CO_2 concentration.
- (F_ACO_2) = end expiratory CO_2 concentration (i.e. alveolar concentration).

$V_TF_ECO_2 = V_AF_ACO_2$. $V_A = V_T - V_{pD}$, therefore:
$V_TF_ECO_2 = V_TF_ACO_2 - V_{pD}F_ACO_2$. Therefore, $V_{pD} = \dfrac{V_TF_ACO_2 - V_TF_ECO_2}{F_ACO_2}$

- **Define all lung volumes and capacities, giving normal values. State the significance of each volume and capacity.**
- **Name four methods for measuring lung volume.**
- **Describe how a spirometer works.**
- **Outline the helium dilution method for measuring lung volumes.**
- **Define minute ventilation and alveolar ventilation.**
- **Define anatomical dead space, quoting its normal value. Describe two methods of measuring anatomical dead space.**
- **Define the terms physiological dead space, wasted ventilation, and describe how these may be measured using the Bohr equation.**
- **Outline the regional variations in ventilation of the lung and how this might be measured.**

MECHANICS OF BREATHING

General concepts in breathing and intrapleural pressure

Intrapleural pressure

In the previous section, we saw that at FRC elastic recoil of the lungs is exactly balanced by the elastic recoil of the chest wall trying to expand the chest. These two opposing forces create a subatmospheric (negative) pressure within the intrapleural space.

Intrapleural pressure varies during breathing (Fig. 3.9); it is about –0.5 kPa at the end of quiet expiration. On inspiration, intrathoracic volume is increased; this lowers intrapleural pressure making it more negative, causing the lungs to expand and air to enter. On expiration, the muscles of the chest wall relax and the lungs return to their original size by elastic recoil, with the expulsion of air.

It should be noted that during quiet breathing, intrapleural pressure is always negative. In forced expiration, however, the intrapleural pressure becomes positve, forcing a reduction in lung volume with the expulsion of air.

Differences in intrapleural pressure between apex and base

The lungs are not rigid and therefore not self-supportive. As we pass vertically down the lung, each layer of lung hangs down from the layer of lung above and sits on the layer of lung below. Thus, at the apex, there is a larger weight of lung pulling away from the chest wall causing the intrapleural pressure to be more negative at the apex than at the base. For an upright subject at functional residual capacity (before inspiration) the intrapleural pressure at the apex is –0.8 kPa and at the base about –0.2 kPa. The lung base is compressed compared with the apex.

It should be noted that:

- Alveolar volumes at the base and the apex of the lung are of different values before inspiration.
- However, intrapleural pressure changes at lung base and apex during breathing are of equal magnitude.

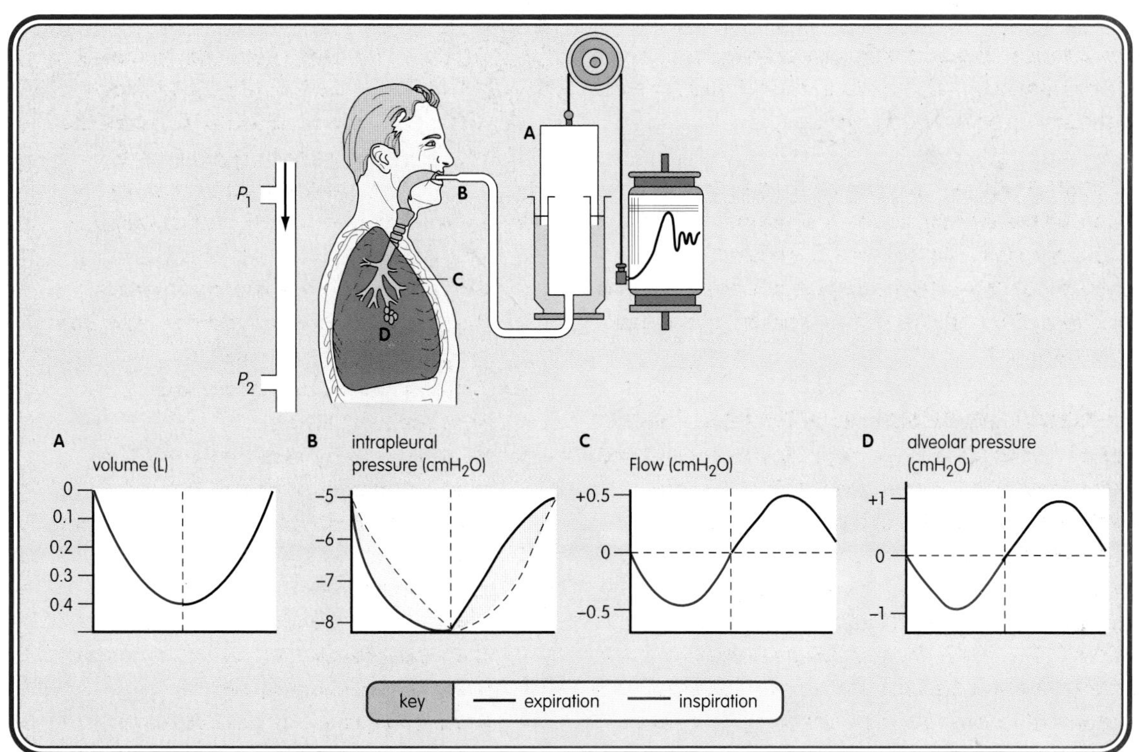

Fig. 3.9 Negative pressure within the intrapleural space and during breathing. Lung volume (A), change in intrapleural pressure (B), air flow (C), and alveolar pressure (D). All measurements are relative to inspiration and expiration.

These two factors will be important later when we look at why ventilation varies from lung base to apex.

General mechanics of breathing

To achieve air flow into the lungs, we require a driving pressure (remember air flows from high pressure to low pressure). Pressure outside the chest is atmospheric (P_{atm}). Pressure inside the lungs is alveolar pressure (P_A).

Therefore:

- If $P_A = P_{atm}$, no air flow occurs (e.g. at functional residual capacity).
- If $P_A < P_{atm}$, air flows into the lungs.
- If $P_A > P_{atm}$, air flows out of the lungs.

Because we cannot change atmospheric pressure, alveolar pressure must be altered to achieve air flow. Thus, if the volume inside the lungs is changed, Boyle's law predicts that pressure inside the lungs will also change. How can this be achieved? (Fig. 3.10)

- The lungs contain no muscle that can actively expand or contract.
- Therefore the chest must be expanded, which lowers intrapleural pressure, expanding the lungs.
- The majority of chest expansion in quiet breathing is caused by contraction of the diaphragm.
- Relaxation of the muscles of the chest wall allows the elastic recoil of the lungs to cause contraction of the lungs and expulsion of gas.

Muscles of respiration

Thoracic wall

The thoracic wall is made up of (from superficial to deep):

- Skin and subcutaneous tissue.
- Ribs, thoracic vertebra, sternum, and manubrium.
- Intercostal muscles: external, internal, and thoracis transversus.
- Parietal pleura.

Situated at the thoracic outlet is the diaphragm, which attaches to the costal margin, xyphoid process, and lumbar vertebrae.

Intercostal muscles

The action of the intercostal muscles is to pull the ribs closer together. There are therefore two main actions:

- If the first rib is fixed by scalene muscle, the external intercostal muscles pull the ribs upwards.

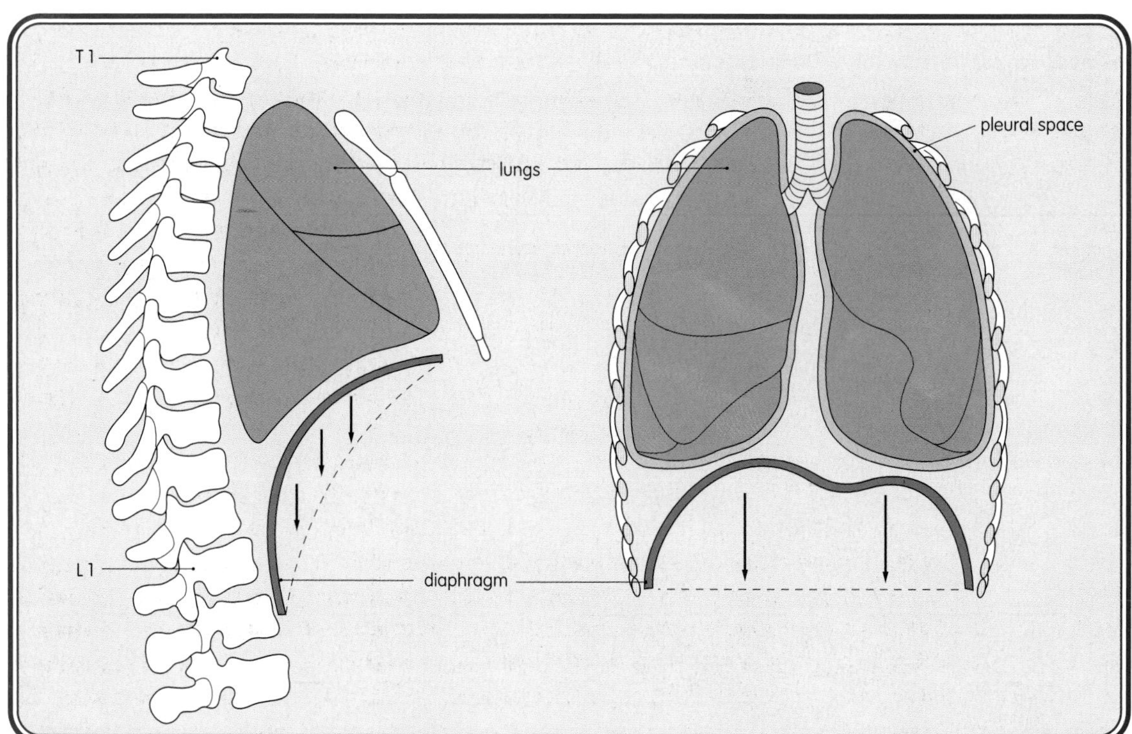

Fig. 3.10 Expanding the lungs to draw in air. Flattening the diaphragm increases the thoracic volume, lowering the intrapleural pressure and expanding the lungs.

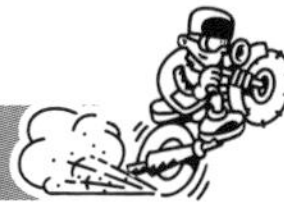

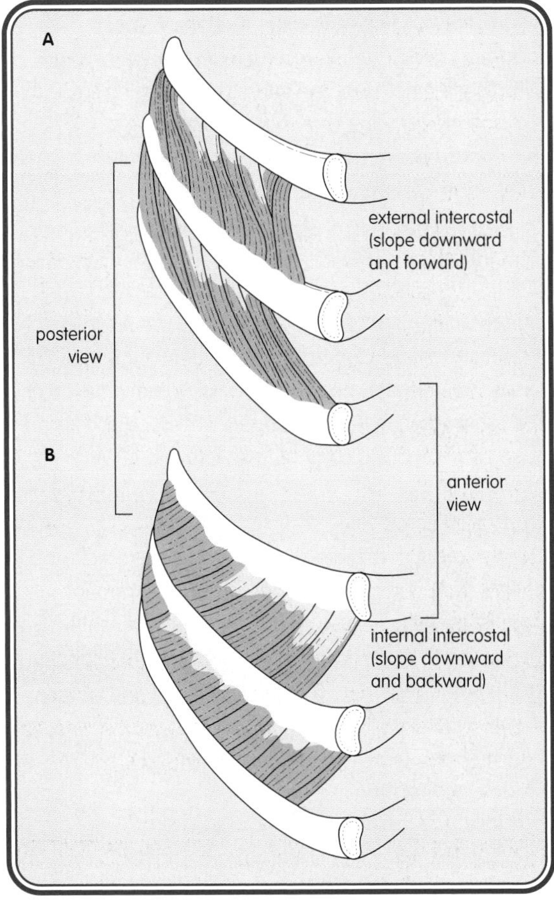

Fig. 3.11 Intercostal muscles. (A) External intercostal muscles; (B) internal intercostal muscles.

- If the last rib is fixed by quadratus lumborum, the internal intercostal muscles pull the ribs downwards.

Their action during respiration is discussed in function of the respiratory muscles.

External intercostal muscles

External intercostal muscles span the space between each rib and originate from the inferior border of the upper rib, attaching to the superior border of the rib below. The muscle attaches along the length of the rib, from the tubercle to the costal chondral junction and its fibres run forward and downward (Fig. 3.11A).

Internal intercostal muscles

Internal intercostal muscles span the space between each rib and originate from the subcostal groove of the rib above and attach to the superior border of the rib below. The muscle attaches along the length of the rib from the angle of the rib to the sternum and its fibres run downward and backward (Fig. 3.11B).

Thoracis transversus

Thoracis transversus muscle is incomplete and has the parietal pleura and neurovascular bundle as its relations.

Diaphragm

The diaphragm is the main muscle of respiration (Fig. 3.12). The central region of the diaphragm is tendinous; the outer margin is muscular, originating from the borders of the thoracic outlet.

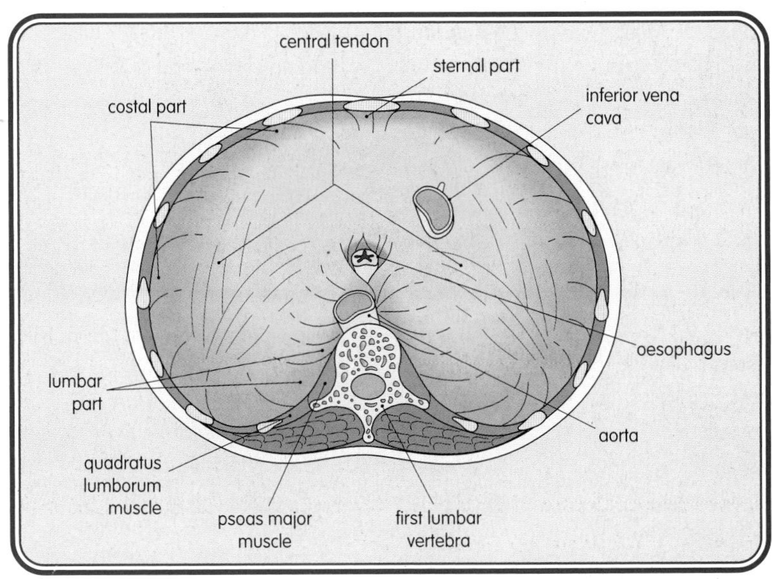

Fig. 3.12 The diaphragm. Many structures pass through the diaphragm notably the inferior vena cava, the aorta and the oesophagus.

The diaphragm has right and left domes. The right dome is higher than the left to accommodate the liver below. There is a central tendon that sits below the two domes, attaching to the xiphisternum anteriorly and the lumbar vertebrae posteriorly.

Several important structures pass through the diaphragm:

- The inferior vena cava passes through the right dome at the level of the eighth thoracic vertebra (T8).
- The oesophagus passes through a sling of muscular fibres from the right crus of the diaphragm at the level of the tenth thoracic vertebra (T10).
- The aorta pierces the diaphragm anterior to the twelfth thoracic vertebra (T12).

The diaphragm attaches to the costal margin anteriorly and laterally. Posteriorly, it attaches to the lumbar vertebrae by the crura (left crus at L1 and L2, right crus at L1, L2, and L3). In addition, the position of the diaphragm changes relative to posture: it is lower when standing than sitting.

The motor and sensory nerve supply of the diaphragm is from the phrenic nerve. Blood supply of the diaphragm is from pericardiophrenic and musculophrenic branches of the internal thoracic artery.

Function of the muscles of respiration

Breathing can classified into inspiration and expiration, quiet or forced.

Quiet inspiration

In quiet inspiration, contraction of the diaphragm flattens its domes. This action increases the length of the thorax and thus its volume. This lowers intrapleural pressure and draws air into the lungs. At the same time, the abdominal wall must relax to allow the abdominal contents to be displaced as the diaphragm moves down.

The main muscle in quiet breathing is the diaphragm, but the intercostal muscles are involved. With the first rib fixed, the intercostal muscles can expand the rib cage by two movements:

- Forward movement of the lower end of the sternum—pump-handle action (Fig. 3.13A).
- Upward and outward—bucket-handle action (Fig. 3.13B).

During quiet inspiration, these actions are small and the intercostal muscles mainly prevent deformation of the tissue between the ribs, which would otherwise lower the volume of the thoracic cage (Fig. 3.14). The internal intercostal muscles carry out this role.

Quiet expiration

Quiet expiration is passive and there is no direct muscle action. During inspiration, the lungs are expanded against their elastic recoil. This recoil is sufficient to drive air out of the lungs in expiration. Thus, quiet expiration involves the controlled relaxation of the intercostal muscles and the diaphragm.

Forced inspiration

In addition to the action of the diaphragm:

- Scalene muscles and sternocleidomastoids raise the ribs anteroposteriorly, producing movement at the manubriosternal joint.
- Intercostal muscles are much more active and raise the ribs to a much greater extent than in quiet inspiration.
- The twelfth rib, which is attached to quadratus lumborum, allows forcible downward movement of the diaphragm.
- Arching the back using erector spinae also increases thoracic volume.

The phrenic nerve supplies the diaphragm (60% motor, 40% sensory). Remember, 'nerve roots 3, 4, and 5 keep the diaphragm alive'. Thus, if you break your neck at C3, you die.

The change in intrathoracic volume is mainly caused by the movement of the diaphragm downwards. Contraction of the diaphragm comprises 75% of the energy expenditure during quiet breathing.

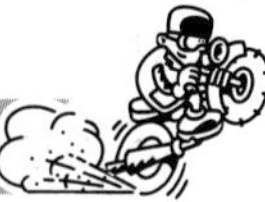

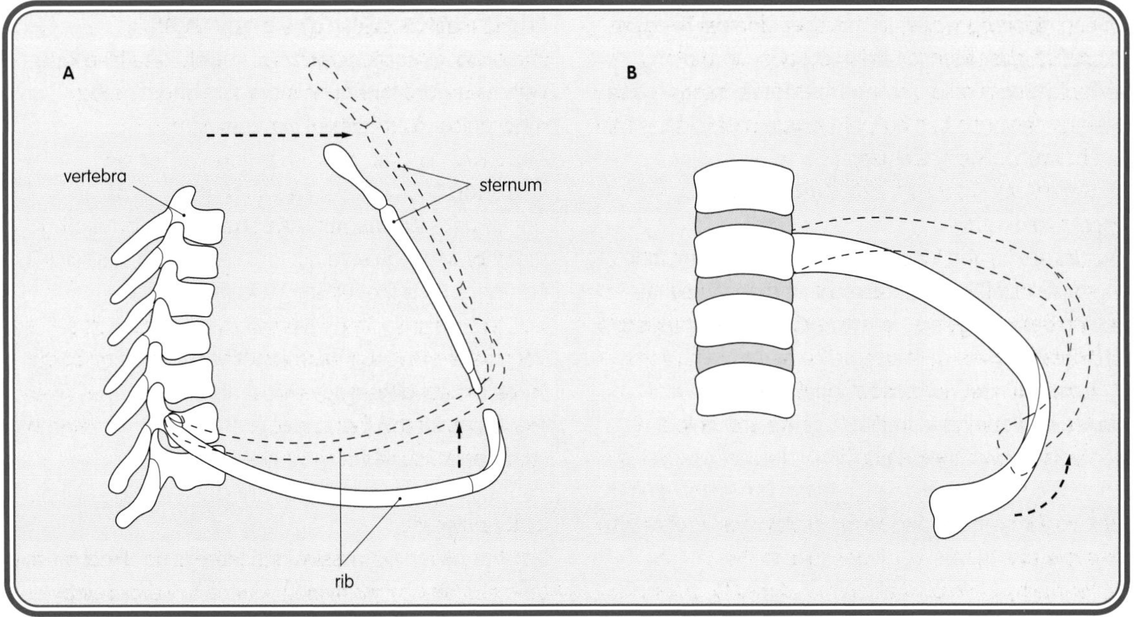

Fig. 3.13 Posterior (A) and lateral (B) expansion of the chest. (A) Note the expansion of the chest in a forward and upward movement (pump-handle action) and (B) an outward and upward movement (bucket-handle action).

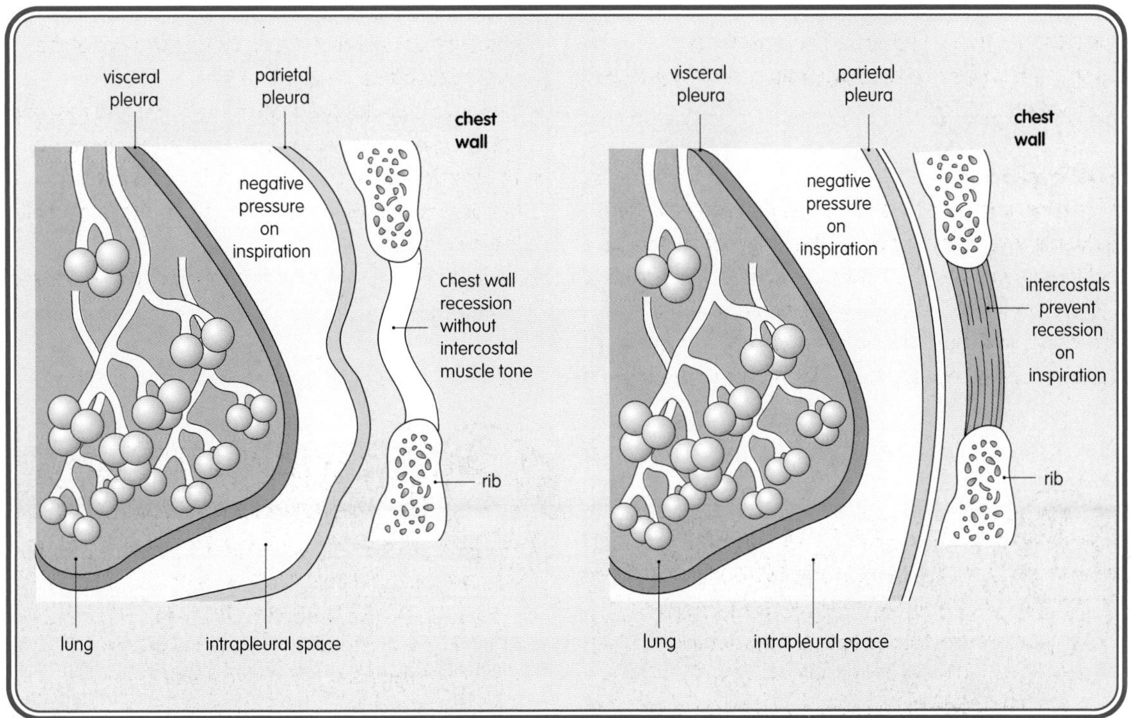

Fig. 3.14 The intercostal muscles: they prevent deformation of the thoracic wall in quiet breathing, thus maintaining thoracic volume.

During respiratory distress, the scapulae are fixed by trapezius muscles, rhomboid muscles, and levator scapulae; pectoralis minor and serratus anterior raise the ribs; the arms can be fixed (e.g. by holding the back of a chair), allowing the use of pectoralis major.

Forced expiration

Elastic recoil of the lungs is reinforced by contraction of the muscles of the abdominal wall. These force the abdominal contents against the diaphragm, pushing it up (Fig. 3.15).

In addition, quadratus lumborum pulls the ribs down, thus adding to the force of the abdominal contents against the diaphragm. Intercostal muscles prevent outward deformation of the tissue between the ribs. Latisimus dorsi and serratus posterior inferior also may play some role.

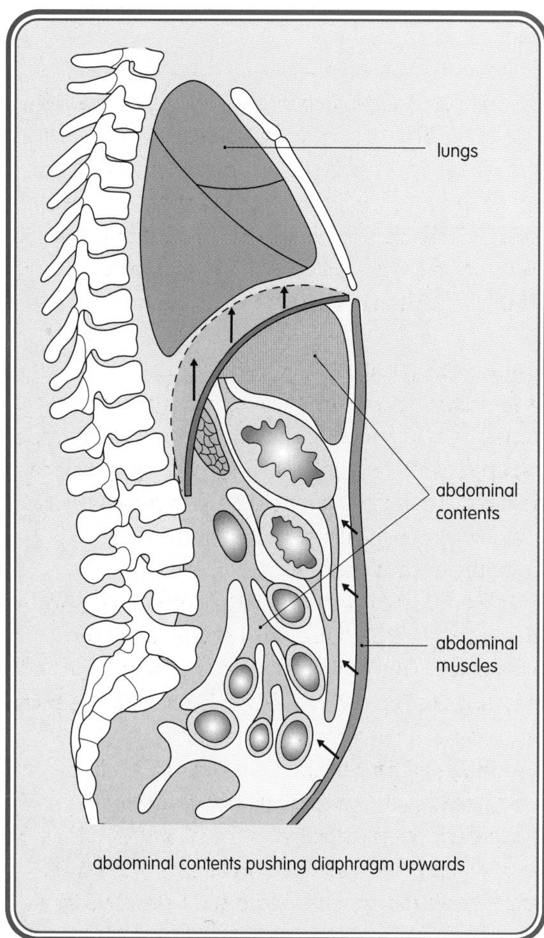

Fig. 3.15 Forced expiration. Note the abdominal contents pushing the diaphragm upwards.

Mechanics of lung ventilation

The previous section describes ventilation of the lung without regard for how it is brought about or the mechanical properties of lung tissue.

Compliance

Compliance (C) describes the ease of stretch of a material when an external force is applied to stretch it. Elastance (E) is the resistance to that stretch:

Therefore, $C = \frac{1}{E}$

In respiratory physiology, we deal with:

- Compliance of the lung (C_L).
- Compliance of the chest wall (C_W).
- Total compliance (C_{TOT}) of the chest wall and lung together.

Lung compliance is measured experimentally and refers to the change in lung volume (ΔV) caused by a change in inflation pressure (ΔP).

$$C = \frac{\Delta V}{\Delta P}$$

In life, the inflation pressure can be considered as the transmural pressure (Fig. 3.16).

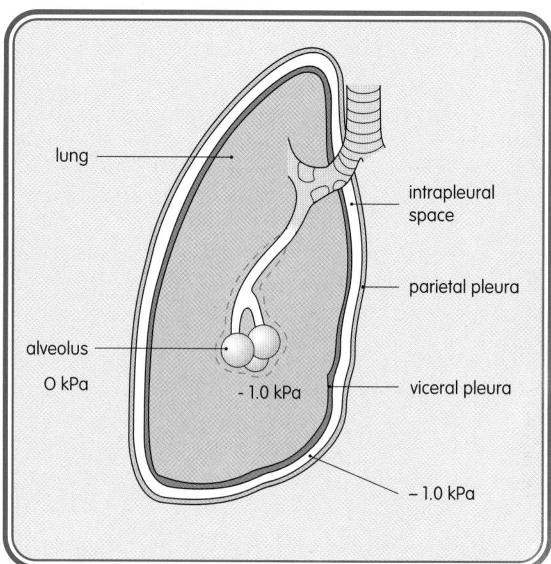

Fig. 3.16 Transmural pressure and inflation pressure. The transmural pressure is the difference in pressure across the walls of the airways. There is a slight difference in pressure between the intrapleural space and the outside of the airway, but this has been ignored in this example and the inflation pressure can be considered as the pressure difference between the intrapleural pressure and the pressure inside the alveoli (–1.0 kPa).

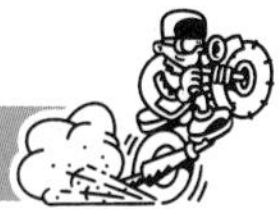

Lung compliance can be looked at in two ways:

- Static lung compliance.
- Dynamic lung compliance.

Dynamic lung compliance is a measure of the change in volume of the lung during breathing and will thus include the work required to overcome airway resistance. This will be discussed later.

Static lung compliance involves the inflation of the lungs in steps of various inflating pressures and recording the volume at the new inflation pressure. The lungs are expanded from complete collapse to total lung capacity, and measurements are also taken in deflation (see dotted line in Fig. 3.17A). This is carried out *in vitro* because, in life, we cannot completely deflate the lungs. Compliance is the change in volume divided by the change in pressure; in other words, the gradient of the pressure–volume curve.

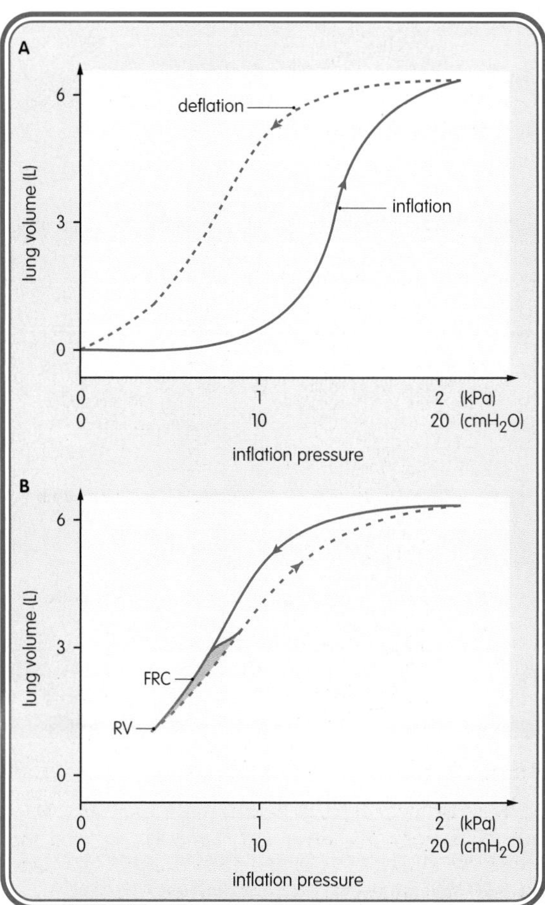

Fig. 3.17 Pressure–volume curves for inflation of the lungs (A) in vitro. (B) in life from residual volume to total lung capacity. Note the curve still shows hysteresis but to a lesser extent.

Why is there a difference between inflation and deflation curves? This difference is called hysteresis and will be explained later.

Fig. 3.17B also shows the pressure–volume curve for inflation of the lungs from functional residual capacity to total lung capacity. The curve still shows hysteresis, but not to the extent of the pressure–volume curve from complete lung collapse to total lung capacity. The slope of the curve (i.e. compliance) varies with lung volume. It can be seen that compliance is greatest at the lower lung volumes and is smallest at higher lung volumes. For these reasons, lung compliance is sometimes quoted as specific lung compliance (sp.C_L).

$$\text{sp.}C_L = \frac{C_L}{V_L}$$

This change in lung compliance helps explain the difference in ventilation of the lung between apex and base.

The lung volume in the base is less (because it is compressed) relative to the apex (see p. 37). Thus, the base of the lung has greater initial compliance than that of the apex. Because both base and apex are subject to intrapleural pressure changes of the same magnitude during inspiration, the base of the lung will therefore expand to a greater extent than the apex. This explains in part the regional difference of ventilation.

Chest wall compliance

As we have discussed before, the chest wall has elastic properties; at functional residual capacity, these are equal and opposite to those in the lung (i.e. tending to expand the chest). If the sternum were cut (e.g. in surgery) or if air were introduced into the intrapleural space then this would cause the chest wall to spring open.

As we breathe in, elastic forces (tending to expand the chest wall) aid inflation; however, at about two-thirds of total lung capacity, the chest wall has reached its resting position and any expansion beyond this point requires a positive pressure to stretch the chest wall.

Below this resting position, the chest wall is being compressed by the pressure difference between atmospheric pressure and intrapleural pressure. Thus, if we plot inflation pressure against volume of the chest wall, the inflation pressure is negative below two-thirds of total lung capacity (the dashed line in Fig. 3.18). However, compliance (the slope of the pressure–volume curve for the chest wall) remains positive, because we

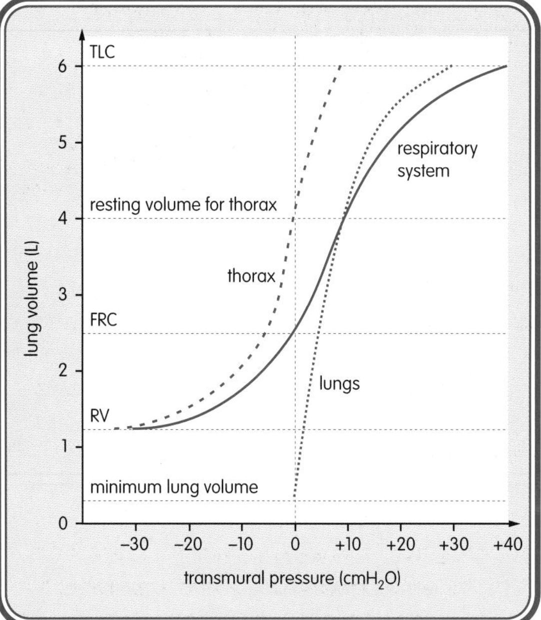

Fig. 3.18 Pressure–volume curve of the entire respiratory system. Only at functional residual capacity does the passively inflated lung–thorax system (respiratory system) have no pressure difference between the alveoli and the body surface.

are looking at the change in volume caused by a change in inflation pressure. Above the resting position the inflation pressure required to expand the chest is positive. Compliance of the lung is also plotted (dotted line in Fig. 3.18). Total compliance is plotted on the same graph and is derived from:

$$1/C_{TOT} = 1/C_L + 1/C_W$$

Elastic properties of the lung

The elastic properties of the lung are caused by:

- Elastic properties of the tissues in the lung (collagen and elastic fibres).
- Surface tension forces in the lung caused by the alveolar–liquid interface.

Therefore, we need to consider the principles of surface tension.

Surface tension

Molecules within a liquid are attracted to each other by very strong forces (van der Waal's forces of attraction). Molecules in the liquid are pulled in all directions; however, molecules on the surface only have components towards the liquid and towards the adjacent molecule (the force of attraction towards air molecules above the surface is minute in comparison). Molecules on the surface are therefore pulled close together and act like a skin. This phenomenon is known as surface tension (Fig. 3.19).

When molecules of liquid lie on a curved surface (e.g. in a bubble), they are attracted to adjacent molecules (Fig. 3.20). If the force of attraction is split into its individual vector components it can be seen that there are two components:

- Tangential component.
- Radial component (pulling inward, tending to collapse the bubble).

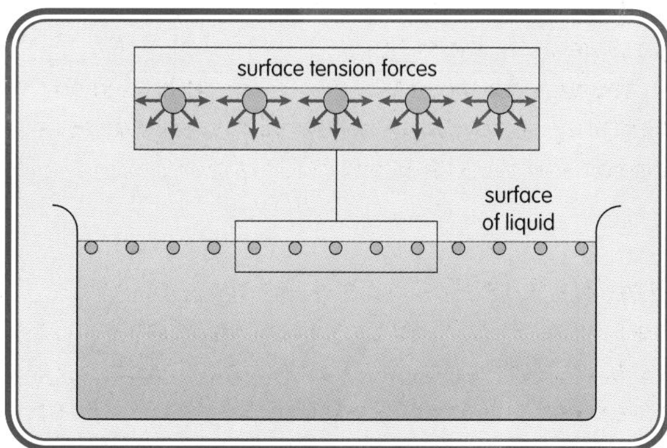

Fig. 3.19 Surface tension. (Adapted with permission from *Physiology* 3e, by R.M.Berne and M.N.Levy. Mosby Year Book, 1993.)

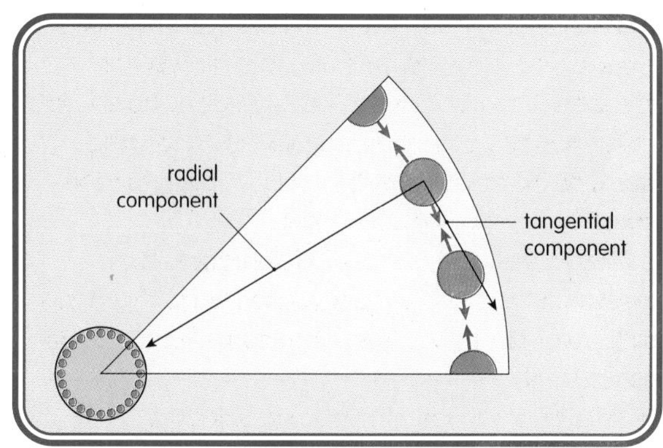

Fig. 3.20 Surface tension of a bubble. The summation of radial components tends to collapse the bubble and there must be a positive pressure inside the bubble to prevent it from collapsing.

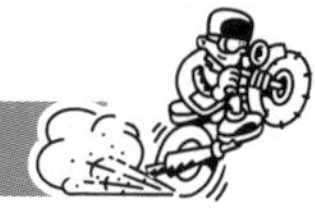

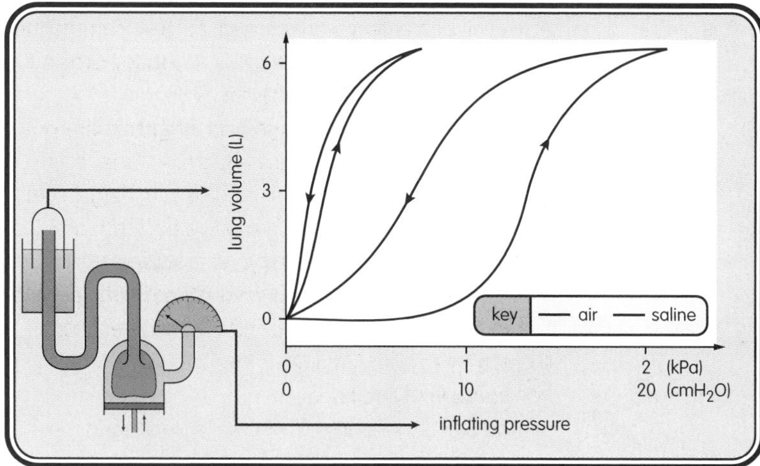

Fig. 3.21 Note the marked difference between the pressure–volume curves of air-filled and saline-filled lungs. It is much easier to inflate the lung without air. (Adapted with permission from *Physiology* 3e, by R.M. Berne and M.N. Levy. Mosby Year Book, 1993.)

Thus, if the bubble is to be prevented from collapsing, there must be an equal and opposite force tending to expand the bubble. This is provided by a positive pressure within the bubble.

This was described by Laplace, whose law stated that 'The pressure (P) within a bubble is equal to twice the surface tension (T) divided by the radius (r).'

$$P = \frac{2T}{r}$$

Therefore, the smaller a bubble (i.e. the more curved the surface) then the larger the radial component and the tendency to collapse. Hence, smaller bubbles must have a greater internal pressure to keep them inflated.

Surface tension within the lung

Surface tension is a physical property of liquids. The alveoli are lined with liquid and therefore can be considered similar to bubbles. If a bubble of about the same size as an alveolus was made of interstitial fluid and filled with air it would require an internal pressure in the order of 3 kPa to prevent it from collapsing. The lungs would have a very low compliance and the forces involved in breathing would be extremely large. This would suggest that the alveoli do not contain a liquid lining.

This was investigated by von Neergaard, who measured the compliance of excised lungs, first using air to inflate them and then using saline (Fig. 3.21). He noticed that:

- Inflating the lungs with saline doubles the compliance.
- The pressure required to inflate the lungs with air was greater during inflation than during deflation. Plotting the pressure of inflation against lung volume forms a loop. This phenomenon is called hysteresis.

His conclusions from this were:

- There was a liquid lining in the alveolus and there existed an air–liquid interface. This interface was responsible for one-half of the elastance of the lungs because inflating the lungs with saline abolished this interface and halved the elastic recoil of the lungs.
- The lining fluid in the lungs must have a very low surface tension because the pressures required to inflate the lung were low. Therefore the liquid could not be interstitial fluid.

This leads us to three questions:

- How is this low surface tension achieved?
- Laplace's law says that small bubbles have higher internal pressure than larger ones. If two bubbles of different sizes were connected, air would flow from the small bubble to the large, causing the small bubble to collapse (Fig. 3.22). Why does this not happen to alveoli?

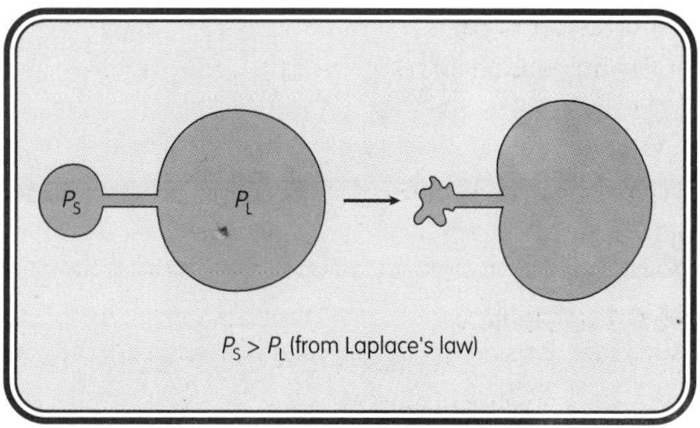

Fig. 3.22 Laplace's law. $P_s > P_l$ from Laplace's law. The smaller bubble collapses emptying into the larger lower pressure bubble.

- How does the phenomenon of hysteresis of the pressure–volume curve occur?

The answers to all these questions are linked to surfactant.

Surfactant

Surfactant is secreted by type II pneumocytes and contains a phospholipid (dipalmitoyl phosphatidyl choline). Surfactant has three functions:

- Prevention of alveolar collapse (gives alveolar stability).
- Increase in lung compliance by reducing surface tension of alveolar lining fluid.
- Prevention of transudation of fluid into alveoli.

Prevention of alveolar collapse

Because of two factors, alveoli of different sizes do not collapse:

- Surface tension of the alveolar lining fluid varies with surface area. This is because surfactant reduces surface tension in proportion to its surface concentration. Surfactant is insoluble in water and floats on the surface of the alveolar lining fluid. In larger alveoli the surfactant is more spread out (dilute) and the surface tension is higher (Fig. 3.23).
- There is interaction between adjacent groups of alveoli. Therefore, collapsing alveoli pull on adjacent alveoli preventing further collapse. This is termed alveolar interdependence.

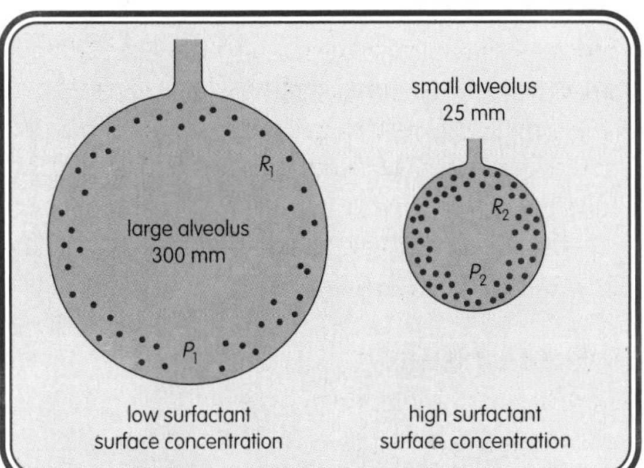

Fig. 3.23 The surface tension (T_1) within the larger alveolus (with radius R_1) is greater than the surface tension (T_2) within the smaller alveolus (with radius R_2). This is because the surfactant is more spread out in the larger alveolus. Thus, the T:R ratio remains constant and the same pressure is required to inflate alveoli of all sizes ($P_1 = P_2$).

Prevention of transudation of fluid into alveoli

Surfactant reduces the surface tension in the alveolar lining fluid, which reduces the tendency for the alveolus to collapse. If the alveoli were lined with interstitial fluid, their collapse would cause a more negative pressure in the interstitial space. This would lead into an increase in hydrostatic presssure difference between the pulmonary capillary and the interstitial space, leading to transudation of fluid.

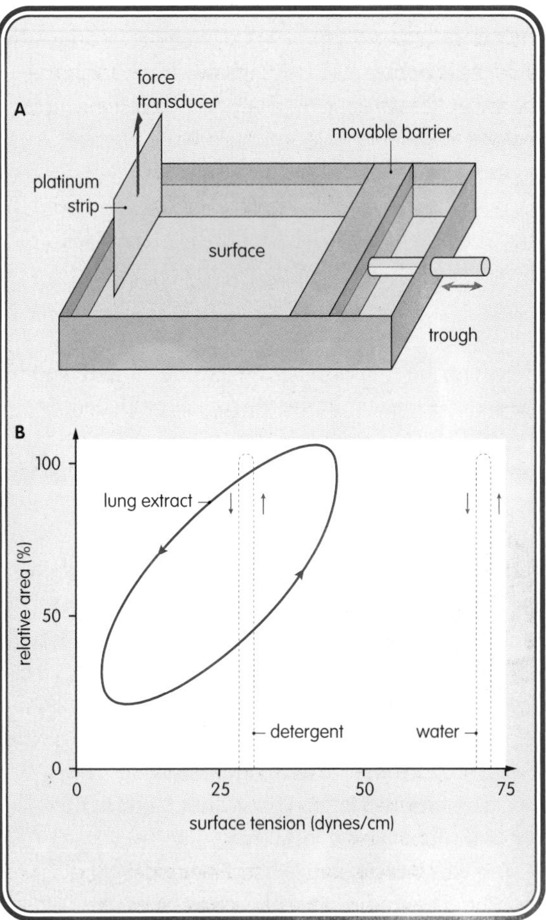

Fig. 3.24 (A) Surface balance. The area of the surface is altered and the surface tension is measured from the force exerted on a platinum strip dipped into the surface. (B) Plots of surface tension and area obtained with a surface balance. Note that lung washings show a change in surface tension with area and that the minimum tension is very small. (Adapted with permission from *Respiratory Physiology* 5e, by J. West. Williams & Wilkins, 1994.)

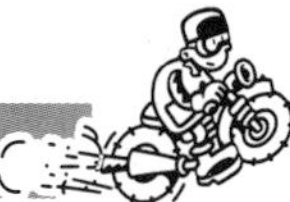

Hysteresis

Hysteresis of the pressure–volume curve is explained by a property of surfactant. The surface tension of surfactant shows different values when being expanded (e.g. during inspiration) or compressed (e.g. during expiration) (Fig. 3.24). Because lung compliance is dependent upon surface tension, this explains why hysteresis of the pressure–volume curve occurs.

Respiratory distress syndrome

Respiratory distress syndrome (RDS) occurs in premature babies of less than 32 weeks' gestation; it is caused by a deficiency of surfactant production by type II pneumocytes. Difficulty in breathing occurs; breathing is rapid and laboured, often with an expiratory grunt. There is diffuse damage to alveoli with hyaline membrane formation. Treatment is with high-concentration oxygen therapy, which reverses the hypoxaemia.

- **Explain why intrapleural pressure is negative. Describe its variation during breathing.**
- **Describe how breathing is brought about, naming the muscles involved and their actions.**
- **Define lung compliance and explain what is meant by static and dynamic lung compliance, including a description of the pressure–volume curve.**
- **Explain what is meant by hysteresis of the pressure–volume curve.**
- **Describe the role of surfactant.**

DYNAMICS OF VENTILATION

The previous section discusses the elastic properties of the lungs (i.e. those caused by surface tension and tissue elasticity). These were looked at under static conditions; however, if we inflate the lungs, dynamic conditions exist. So, in addition to overcoming the elastic properties of the lung during breathing, we must also overcome the dynamic resistance to inflation of the lungs.

Dynamic resistance comprises of:

- Resistance presented by the airways to flow of air into the lungs—airway resistance.
- Resistance to tissues as they slide over each other—viscous tissue resistance.

Viscous tissue resistance comprises approximately 20% of the total dynamic resistance.

Inflation pressure

The total pressure difference (P_{TOT}) required to inflate the lungs can be calculated by:

$$P_{TOT} = P_{COM} + P_{DYN}$$
$$P_{DYN} = P_{AR} + P_{VTR}$$

P_{AR} = pressure to overcome airways resistance;
P_{COM} = pressure to overcome lung compliance;
P_{DYN} = pressure to overcome the dynamic resistance;
P_{VTR} = pressure to overcome viscous tissue resistance.

Dynamic lung compliance

If a pressure–volume curve is plotted under dynamic conditions, the pressure volume loop is widened when compared with the curve under static conditions (Fig. 3.25). Dynamic lung compliance is the slope of this curve at any one point. Dynamic lung compliance is less than static lung compliance.

Before we discuss airway resistance, it is important to outline pattern of flow.

Pattern of flow

The pattern of fluid flowing through a tube (e.g. an airway or blood vessel) varies with the velocity and physical properties of the fluid. This was established by a French engineer, Reynolds, who injected a coloured dye into the centre of a clear pipe of water flowing at various velocities. He discovered two phenomena, which he described as laminar flow (which appeared at low flow rates; Fig. 3.26) and turbulent flow (which

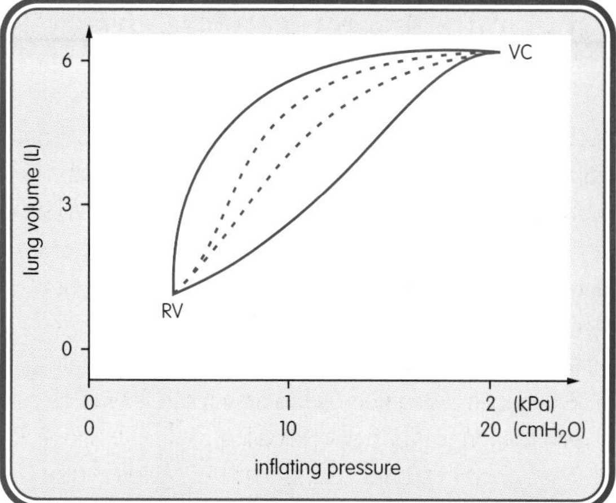

Fig. 3.25 Difference in pressure–volume relationships in lungs inflated and deflated (measurements made under static conditions with no air flowing—dotted lines; dynamic conditions with air flowing continuously into or out of the lung—full lines).

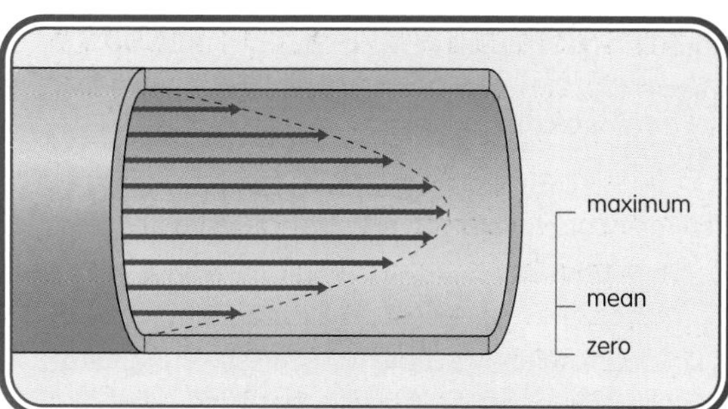

Fig. 3.26 Laminar flow in which the coloured filament remained central. The flow occurs in streamlines, or laminae. The greatest velocity of flow is centrally and the velocity profile is parabolic. (Adapted with permission from *Physiology* 3e, by R.M. Berne and M.N. Levy. Mosby Year Book, 1993.)

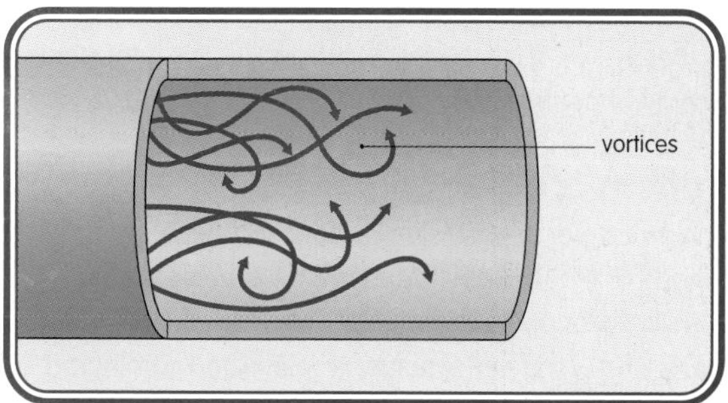

Fig. 3.27 Turbulent flow in which the coloured filament broke up into eddies. (Adapted with permission from *Physiology* 3e, by R.M. Berne and M.N. Levy. Mosby Year Book, 1993.)

appeared at high flow rates; Fig. 3.27). The change between these two flow regimes is not instantaneous and a transition zone exists, where the flow pattern is poorly described by either regime. Reynolds developed a dimensionless number, the Reynolds number (Re):

$$Re = 2\,r \cdot v \cdot d/\eta$$

where, v = velocity, r = radius of pipe, d = density of fluid, and η = viscosity of fluid.

If Re < 1500 usually there is laminar flow; turbulent flow occurs at values much greater than this (usually Re > 2000). Thus turbulent flow is much more likely to occur with:

- High velocities (e.g. within the airways during exercise).
- Larger diameter blood vessels or airways.
- Low-viscosity, high-density fluids.
- Branching or irregular surfaces can also initiate turbulence.

Fig. 3.28 describes some of the differences between laminar and turbulent flow.

Airway resistance

Airway resistance can be defined as 'The resistance to flow of gas within the airways of the lung'. Remember that:

- Airway resistance occurs only during flow within the airways.
- Airway resistance occurs in both laminar and turbulent flow conditions.

Laminar flow is described by Poiseuille's law. In basic terms, Poiseuille's law states that for a fluid under laminar flow conditions, the flow rate (F) is directly related to the pressure drop (P) between the two ends of a tube and the fourth power of the radius (r); however, it is inversely related to the viscosity (η) and the length of pipe (L):

$$F = \frac{P\pi r^4}{8\eta L}$$

From this equation, we can see that as the driving force (P) increases, so does flow. Narrower or longer pipes or a higher fluid viscosity have a higher resistance to flow and so flow rate is reduced.

Resistance to flow (R) can be defined as the ratio of driving force to actual flow achieved.

$$R = \frac{P}{F}$$

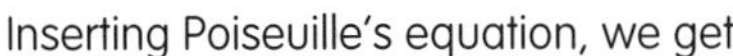

Inserting Poiseuille's equation, we get:

$$R = \frac{8\eta L}{\pi r^4}$$

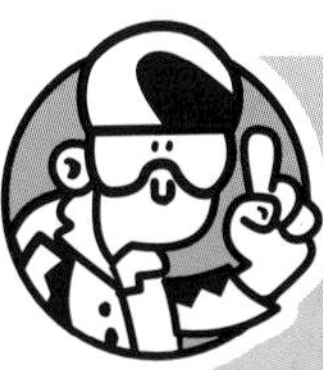

Remembering Poiseuille's law isn't drastically important, but understanding it is! So, remember that in laminar flow:

- **A small change in radius significantly affects either flow rate or pressure drop required to achieve the same flow. An example of this is bronchoconstriction in asthma.**
- **Flow varies directly with pressure drop.**
- **Flow varies inversely with viscosity (e.g. during scuba diving).**

Sites of airway resistance

Considering the whole respiratory system:

- Approximately one-half of the resistance to airflow occurs in the upper respiratory tract when breathing through the nose. This is significantly reduced when mouth breathing.
- Thus, approximately one-half of the resistance lies within the lower respiratory tract.

Assuming laminar air flow, Poiseuille's law would predict that the major resistance to air flow would occur in the smaller radius airways. This is not the case because although the individual diameter of each airway is small, the total cross-sectional area for flow increases (large number of small airways) as we go down the tracheobronchial tree.

In exercise, the airway resistance may increase significantly due to high air flows inducing turbulence. It is normal under these conditions to switch to mouth breathing to reduce airway resistance.

It is important to note that resistance of the smaller airways is difficult to measure. Thus, these small airways may be damaged by disease and it may be some time before this damage is detectable, thus representing a 'silent' zone.

Factors determining airway resistance

Factors affecting airway resistance are:

- Lung volume.
- Bronchial motor tone.
- Altered airway calibre.
- Change in density and viscosity of inspired gas.

Lung volume

Airways are supported by radial traction of lung parenchyma and thus their diameter and resistance to

Differences between laminar and turbulent flow

Laminar	Turbulent
fluid moves parallel to walls only	flow has some movement at right angles
no mixing between fluid other than by diffusion	well-mixed flow eddies and diffusion
non erosive flow regime	flow regime can be erosive
flow is quiet	may account for murmurs heard clinically
poor flow for arterial thrombi but venous stasis may lead to thrombi	arterial thrombi more likely to form
resistance to flow is independent of surface roughness	resistance to flow is dependent on surface roughness
flow is proportional to the radius to the power 4	flow is proportional to diameter to the power 5

Fig. 3.28 Differences between laminar and turbulent flow.

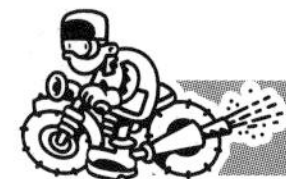

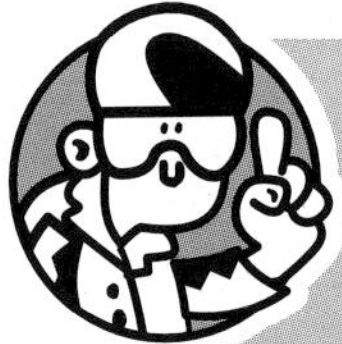

Things to remember:

- **The major site of airway resistance is medium-sized bronchi.**
- **80% of the resistance of the lower respiratory tract is presented by the trachea and bronchi.**
- **Less than 20% of airway resistance is caused by airways less than 2 mm in diameter.**

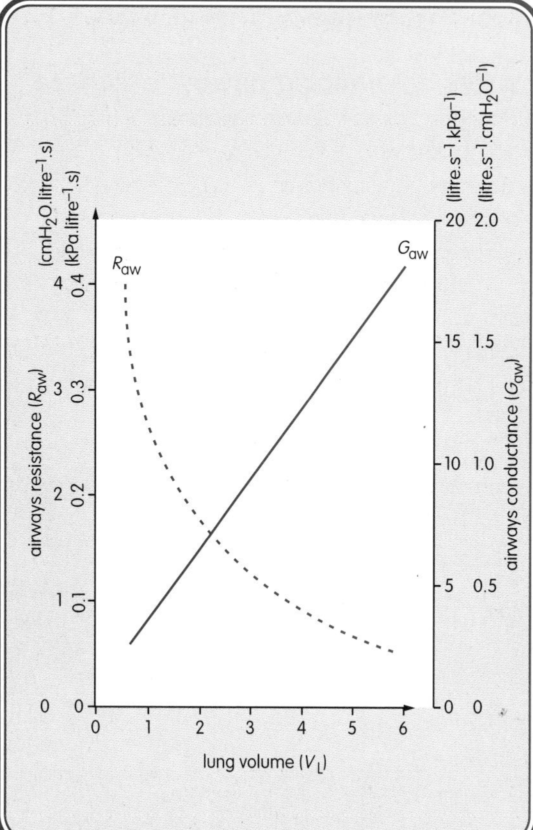

Fig. 3.29 The relationship between lung volume (V_L) and airway resistance (R_{aw}) and conductance (G_{aw}). Note that at low lung volumes, R_{aw} is high and G_{aw} is low. (Adapted with permission from *Respiratory Physiology* 2e, by J. Widdicombe and A. Davies. Edward Arnold, 1991.)

flow are affected by lung volume (Fig. 3.29):

- Low lung volumes tend to collapse and compress the airways, reducing their diameter and thus increasing resistance to flow.
- High lung volumes tend to increase radial traction, increasing the length and diameter of airways.
- The increase in diameter reduces airway resistance. The increase in length has a much smaller effect of increasing resistance, which is explained by Poiseuille's law.

Bronchial motor tone

Bronchial motor tone is affected by eight factors (Fig. 3.30):

- Irritant cough, C fibre reflex.
- Pulmonary stretch receptors.
- Carbon dioxide concentration.
- Oxygen concentration.
- Mediator release.
- Catecholamine release.
- Sympathetic activity.
- Other nerves.

Reduced airway calibre can be caused either by disease or by an inhaled foreign body. A change in density and viscosity of gas occurs in scuba diving (Chapter 5).

Dynamic compression of airways

The pressure difference between the gas in the airway and the pressure outside the airway is known as the transmural pressure difference. The pressure

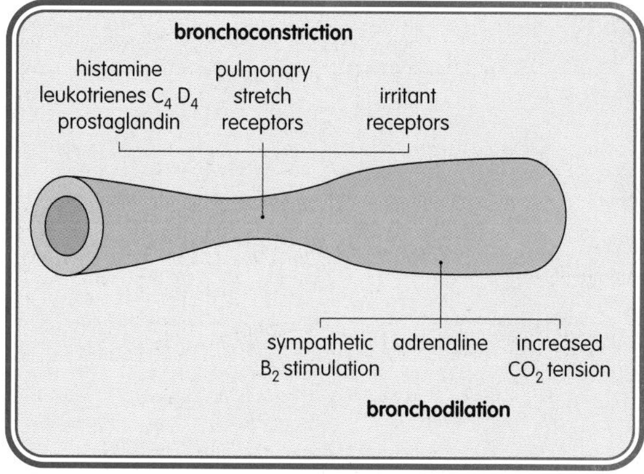

Fig. 3.30 Factors affecting bronchial motor tone. (Adapted with permission from *Physiology* 3e, by R.M. Berne and M.N. Levy. Mosby Year Book, 1993.

outside the airway reflects the intrapleural pressure (Fig. 3.31).

During inspiration

The pressure within the pleural cavity is always negative and the alveolar pressure is greater than intrapleural pressure. The transmural pressure difference is always positive thus the airway is distended (radial traction).

During expiration

The pressure within the alveolus is positive with respect to the intrapleural pressure; hence, the alveolus stays open. The transmural pressure difference, however, is dependent upon expiratory flow rate and intrapleural pressure.

During forced expiration, the positive intrapleural pressure is transmitted through the lungs to the external wall of the airways. In addition, there is a dynamic pressure drop from alveolus to the airway caused by airway resistance. This is greater at high expiratory flow rates. Thus, the pressure in the lumen of the airway may be lower than the external wall pressure (negative transmural pressure), leading to collapse of the airways.

Thus, the harder the subject tries to exhale forcibly, the more the airways are compressed, so the rate of expiration does not rise as the increased pressure gradient (from alveoli to atmospheric pressure) is offset by the reduced calibre of the airways. This phenomenon is known as the dynamic compression of airways.

Dynamic compression of airways is greater at lower lung volumes because the effect of radial traction holding the airways open is less. Thus it can be seen that for a specific lung volume there is a maximum expiratory flow rate caused by dynamic compression of the airways (Fig. 3.32). Any rate of expiration below this flow rate is dependent on how much effort is made to expel the air from the lungs and the flow is said to be effort dependent. At maximum expiratory flow rate, any additional effort does not alter the expiratory flow rate (because of dynamic compression of airways) and the flow is said to be effort independent.

Work done by breathing

The work done (*W*) to change a volume (ΔV) of gas at constant pressure (*P*) is shown by the relationship below:

$$W = P \cdot \Delta V$$

Work done is measured in joules; a volume change of 10 L at a pressure of 1 cmH_2O = 1 J of energy.

An increase in tidal volume will increase the volume change and hence the work done. An increase in the ventilation rate not associated with a change in tidal volume will increase the rate of work done (power).

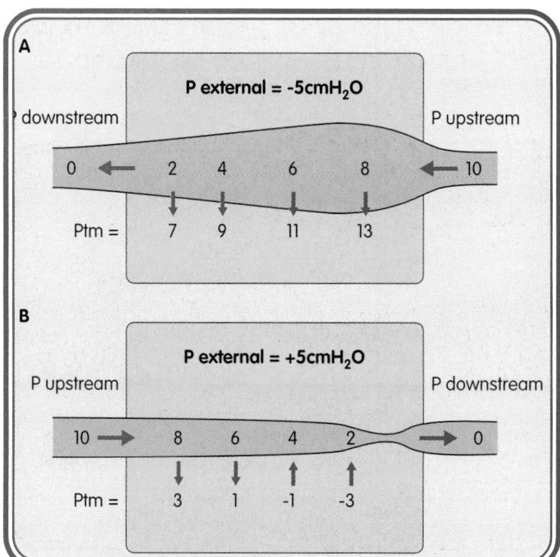

Fig. 3.31 Transmural pressure. (A) during inspiration. (B) during expiration. Ptm = transmural pressure.

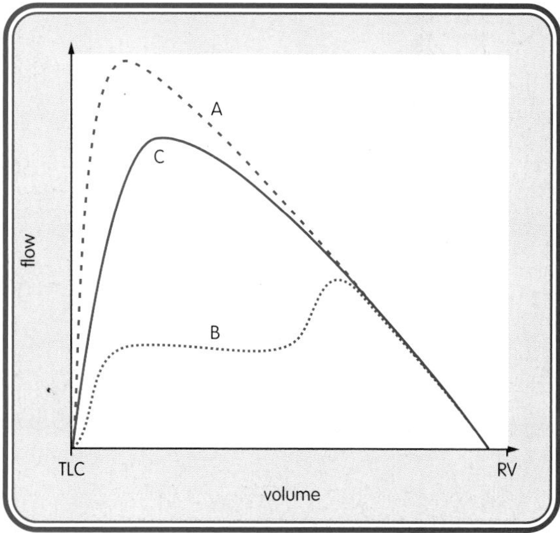

Fig. 3.32 Flow–volume curves made with a spirometer. (A) Maximum inspiration and forced expiration. (B) Slow expiration initially then forced. (C) Expiratory flow almost to maximum effort. Note that the three descending curves are almost superimposed.

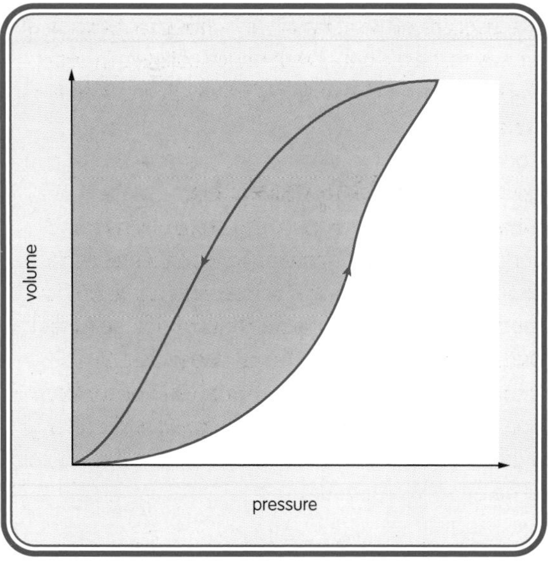

Fig. 3.33 Graph of normal lung volume against trans-lung pressure. The shaded area is the inspiratory work of breathing. (Adapted with permission from *Respiratory Physiology* 2e, by J. Widdicombe and A. Davies. Arnold, 1991.)

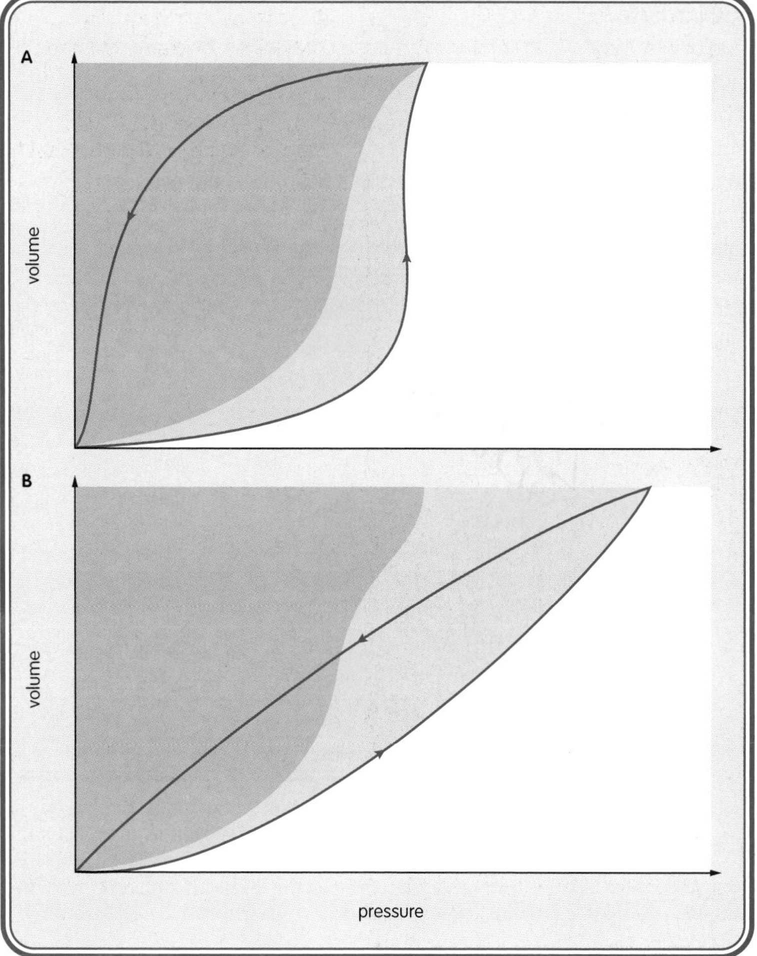

Fig. 3.34 Changes to breathing work during diseased states. Paler shading denotes disease state; dark shading shows the normal work prefills from Fig. 3.35. (A) Increased airway resistance (e.g. in asthma); (B) decreased compliance (e.g. in fibrotic lung disease). (Adapted with permission from *Respiratory Physiology* 2e, by J. Widdicombe and A. Davies. Arnold, 1991.)

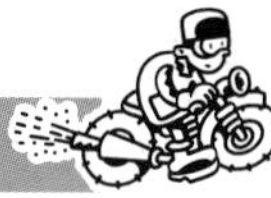

Fig. 3.33 shows a graph of lung volume against trans-lung pressure. In expiration, less work is required than in inspiration because of hysteresis. This additional free energy that was stored in the elastic recoil of the lungs during inspiration is used to pull the chest wall back to its resting position at functional residual capacity.

The work of breathing can be changed during diseased states (Fig. 3.34). The work required to inflate the lungs will increase if:

- Lungs are inflated to a larger volume.
- Lung compliance decreases (e.g. fibrotic lungs).
- Airway resistance increases (e.g. chronic obstructive pulmonary disease and asthma).
- Turbulence is induced in the airways (e.g. in high flow rates experienced during severe exercise).

The opposite of these factors will decrease the work of breathing; hence, the use of bronchodilators in asthma. The work done in breathing is altered by the pattern of breathing (Fig. 3.35).

Efficiency of lung ventilation

Efficiency (*e*) of any system is the amount of work performed divided by the energy expenditure. The efficiency of the respiratory systems during ventilation can be assessed by comparing the amount of work done by the respiratory muscles during breathing (metabolic energy required: *Q*) with the mechanical work performed on expanding the chest and the lungs ($P \cdot \Delta V$).

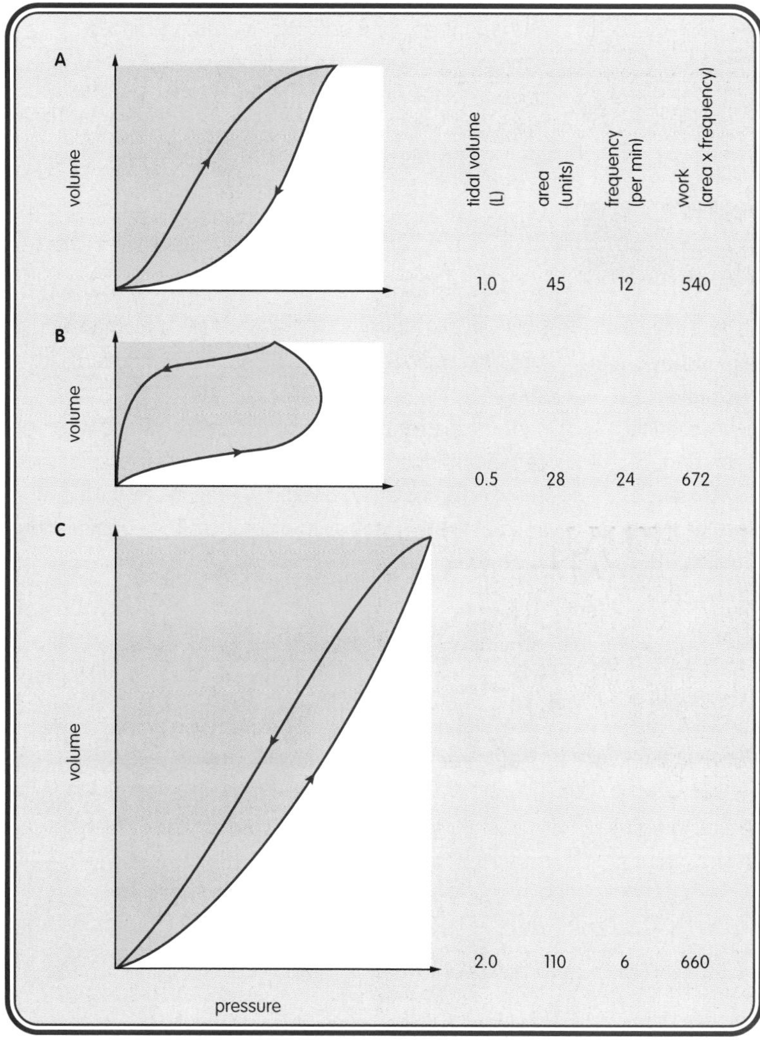

Fig. 3.35 The work done in breathing is altered by the pattern of breathing. (A) Optimal pattern; (B) increased frequency and decreased volume; (C) decreased frequency and increased volume. (Adapted with permission from *Respiratory Physiology* 2e, by J. Widdicombe and A. Davies. Arnold, 1991.)

Thus, if e is measured as a percentage:

$$e = \left(\frac{P \cdot \Delta V}{Q}\right) \times 100$$

The efficiency of normal quiet breathing is only 10%. In disease, efficiency may decrease (e.g. in chronic obstructive pulmonary disease) and work done may increase so much that all the oxygen supplied from increasing ventilation is consumed by the respiratory muscles, thus leading to a maximum ventilation rate.

- **Define airway resistance and viscous tissue resistance.**
- **List the factors determining airway resistance.**
- **Explain what is meant by dynamic compression of the airways.**

GASEOUS EXCHANGE IN THE LUNGS

This section discusses how gas is transferred from the alveoli to the bloodstream and from the bloodstream to the alveoli. A brief outline of how the laws of diffusion apply to the diffusion of gas from the airways to the circulation is given below. Time for diffusion and diffusion–perfusion limitations are also discussed.

Diffusion is the process in which molecules move due to their random motion (Brownian motion). The process of diffusion is seen to be a net movement of particles:

- Diffusion occurs from an area of concentration to an area of low concentration. Thus, the driving force for diffusion is concentration difference (ΔC).
- Diffusion will occur until the concentration in the two areas is equalized (i.e. net movement has ceased). Random movement of particles continues to occur and this is known as dynamic equilibrium.

Gaseous exchange between alveolar air and blood in pulmonary capillaries

Gas exchange within the lungs takes place by diffusion

Diffusion through a membrane was first described by Fick. Fick's law of diffusion states that the rate of diffusion (flux, J) of a substance through a membrane is proportional to the surface area of the membrane (A), the solubility (S) of the substance in the membrane, and the concentration difference (ΔC) between both sides of the membrane, and that it is universely proportional to the thickness of the membrane (t) and the square root of the molecular weight (wt_{mol}):

$$J = \frac{(A \times S \times \Delta C)}{(t \times wt_{mol})}$$

The equation can be simplified by using the term diffusivity (K). The diffusivity or diffusion coefficent (K) is dependent upon the substance and also the membrane, and is constant for a particular membrane and a particular substance. The coefficient is proportional to the solubility of the gas divided by the square root of its molecular weight (Fig. 3.36).

$$J = \frac{K \times A \times \Delta C}{t}$$

where

$$K = \frac{S}{wt_{mol}}$$

Because alveolar gas diffuses through a membrane and then dissolves into the blood, the driving force for transfer is the partial pressure of gas.

Thus, the rate of diffusion across the alveoli is directly dependent upon the difference in partial pressures between a gas in the alveoli (P_A) and in arterial blood (P_a), not the concentration difference. The equation can be rewritten as:

Henry's law states that at equilibrium, the amount of gas dissolved in a given volume of liquid at a given temperature is proportional to the partial pressure (P) of the gas in the gas phase and its solubility in the liquid (S).

$$C = S \cdot P$$

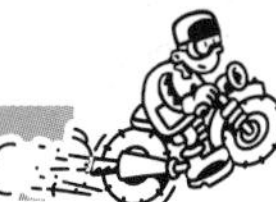

$$J = \frac{K \times A \cdot (P_A - P_a)}{t}$$

Thus, it can be seen why the blood–gas interface (Chapter 2), with its large surface area of 50–100 m^2 and average thickness of 0.4 µm permits the high rate of diffusion required by the body.

Partial pressures of respiratory gases

The partial pressure of a gas can be calculated by Dalton's law. Dalton's law states that 'The pressure exerted by a mixture of nonreacting gases is equal to the sum of the partial pressures of the separate components.' In other words, each gas in a mixture of gases exerts the same pressure as it would if it were present alone in the volume occupied by the mixture (Fig. 3.37).

$$P_{atm} = PO_2 + PN_2 + PCO_2 + PH_2O$$
$$PN_2 = FN_2 \times P_{atm}$$

where P_{atm} = barometric pressure (about 761 mmHg at sea level), PO_2 = partial pressure of oxygen, and FN_2 = fractional concentration of nitrogen in atmospheric air. The partial pressure of a gas in a system will alter with total pressure. If atmospheric pressure is reduced (e.g. when climbing Mount Everest), so will the partial pressure of oxygen.

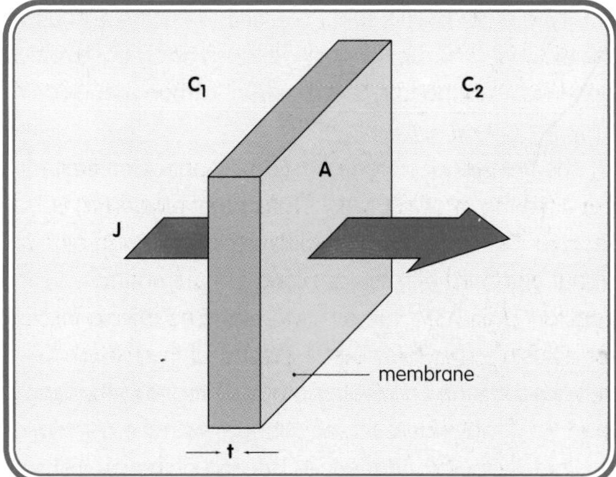

Fig. 3.36 Diffusion—Fick's law. Fick stated that the rate of diffusion (J) of a gas through a membrane was:

$$J = \frac{K \times A \times \Delta C}{t}$$

where

$$K = \frac{S}{wt_{mol}}$$

A = surface area; t = thickness of membrane; ΔC = concentration difference; S = solubility of substance in the membrane; wt_{mol} = molecular weight.

Partial pressures of respiratory gases			
Gas	**PO_2 (kPa)**	**PCO_2 (kPa)**	**PH_2O (kPa)**
atmosphere	21	0	variable
trachea (inspiration)	20	0	6.3*
alveolar gas	13.5	5.3	6.3
exhaled breath	16	3.5	variable

*note inspired air is fully saturated with water vapour before it enters the lungs

Fig. 3.37 Partial pressures of respiratory gases.

Water vapour pressure

The water vapour pressure of a gas depends on:

- Saturation of the gas.
- Temperature of the gas.

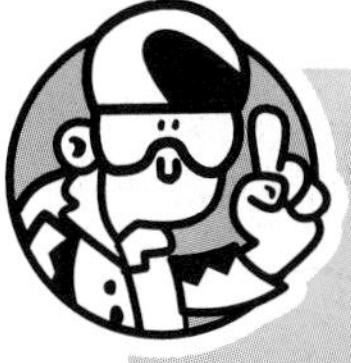

The following will increase the rate of oxygen diffusion into the blood:

- **Increased surface area of the alveolus.**
- **Decreased thickness of the alveolar wall.**
- **Increased alveolar partial pressure of oxygen (oxygen therapy).**

The following will decrease the rate of oxygen diffusion into the blood:

- **Reduction in the overall alveolar surface area (e.g. emphysema).**
- **Increased distance for diffusion (e.g. emphysema).**
- **Increased thickness of the alveolar wall (e.g. fibrosing alveolitis).**
- **Reduction in the alveolar partial pressure of oxygen (e.g. altitude).**

Saturation depends on the condition to which the dry gas has been exposed (i.e. water contact and temperature of contact). Saturation is quoted as percentage saturation. Water vapour pressure increases with rising temperature. It is important to know that for fully (100%) saturated air, the water vapour pressure at 37°C is 47 mmHg.

Perfusion and diffusion limitation

At the gas exchange surface, gas transfer occurs through a membrane into a flowing liquid. There are two processes (Fig. 3.38) occurring:

- Diffusion across the alveolar capillary membrane.
- Perfusion of blood through pulmonary capillaries.

Uptake of a gas into the blood is dependent on its solubility and the chemical combination of a gas (e.g. with haemoglobin: Hb). If the chemical combination is strong, the gas is taken up by the blood with little rise in arterial partial pressure.

The solubility of nitrous oxide (N_2O) in the blood is low, and it does not undergo chemical combination with any component of the blood. Thus, rate of transfer of gas into the liquid phase is slow and partial pressure of the gas in the blood rises rapidly (Fig. 3.39). This reduces the partial pressure difference between alveolar gas and the blood and hence the driving force for diffusion. Nitrous oxide is, therefore, an example of a gas that is said to be perfusion limited. Thus, the amount of nitrous oxide taken up by the blood is dependent almost solely upon the rate of blood flow through the pulmonary capillaries.

In the case of carbon monoxide (CO), the gas is taken up rapidly and bound tightly by haemoglobin; the arterial partial pressure rises slowly (Fig. 3.39). Thus, there is always a driving force (partial pressure difference) for diffusion (even at low perfusion rates), and the overall rate of transfer will be dependent on the rate of diffusion. This type of transfer is said to be diffusion limited. Thus the amount of carbon monoxide taken up by the blood is dependent on the rate of diffusion of carbon monoxide from the alveoli to the blood.

The transfer of oxygen is normally perfusion limited because the arterial partial pressure of oxygen (P_aO_2) reaches equilibrium with the alveolar gas (P_AO_2) by about one-third of the way along the pulmonary capillary (Fig. 3.39); there is, therefore, no driving force for diffusion after this point. However, if the diffusion is slow because of emphysematous changes to the lung, then P_aO_2 may not reach equilibrium with the alveolar gas before the blood reaches the end of the capillary. Under these conditions, the transfer of oxygen is diffusion limited.

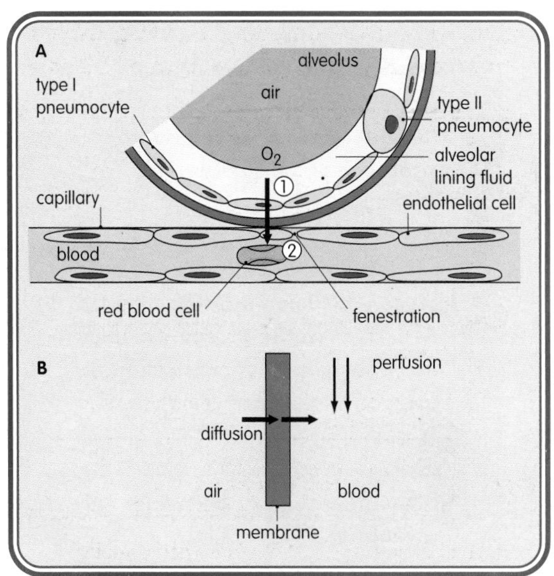

Fig. 3.38 Gas transfer across alveolar capillary membrane. (A) Diffusional process; (B) uptake process.

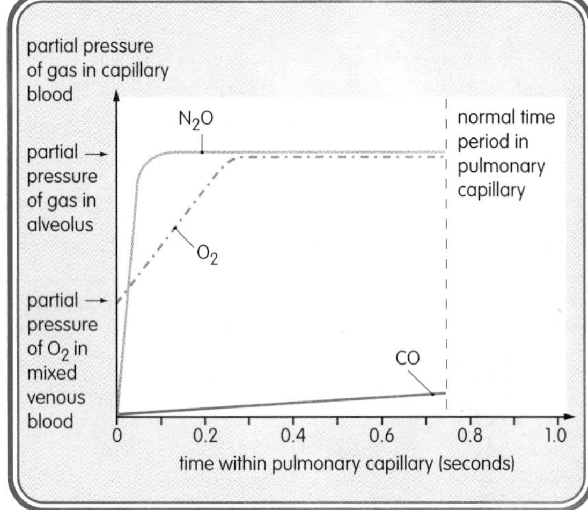

Fig. 3.39 Graph of partial pressure of respiratory gases against time within the pulmonary capillary bed. Transfer of N_2O is perfusion limited, transfer of CO is diffusion limited. Transfer of O_2 is usually perfusion limited but may change with diseased states.

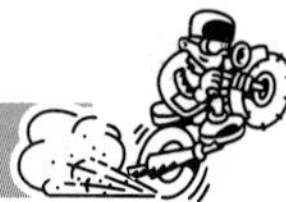

Oxygen uptake in the capillary network

The time taken for the partial pressure of oxygen to reach its plateau is approximately 0.25 secs. The pulmonary capillary volume under resting conditions is about 75 mL, which is approximately the same size as the stroke volume of the right ventricle. Pulmonary capillary blood is therefore replaced with every heart beat, approximately every 0.75 seconds. This far exceeds the time for transfer of oxygen into the bloodstream.

During exercise, however, the cardiac output increases and the flow rate though the pulmonary capillaries also increases. Because the lungs have the ability to recruit new capillaries and distend already open capillaries (see Chapter 4), the effect of increased blood flow rate on the time allowed for diffusion is not as great as one might expect. In severe exercise, the pulmonary capillary network volume may increase by up to 200 mL. This helps maintain the time allowed for diffusion, although it cannot keep it to the same value as at rest (Fig. 3.40).

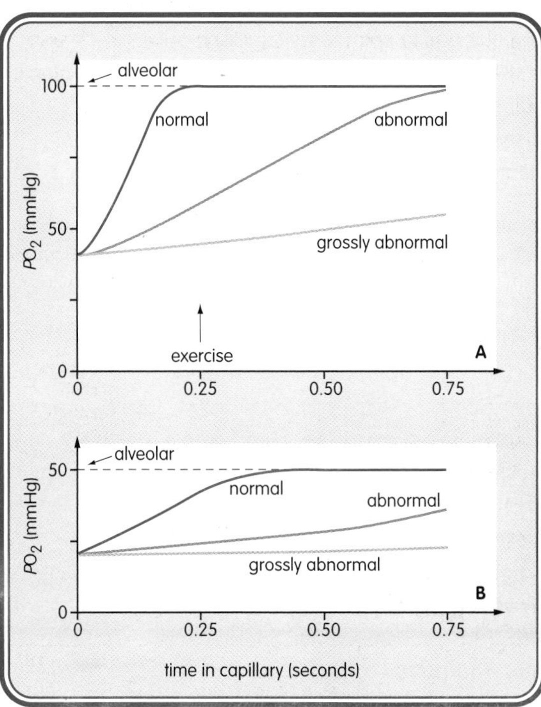

Fig. 3.40 Pulmonary capillary partial pressure of oxygen vs time in the pulmonary capillary network. (A) Alveolar PO_2 normal (B) low alveolar PO_2. Curves are for normal blood gas interface and abnormal in diseased state. (Adapted with permission from *Respiratory Physiology* 5e, by J. West. Williams & Wilkins, 1994.)

Carbon dioxide transfer

Diffusion within the gaseous state is described by Graham's law, which states that 'The rates of diffusion (*D*) of two gases under the same conditions of temperature and pressure are inversely proportional to the square roots of their molecular weights ($wt_{mol.}$).'

$$D_1/D_2 = wt_{mol2}/\ wt_{mol1}$$

However, diffusion in liquids is directly dependent upon the solubility of the gas, but inversely proportional to the square root of its molecular weight. Carbon dioxide diffuses 20 times more rapidly than oxygen, but has a similar molecular weight. Thus, the difference in rates of diffusion is caused by the much higher solubility of carbon dioxide.

Under normal conditions, the transfer of carbon dioxide is not diffusion limited (Fig. 3.41).

Measuring diffusion

As we have already seen (p 54), gas transfer (*J*) can be calculated:

$$J = K \cdot A \cdot (P_A - P_a)/t$$

It is not possible to measure the area and thickness of a complex structure like the blood–gas barrier, so the equation is rewritten:

$$J = D_L(P_A - P_a)$$

Where D_L is the diffusing capacity of the lung, defined as the ease of diffusion of gas into the blood (the rate

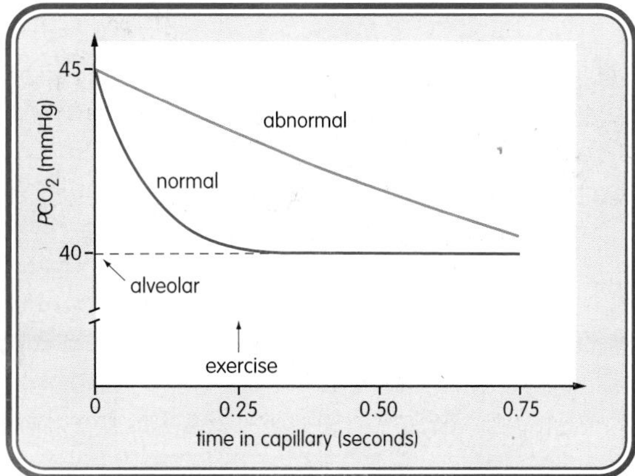

Fig. 3.41 Change in P_aCO_2. Calculate when alveolar capillary membrane normal or abnormal. (Adapted with permission from *Respiratory Physiology* 5e, by J. West. Williams & Wilkins, 1994.)

of uptake of a gas divided by the partial pressure difference between alveoli and blood).

$$D_L = J/(P_A - P_a)$$

Because carbon monoxide is taken up into the liquid phase very quickly, the rate of perfusion of pulmonary capillaries does not significantly affect the partial pressure difference between alveolar gas and the bloodstream. In addition, carbon monoxide binds irreversibly to haemoglobin and is not taken up by the tissues. Carbon monoxide is therefore a suitable gas for measuring diffusing capacity.

$$D_{L(CO)} = J_{(CO)}/(P_{A(CO)} - P_{a(CO)})$$

The partial pressure of carbon monoxide in the blood ($P_{a(CO)}$) is negligible, so the equation can be rewritten:

$$D_{L(CO)} = J_{(CO)}/P_{A(CO)}$$

One of the methods used to measure diffusion across the blood–gas interface is the single-breath method. A single breath of a mixture of carbon monoxide and air is taken. The breath is then held for approximately 10 secs. The difference between inspiratory and expiratory concentrations of carbon dioxide is measured. The lung volume is also measured by the helium dilution method. Thus, the amount of carbon monoxide taken up by the blood in 10 secs is known. The rate of transfer can then be calculated; this is a measure of the non-steady-state gas transfer (units: mL/min/mmHg).

Low values are caused by a reduced rate of diffusion because of:

- Thickening of the alveolar capillary membrane (e.g. in fibrosing alveolitis).
- Oedema of the alveolar capillary walls.
- Increased lining fluid within the alveoli.
- Increased distance for gaseous diffusion (e.g. in emphysema).
- Reduced area of alveolar capillary membrane (e.g. in emphysema).
- Reduced flow of fresh air to the alveoli from terminal bronchioles.
- Hypoventilation.

Oxygen is not a good candidate for calculating diffusing capacity because it binds reversibly to haemoglobin; thus, mixed venous partial pressure may not be the same as that of blood entering the pulmonary capillary bed.

Perfusion also affects the rate of transfer from alveolar gas to pulmonary capillary.

Because there can be many causes of a reduction in diffusing capacity, it is not a specific test for lung disease. It is, however, a sensitive test; it is able to demonstrate minor impediments to gas diffusion.

- **Which factors affect the rate of diffusion across the blood–air interface? What is the driving force for diffusion?**
- **Give the normal values of the partial pressures of carbon dioxide and oxygen within the respiratory system.**
- **Explain the terms 'partial pressure of a gas' and 'vapour pressure'.**
- **Name three conditions that lower the transfer of oxygen to the blood. How do these conditions affect diffusion?**
- **Using examples, define perfusion limition and diffusion limitation.**
- **Define diffusing capacity. How can diffusing capacity be measured?**

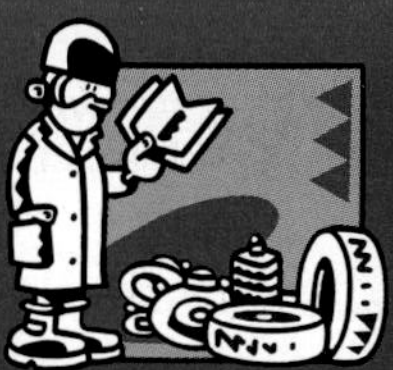

4. Perfusion and Gas Transport

PULMONARY BLOOD FLOW

Outline of pulmonary circulation

An outline of the pulmonary blood flow was given in Fig. 2.22. Venous blood returning from the body enters the right atrium and passively fills the right ventricle during diastole. During systole, the right ventricle contracts, ejecting its contents into the pulmonary artery (note the pulmonary artery contains deoxygenated blood).

Blood flows along the pulmonary arteries and arterioles, which closely follow the course of the airways. Blood enters the pulmonary capillaries (situated within the walls of the alveoli) and gaseous exchange takes place. Blood that returns to enter the left atrium through postcapillary venules and pulmonary veins (which contain oxygenated blood).

Mechanics of the circulation

The flow of blood through the pulmonary vasculature is slightly less than the systemic output of the left ventricle. This is because a proportion of the coronary circulation from the aorta drains directly into the left ventricle. In addition, the bronchial circulation from the aorta drains into pulmonary veins, thus bypassing the lungs. However, we can consider the flow through the pulmonary artery to be equal to cardiac output.

Pressures within the pulmonary circulation are much lower than those equivalent regions within the systemic circulation (Fig. 4.1). Because the volume of blood flowing through both circulations is approximately the same, the pulmonary circulation must offer lower resistance.

Pulmonary capillaries and arterioles cause the main resistance to flow in the pulmonary circulation. This low resistance is achieved in two ways:

- A large number of resistance vessels exist, which are usually dilated; thus, the total area for flow is very large.
- Small muscular arteries contain much less smooth muscle than equivalent arteries in the systemic circulation; they are more easily distended.

Many other factors affect pulmonary blood flow and pulmonary vascular resistance. These are discussed below.

Normal pressures in the pulmonary circulation

Site	Pressure (mmHg)	Pressure (cmH_2O)
pulmonary artery systolic/diastolic pressure	24/9	33/11
mean pressure	14	19
arteriole (mean pressure)	12	16
capillary (mean pressure)	10.5	14
venule (mean pressure)	9.0	12
left atrium (mean pressure)	8.0	11

Fig. 4.1 Pressures within the pulmonary circulation. The pulmonary arterial and left atrial pressures are measured during cardiac catheterization, the former directly, the latter by wedging the arterial catheter into a branch of the pulmonary artery. The capillary pressure is computed by a standard equation. (Adapted with permission from *Physiology* 3e, by R.M. Berne and M.N. Levy. Mosby Year Book, 1993.)

Hydrostatic pressure

Hydrostatic pressure has three effects.

- It distends blood vessels; as hydrostatic pressure rises, distension of the vessel increases.
- It is capable of opening previously closed capillaries (recruitment).
- It causes flow to occur; in other words, a pressure difference (ΔP) between the arterial and venous ends of a vessel provides the driving force for flow (see Fig. 4.7).

In situations where increased pulmonary flow is required (e.g. during exercise), the cardiac output is increased, which raises pulmonary vascular pressure. This causes recruitment of previously closed capillaries and distension of already open capillaries (Fig. 4.2). In turn, this reduces the pulmonary vascular resistance to flow; it is for this reason that resistance to flow through the pulmonary vasculature decreases with increasing pulmonary vascular pressure.

Remember, any resistance to flow causes a drop in pressure; therefore, the hydrostatic pressure in postcapillary venules will be less than that within the capillaries.

Pressure outside pulmonary blood vessels

Pressure outside a vessel can tend either to compress or collapse the vessel if the pressure is positive, or to aid the distention of the vessel if the pressure is negative.

The tendency for a vessel to distend or collapse is also dependent on the pressure inside the lumen. Thus, it is the pressure difference across the wall, which is the determinant factor (transmural pressure) (Fig. 4.3).

Pulmonary vessels can be considered in two groups (Fig. 4.4): alveolar and extra-alveolar vessels.

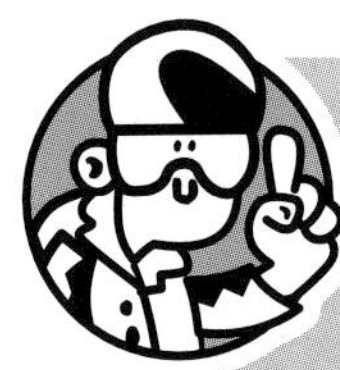

Pulmonary ΔP is small compared with the systemic circulation, so R must be small to achieve the same flow rate.

Flow = driving force/resistance = $\Delta P/R$

Poiseuille's law describes lamina flow and shows the importance of radius to the flow rate within a vessel.

$$Q = \frac{\pi(P_1 - P_2)r^4}{8\eta l} \qquad R = \frac{8\eta l}{\pi r^4}$$

Thus, it can be seen that the calibre of a vessel significantly affects resistance to flow and hence the flow rate through a vessel when a particular pressure difference is applied.

The pulmonary circulation is therefore a low-pressure, low-resistance system.

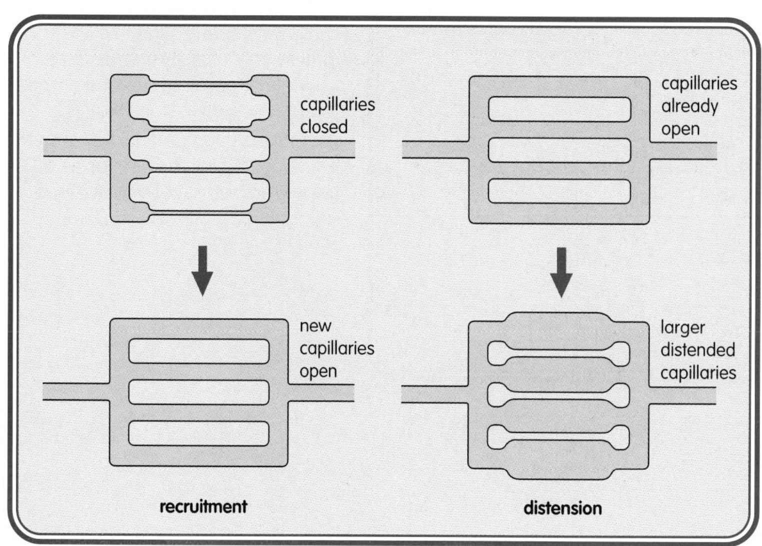

Fig. 4.2 Recruitment and distension of pulmonary capillaries to lower pulmonary vascular resistance.

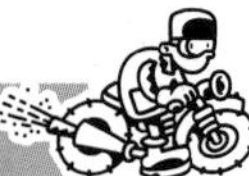

Alveolar vessels

Alveolar vessels are contained in the alveolar wall (capillaries and slightly larger vessels). External pressure is alveolar pressure (normally atmospheric pressure). As the lungs expand, these vessels are compressed.

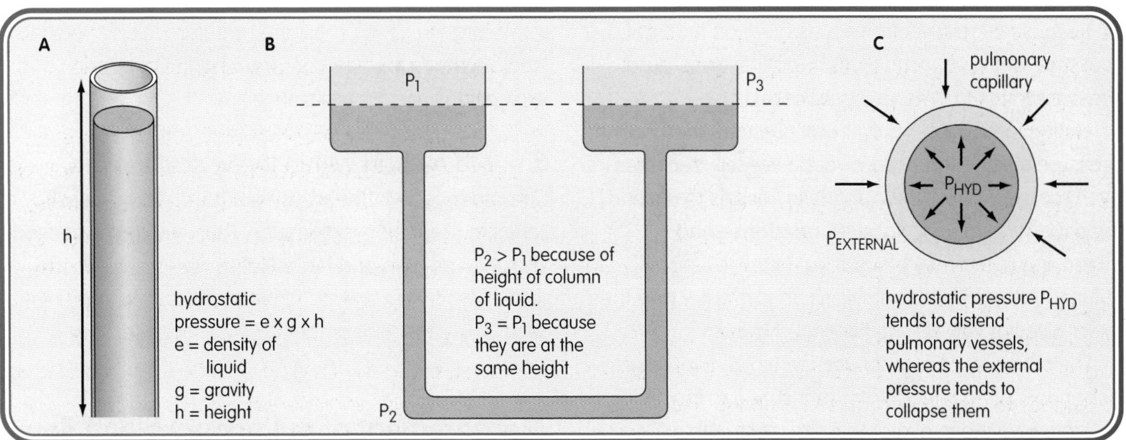

Fig. 4.3 Hydrostatic pressure. (a) Hydrostatic pressure = $\rho \cdot g \cdot h$ [ρ = density of liquid; g = gravity; h = height]. (b) $P_2 > P_1$ because of height of column of liquid. $P_3 = P_1$ because they are at the same height. (c) Hydrostatic pressure tends to distend pulmonary vessels, whereas the external pressure tends to collapse them.

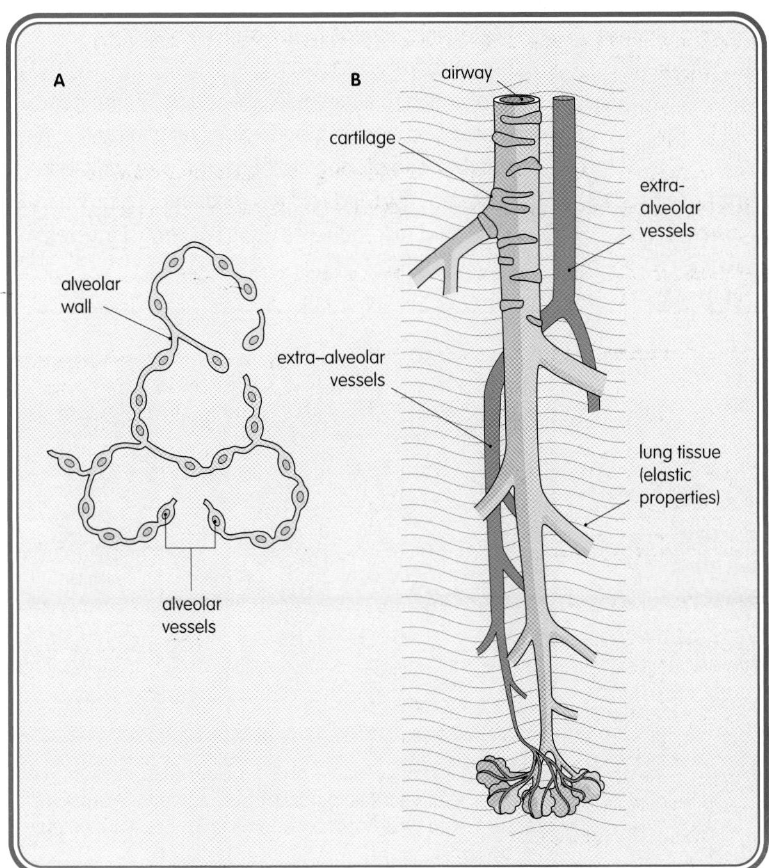

Fig. 4.4 Diagram of (A) alveolar vessels, which are subject to external pressures of alveolar gas, and (B) extra-alveolar vessels contained within lung tissue, subject to intrapleural pressure.

Extra-alveolar vessels

Extra-alveolar vessels are arteries and veins contained within the lung tissue. As the lungs expand, these vessels are distended by radial traction. The external pressure is similar to intrapleural pressure (subatmospheric—negative).

Because extra-alveolar vessels have an external pressure that is almost always negative, transmural pressure tends to distend these vessels.

During inspiration, intrapleural pressure and thus the pressure outside the extra-alveolar vessels becomes even more negative, causing these vessels to distend even further, reducing vascular resistance and increasing pulmonary blood flow. At large lung volumes, the effect of radial traction is greater and the extra-alveolar vessels are distended more.

The diameter of alveolar vessels (capillaries) is also dependent on the transmural pressure (i.e. the difference between hydrostatic pressure within the capillary lumen and pressure within the alveolus). If the alveolar pressure is greater than capillary hydrostatic pressure, the capillary will tend to collapse.

Vessels in the top of the lung may collapse as the alveoli expand. This is much more likely during diastole when the venous (capillary) pressure falls below alveolar pressure (Fig. 4.3).

Lung volume

Extra-alveolar vessels are distended by increased radial traction associated with increased lung volumes. The capillary, however, is affected in several ways.

Hydrostatic pressure within the capillaries during deep inspiration is lowered. This is caused by a negative intrapleural pressure around the heart. This changes the transmural pressure and the capillaries tend to be compressed, increasing pulmonary vascular resistance (Fig. 4.5).

At large lung volumes, the alveolar wall is stretched and becomes thinner, compressing the capillaries and increasing vascular resistance.

Smooth muscle within the vascular wall

Smooth muscle in the walls of extra-alveolar vessels tends to reduce their diameter. Thus, the forces caused by radial traction and hydrostatic pressure within the lumen are trying to distend these vessels, whereas the tone of the vascular smooth muscle opposes this action.

Measurement of pulmonary blood flow

Pulmonary blood flow can be measured by three methods:

- Fick principle (Fig. 4.6).
- Indicator dilution method: a known amount of dye is injected into venous blood and its arterial concentration is measured.
- Uptake of inhaled soluble gas (e.g. N_2O): the gas is inhaled and arterial blood values measured.

Both the first and second methods give average blood flow, whereas the third method measures instantaneous flow. The third method relies upon N_2O transfer across

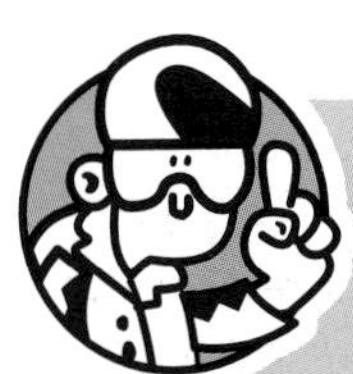

The factors affecting the capillary blood flow are:

- **Hydrostatic pressure.**
- **Alveolar air pressure.**
- **Lung volume.**

The factors affecting extra-alveolar vessels are:

- **Hydrostatic pressure.**
- **Intrapleural pressure.**
- **Lung volume.**
- **Smooth muscle tone.**

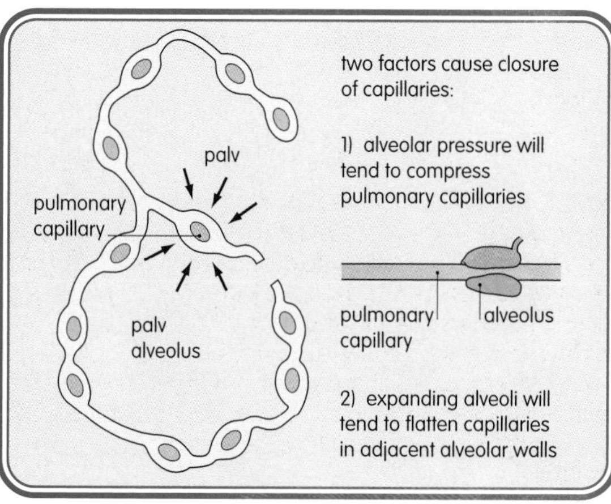

Fig. 4.5 Alveolar pressure and capillary compression. The transmural pressure is the difference between hydrostatic pressure inside the capillary and alveolar pressure outside the capillary.

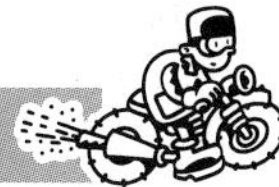

the gas exchange surface being perfusion limited.

Fick theorized that because of the laws of conservation of mass, the difference in oxygen concentration between mixed venous blood returning to the pulmonary capillary bed $[O_2]_{pv}$ and arterial blood leaving the heart $[O_2]_{pa}$ must be caused by uptake of oxygen within the lungs. This uptake must be equal to the body's consumption of oxygen (see Fig. 4.6).

Distribution of blood within the lung

Blood flow within the normal, healthy upright lung is not uniform. Blood flow at the base of the lung is greater than at the apex. Why is this the case?

The hydrostatic pressure exerted by a vertical column of fluid and given by the relationship:

$$P = \rho \cdot g \cdot h$$

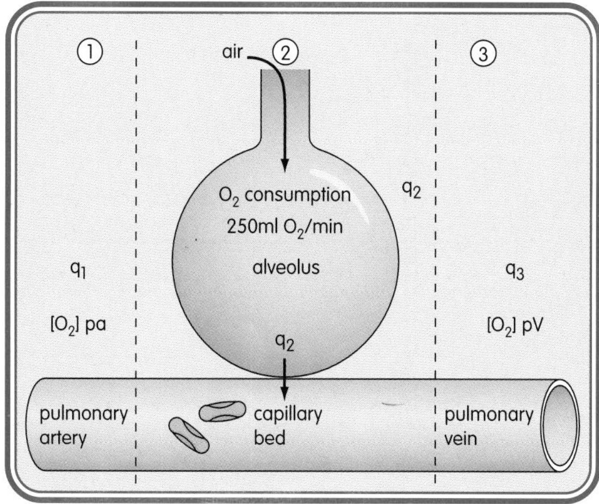

Fig. 4.6 Fick principle for measuring pulmonary blood flow. The amount of oxygen delivered to the lungs in pulmonary artery blood is: $q_1 = Q[O_2]_{pa}$. The amount of oxygen leaving the lungs pulmonary veins is: $q_3 = Q[O_2]_{pa}$. Q = blood flow rate in pulmonary artery + vein.
Fick theorised that the difference in oxygen content between pulmonary venous blood and pulmonary arterial blood must be due to uptake of oxygen in the pulmonary capillaries, therefore $q_3 - q_1 = q_2$ (uptake of oxygen in pulmonary capillaries).
Therefore $Q[O_2]_{pa} + q_2 = Q[O_2]_{pv}$

$$Q = \frac{q_2}{([O_2]_{pv} - [O_2]_{pa})}$$

thus the pulmonary blood flow can be calculated.

Where ρ = density of the fluid, h = height of the column and g = acceleration due to gravity.

Because the lungs are vertical in an upright human, they are under the influence of gravity and the pulmonary vessels at the lung base will therefore have a greater hydrostatic pressure than vessels at the apex.

From the equation above, it can be seen that:

- Vessels at the lung base are subjected to a higher hydrostatic pressure (therefore, increased driving force for flow).
- In addition, the increase in hydrostatic pressure will distend these vessels lowering the the resistance to blood flow. Thus, pulmonary blood flow in the bases will be greater than in the apices.

Ventilation also increases from apex to base, but is less affected than blood flow because the density of air is much less than blood. In diastole, the hydrostatic pressure in the pulmonary artery is 11 cmH_2O. The apex of each lung is approximately 15 cm above the right ventricle, and the hydrostatic pressure within these vessel is lowered or even zero. Vessels at the apex of the lung are therefore narrower or even collapse because of the lower hydrostatic pressure within them.

Pattern of blood flow

The distribution of blood flow within the lung can be described in three zones (Fig. 4.9).

Zone 1 (at the apex of the lung)

In zone 1, arterial pressure is less than alveolar pressure: capillaries collapse and no flow occurs. This does not occur under normal conditions.

Zone 2

In zone 2, arterial pressure is greater than alveolar pressure, which is greater than venous pressure. Postcapillary venules open and close depending on hydrostatic pressure (i.e. hydrostatic pressure difference in systole and diastole). Flow is determined by the arterial–alveolar pressure difference (transmural pressure).

Zone 3 (at the base of the lung)

In zone 3, arterial pressure is greater than venous pressure, which is greater than alveolar pressure. Blood flow is determined by arteriovenous pressure difference as in the systemic circulation.

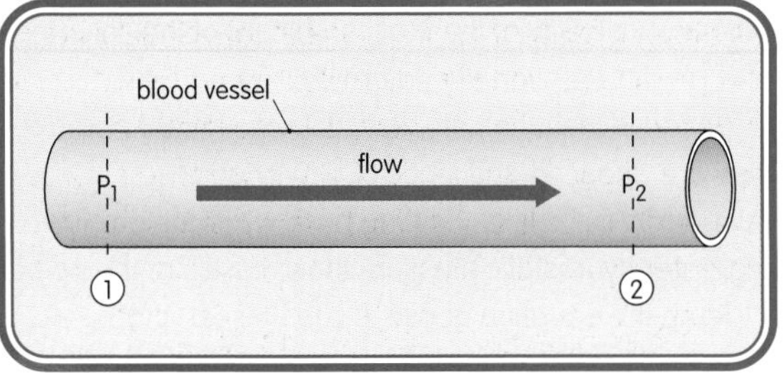

Fig. 4.7 Hydrostatic pressure in terms of driving force.

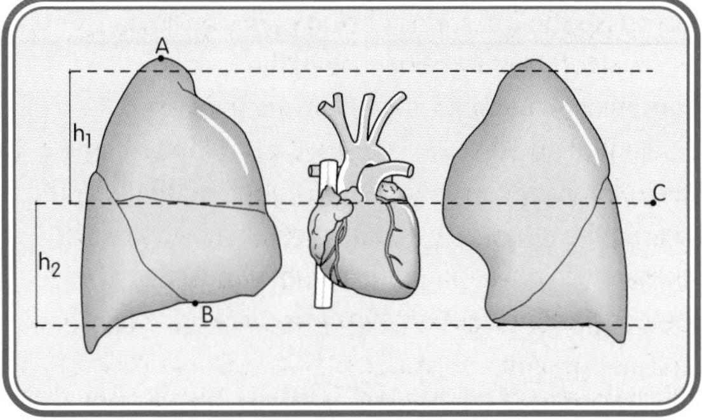

Fig. 4.8 Hydrostatic pressure within the pulmonary circulation.

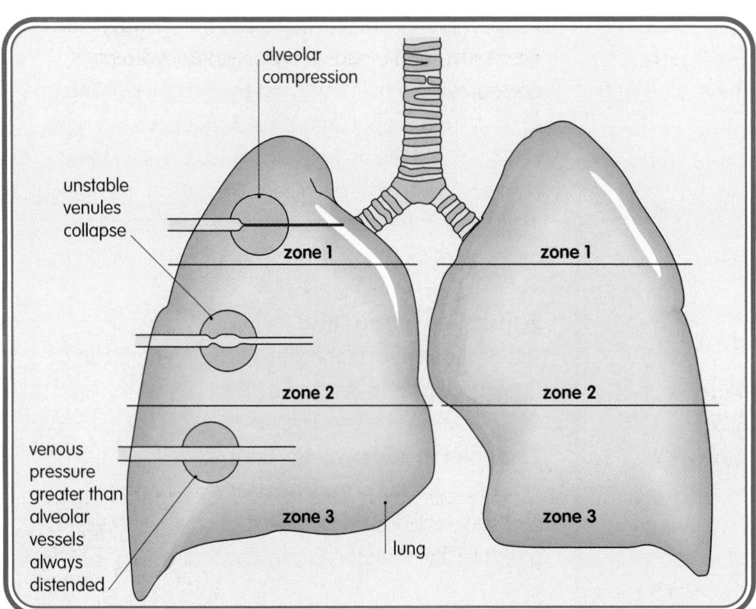

Fig. 4.9 Zones of pulmonary blood flow.

Control of pulmonary blood flow

We have already mentioned how the pulmonary circulation adapts to changes of hydrostatic pressure and how it can recruit capillaries during exercise. These effects are passive and caused by changes in hydrostatic pressure. The pulmonary blood flow can also be controlled by other local mechanisms to improve efficiency of gaseous exchange. Like the systemic circulation, other mediators such as thromboxane, histamine, and prostacylin also alter pulmonary vascular tone.

Contraction and relaxation of smooth muscle contained within the walls of arteries, arterioles, and veins is the mechanism for active control of pulmonary blood flow.

Hypoxic vasoconstriction

The aim of breathing is to oxygenate the blood sufficiently. This is achieved by efficient gaseous exchange between alveolar gas and the bloodstream. If an area of lung is poorly ventilated and the alveolar partial pressure of oxygen (alveolar oxygen tension) is low, perfusion of this area with blood will lead to inefficient gaseous exchange. It would be more beneficial to perfuse an area that is well ventilated. This is the basis behind hypoxic vasoconstriction. Small pulmonary arteries and arterioles are in close proximity to the gas exchange surface, and vessels in and around the alveolar wall are surrounded by alveolar gas. Oxygen passes through the alveolar walls into the smooth muscle of the blood vessel by diffusion. The extremely high oxygen tension to which these smooth muscles are normally exposed acts to dilate the pulmonary vessels. In contrast, if the alveolar oxygen tension is low, pulmonary blood vessels are constricted, which leads to reduced blood flow in the area of lung which is poorly ventilated and diversion to other regions where alveolar oxygen tension is high.

It should be noted that it is the partial pressure of oxygen in the alveolus (P_AO_2) and not in the pulmonary artery (P_aO_2) that causes this response.

The actual mechanism and the chemical mediators involved in hypoxic vasoconstriction are not known. Many mediators have been investigated and nitric oxide has been shown to reverse the vasoconstriction. Nitric oxide causes relaxation of smooth muscle by the synthesis of GMP (Fig. 4.10).

In summary:

- The aim of ventilation is to oxygenate blood sufficiently and blow off carbon dioxide.
- High levels of alveolar oxygen dilate pulmonary vessels.
- Low levels of alveolar oxygen constrict pulmonary blood vessels.
- This aims to produce efficient gaseous exchange.

Higher than normal alveolar carbon dioxide partial pressures also cause pulmonary blood vessels to constrict, thus reducing blood flow to an area that is not well ventilated.

Pulmonary water balance

There is only a tiny membrane between pulmonary capillary blood and the alveolus. It is important to know how liquid is prevented from entering.

Fluids in the pulmonary capillary and interstitial spaces obey Starling's forces (Fig. 4.11). In addition, surfactant lowers the surface tension of the alveolar lining fluid, thus reducing the transudation of liquid into the alveolus by increasing the interstitial pressure from −23 mmHg to −4 mmHg. Hydrostatic pressure within the capillary tends to force fluid out into the interstitial space. The colloid osmotic pressure difference between interstitial space and capillary tends to force fluid into the capillary.

$$\text{Net fluid movement} = K_f(P_c - P_i) - s(p_c - p_i)$$

Where, s = reflection coefficient; P_c = hydrostatic pressure in the capillary; K_f = filtration coefficient; P_i = hydrostatic pressure of interstitial fluid; p_c = colloid osmotic pressure in the capillary fluid; p_i = colloid osmotic pressure of interstitial fluid.

The resultant fluid flow from capillary to interstitial space is small. Fluid drains to lymphatics into the perivascular space. Under pathological conditions, fluid can reside either in the interstitial space (interstitial oedema) or in the alveoli (alveolar oedema).

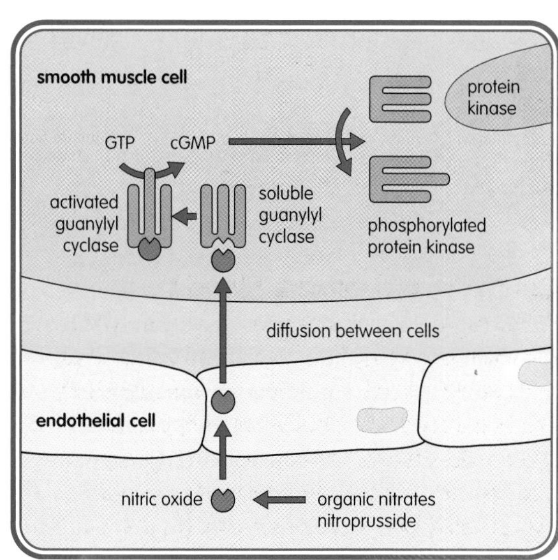

Fig. 4.10 Mechanism of action of nitric oxide.

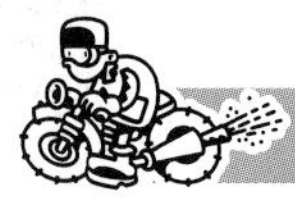

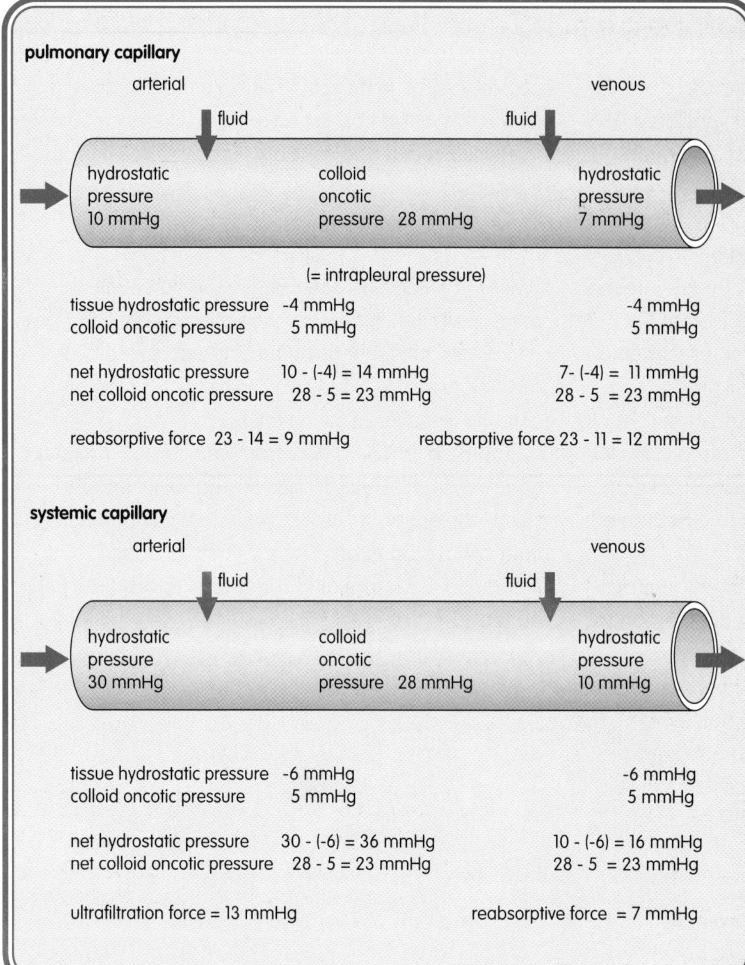

Fig. 4.11 Comparison of Starling's forces between pulmonary and systemic capillary beds. The resorptive force is positive and hence fluid is reabsorbed into the pulmonary capillary. If there was no surfactant in the alveoli the tissue hydrostatic pressure could be −23mmHg and the reabsorptive force would be −10mmHg causing transudation of fluid into the alveolus.

- **What are the normal diastolic and systolic pressures in the pulmonary circulation?**
- **Describe recruitment and distension. How do these affect pulmonary vascular resistance?**
- **Describe Fick's principle of measurement of pulmonary blood flow.**
- **Define alveolar and extra-alveolar vessels.**
- **Outline what factors affect pulmonary blood flow and resistance of the pulmonary vasculature.**
- **Describe the pattern of blood flow through the lungs in terms of three zones.**
- **Explain the term hypoxic vasoconstriction and its importance.**
- **Explain why fluid doesn't build up in the alveolar interstitial space.**

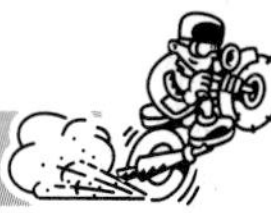

THE VENTILATION:PERFUSION RELATIONSHIP

Basic concepts

Ventilation and perfusion

To achieve efficient gaseous exchange, it is essential that the flow of gas (ventilation: $\dot{V}$) and the flow of blood (perfusion: $\dot{Q}$) are closely matched.

The ideal situation would be where:

- All alveoli are ventilated equally with gas of identical composition and pressure.
- All pulmonary capillaries in the alveolar wall are perfused with equal amounts of mixed venous blood.

Unfortunately, this is not the case. Ventilation is not uniform throughout the lung; neither is perfusion.

The partial pressure of oxygen in the alveoli determines the amount of oxygen transferred to the blood. Two factors affect the partial pressure of oxygen in the alveoli: the amount of ventilation (i.e. the addition of oxygen to the alveolar compartment) and the perfusion of blood through pulmonary capillaries (i.e. the removal of oxygen from the alveolar compartment).

It is the ratio of ventilation to perfusion that determines the concentration of oxygen in the alveolar compartment.

Ventilation:perfusion ratio

By looking at the ventilation:perfusion ratio, we can see how well ventilation and perfusion are matched.

By definition, ventilation:perfusion ratio = $\dot{V}_A / \dot{Q}$

Where $\dot{V}_A$ = alveolar minute ventilation (usually about 4.2 L/min); $\dot{Q}$ = pulmonary blood flow (usually about 5.0 L/min).

Thus, normal $\dot{V}_A / \dot{Q} = 0.84$

This is an average value across the lung. Different ventilation:perfusion ratios are present throughout the lung from apex to base (Fig. 4.12).

Extremes of ventilation:perfusion ratio

Looking at the ventilation:perfusion ratio, it can be seen that there are two extremes to this relationship. Either there is:

- No ventilation (a shunt): $\dot{V}_A / \dot{Q} = 0$
- No perfusion (dead space): $\dot{V}_A / \dot{Q} = \infty$

Right-to-left shunt

A right-to-left shunt is described when the pulmonary circulation bypasses the ventilation process (Fig. 4.13), either by:

- Bypassing the lungs completely (e.g. transposition of great vessels, see Chapter 2).
- Perfusion of an area of lung that is not ventilated.

The shunted blood will not have been oxygenated or been able to given up its carbon dioxide. Therefore, its levels of PO_2 and PCO_2 are those of venous blood. When added to the systemic circulation, this blood is called the venous admixture.

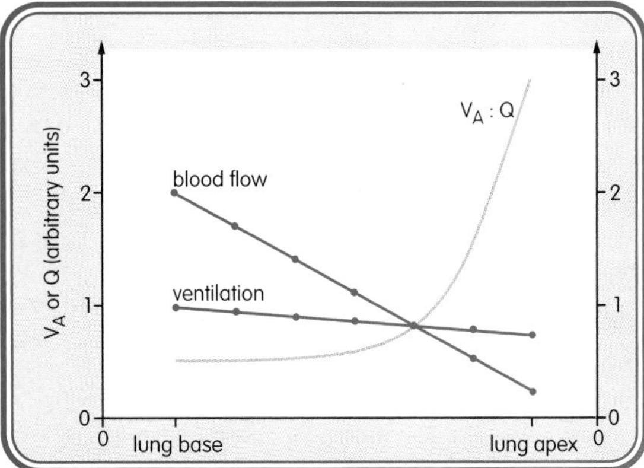

Fig. 4.12 Distribution of ventilation ($\dot{V}_A$) and perfusion ($\dot{Q}$). (Adapted from *Respiratory Physiology* 2e by J. Widdicombe and A. Davies. Edward Arnold, 1991.)

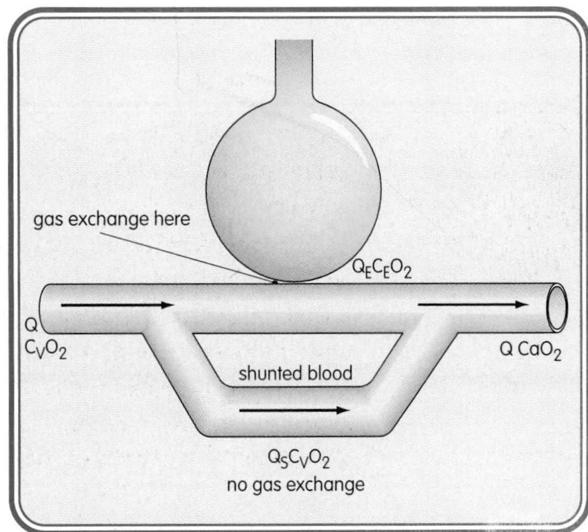

Fig. 4.13 Shunted blood. The shunted blood has a low oxygen concentration (i.e. of venous blood) and is known as the venous admixture.

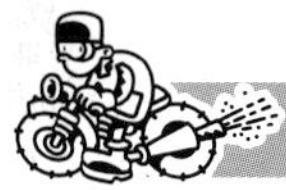

A right-to-left shunt may cause a low arterial PO_2 but a normal PCO_2—how can this be explained? The venous admixture has a low arterial PO_2 and high PCO_2. This initially causes the arterial PO_2 to be lowered and the arterial PCO_2 to be increased. This high PCO_2 causes an increase in ventilation, which reduces PCO_2 in those areas of lung that are well ventilated, giving them a lower than normal PCO_2. This reduction in PCO_2 lowers the arterial PCO_2 to its normal value. This additional ventilation in well-ventilated areas, however, has very little effect on the arterial oxygen content because of the shape of the oxyhaemoglobin dissociation curve (i.e haemoglobin is already saturated in the well-ventilated areas). Only a small increase in oxygen content is seen because of increased dissolved oxygen from the overventilated areas. This small increase in PO_2 from overventilated areas is unable to increase the arterial PO_2 to its normal value. Thus, the mixed blood has a lower PO_2 and normal PCO_2.

Effect of altering the ventilation:perfusion ratio

The easiest way to imagine how the ventilation:perfusion ratio affects the concentration of oxygen in the alveolar compartment (and hence its concentration in the blood) is to look at the extremes of ventilation:perfusion.

If a unit of lung is ventilated but not perfused, that unit will have a PO_2 and PCO_2 of inspired gas, because no gas exchange with the blood has taken place (Fig. 4.14C). If the perfusion of the unit increases (lowering the ventilation:perfusion ratio), PCO_2 will rise and the PO_2 will fall (an example of lung normally perfused is shown in Fig. 4.14A).

If the perfusion is increased further and the ventilation reduced until the unit of lung is perfused but not ventilated, the gas within that unit will be in equilibrium with the blood perfusing the alveolar capillaries (venous blood), because no gas exchange has taken place (Fig. 4.14B). This relationship is also described in Fig. 4.15; read the caption to work throught the figure.

It should be noted that:

- PO_2 varies to a much greater extent than PCO_2 with small changes in ventilation:perfusion ratio.
- Overall, variation in PO_2 is much greater than that of PCO_2
- PCO_2 cannot rise above that of mixed venous blood, assuming the ventilation:perfusion ratio applies to a small area of lung.

Regional variation of ventilation and perfusion

Both ventilation and perfusion increase towards the lung base because of the effects of gravity.

Because the blood has a greater density than air, the gravitational effects on perfusion are much greater than on ventilation. This leads to a regional variation (see Fig. 4.12) in ventilation:perfusion ratio from lung apex (high $\dot{V}/\dot{Q}$) to lung base (low $\dot{V}/\dot{Q}$).

These regional variations in ventilation:perfusion ratio are caused by the lung being upright; thus, changes in posture will alter the ventilation:perfusion

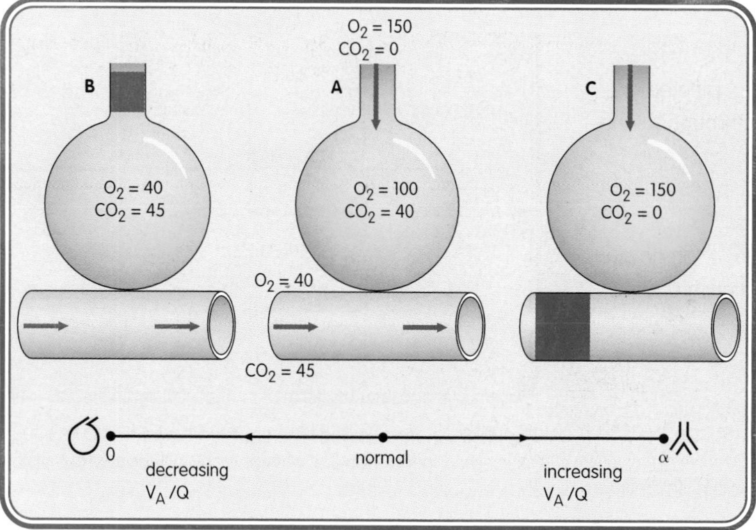

Fig. 4.14 The effect of altering the ventilation:perfusion ratio on the P_AO_2 and P_ACO_2 in a lung unit.

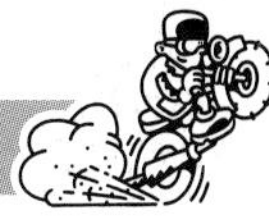

ratio throughout the lung. For example, when lying down, the posterior area of the lung has a low ventilation:perfusion ratio and the anterior area has a high ventilation:perfusion ratio.

The affect of high and low ventilation:perfusion ratios on carbon dioxide and oxygen in the alveolus and blood is highlighted in Fig. 4.16 and described below.

At low ventilation:perfusion ratios (e.g. at the lung base)

Effect on carbon dioxide concentrations

Carbon dioxide diffuses from the blood to alveoli; however, because ventilation is low, carbon dioxide is not taken away as rapidly. Thus, carbon dioxide tends to accumulate in the alveolus until a new, higher steady-state P_ACO_2 is reached.

Diffusion occurs only until equilibrium is achieved, when P_aCO_2 is equal to P_ACO_2. If there were no ventilation, the P_ACO_2 of this lung unit would rise quickly to meet mixed venous P_vCO_2, and no diffusion could take place.

Assuming that the overall lung function is normal, this regional variation in P_aCO_2 will not affect overall P_vCO_2. Thus, reducing the ventilation:perfusion ratio will not increase P_aCO_2 above the mixed venous value.

Effect on oxygen concentrations

Oxygen diffuses from the alveolus into the blood; however, because ventilation is low, oxygen taken up by the blood and metabolized is not replenished fully by new air entering the lungs.

Oxygen in the alveolus is depleted until a new, lower steady-state P_AO_2 is reached. Because diffusion

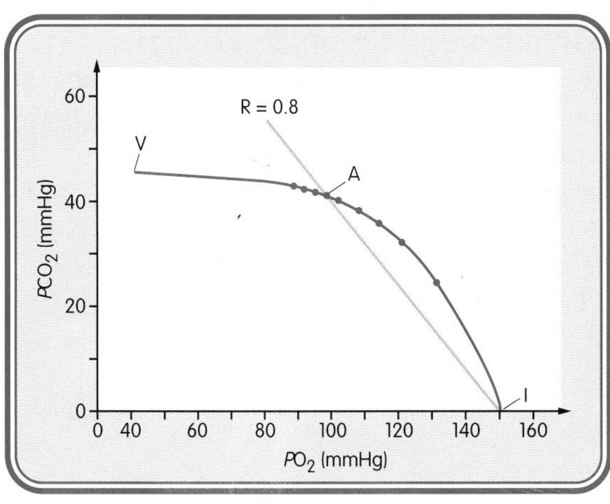

Fig. 4.15 The effect of altering the ventilation:perfusion ratio on both PO_2 and PCO_2. Point A represents normal arterial values of PO_2 and PCO_2 at a value of ventilation:perfusion ratio of 0.84. Increasing ventilation/perfusion ratios reduces PCO_2 but causes a corresponding rise in PO_2. Eventually point I is reached, where PCO_2 is zero and PO_2 is equal to that of inspired gas; this relates to a point of infinite ventilation:perfusion (i.e. there is no perfusion). Point V represents the opposite end of the ventilation:perfusion spectrum where the lung is not ventilated at all. The alveolar end capillary blood partial pressures of oxygen and carbon dioxide are of venous values. Thus values of ventilation:perfusion ratio greater than normal are to the right of point A and those that are less are to the left. (Adapted from *Physiology* 3e by R.M. Berne and M.N. Levy. Mosby Year Book, 1993.)

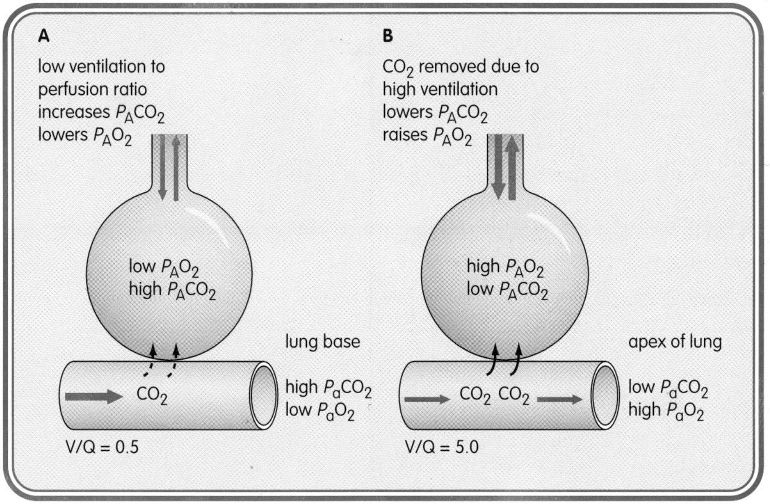

Fig. 4.16 Ventilation and perfusion at lung base (A) and apex (B).

continues until equilibrium is achieved, the P_aO_2 of this unit will also be low (Fig. 4.16A).

At high ventilation:perfusion ratios (e.g. at the lung apex)

Effect on carbon dioxide concentrations

The carbon dioxide diffusing from the blood is nearly all removed; carbon dioxide in the alveolus is depleted until a new, lower steady-state P_ACO_2 is reached. Diffusion continues until equilibrium is achieved: P_aCO_2 will also be low.

If we take this to the extreme, then as ventilation: perfusion ratios tend to zero, P_ACO_2 tends to zero.

Effect on oxygen concentrations

Oxygen diffusing from the alveolar gas is not taken away by the blood in such large amounts because the relative blood flow is reduced; in addition, oxygen is replenished with each breath. Thus, oxygen tends to accumulate in the alveolus until a new steady-state concentration is reached (Fig. 4.16B).

Diffusion occurs until a new higher equilibrium is achieved; thus, P_aO_2 is also higher.

How does ventilation:perfusion inequality affect overall gas exchange?

As mentioned previously, a normal healthy lung is not ventilated or perfused uniformly and ventilation:perfusion ratios vary (Fig 4.17). The actual difference between gaseous exchange in a healthy lung and in an ideal lung is perhaps smaller than one might expect. The ideal lung is capable of only 2–3% more gaseous exchange.

However, if the ventilation:perfusion inequality from lung apex to base becomes more severe, the transfer of oxygen and carbon dioxide will be significantly affected. The majority of the blood will come from poorly ventilated areas at the lung base, where P_AO_2 is low; thus P_aO_2 will be low. P_aCO_2 will similarly be raised at the base of the lung.

The nonlinear shape of the oxyhaemoglobin dissociation curve does not allow areas with high ventilation:perfusion ratios to compensate for areas of low ratio.

Ventilation:perfusion distributions

As we have mentioned, ventilation:perfusion ratios are not uniform within the lung. If we look at the variation in ventilation and blood flow in relation to $\dot{V}/\dot{Q}$ in the normal lung (Fig. 4.18), it should be noted that:

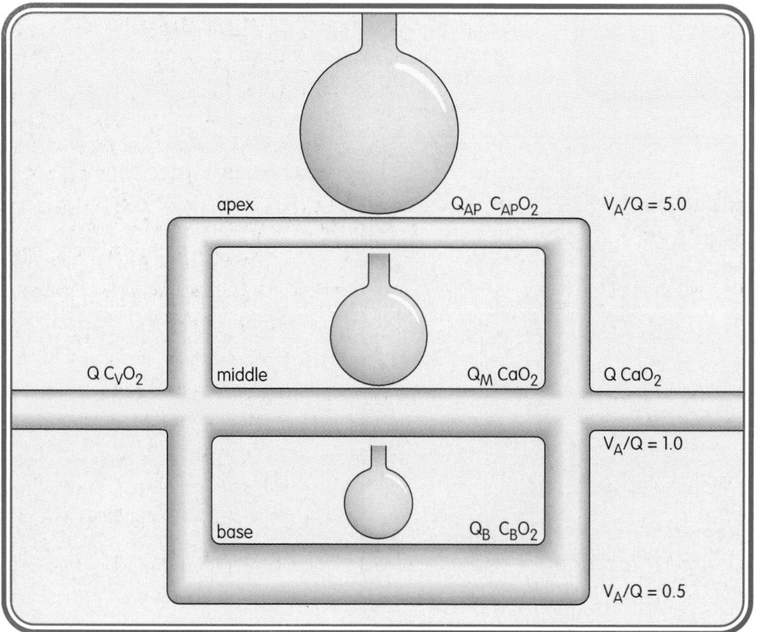

Fig. 4.17 Ventilation and perfusion at the lung apex, middle, and base.

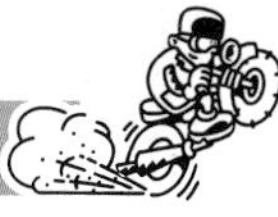

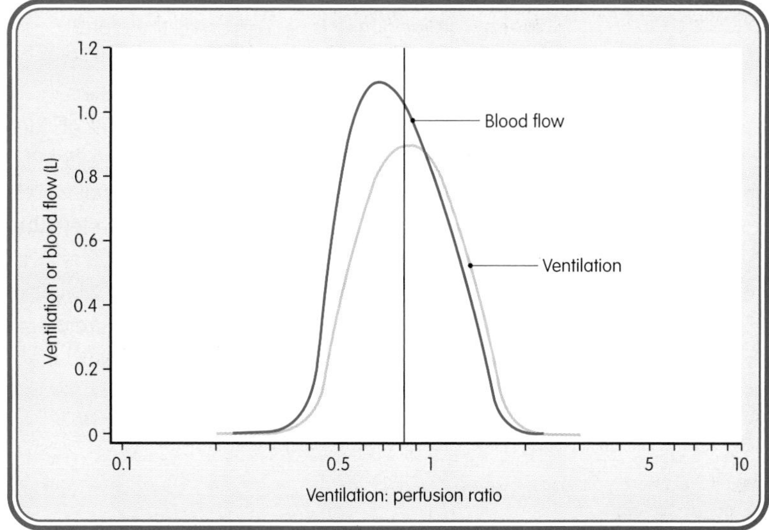

Fig. 4.18 Normal human ventilation:perfusion curves. (Adapted from *Respiratory Physiology* 5e by J. West. Williams & Wilkins, 1995.)

- Where the ventilation:perfusion ratio is high, absolute values of ventilation are low.
- Where the ventilation:perfusion ratio is low, absolute values of blood flow are also low.

Thus, the majority of blood flow and ventilation go to areas of lung that have a ventilation:perfusion ratio that is close to the average value. In the diseased lung, this might not be the case and blood may flow to areas where ventilation:perfusion ratios are extremely low; this is effectively a shunt.

Areas with extremely high ventilation:perfusion ratios may be ventilated to high absolute values and receive very poor blood flow. This is effectively wasted ventilation (Fig. 4.19).

Measurement of ventilation:perfusion ratio

There are two basic methods for measurement of ventilation:perfusion ratio: the multiple inert gas procedure and by radioactive gas.

Multiple inert gas procedure

In the multiple inert gas procedure, six inert gases are infused into the venous blood stream. Each gas has a different partition coefficient in gas and blood (i.e. different solubility in gas and blood).

Steady state is reached by a constant rate of infusion and expiration. From component balances for each gas of amount infused and amount expired the ventilation:perfusion distribution is calculated.

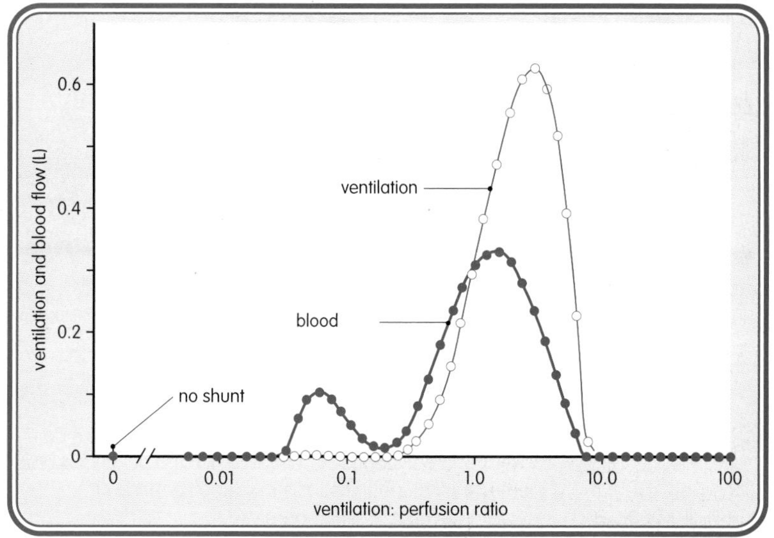

Fig. 4.19 Ventilation:perfusion curves for patient with chronic bronchitis. From J. West: *Respiratory Physiology* 5e. Williams & Wilkins,1995.

Amount infused = $P_{in} \cdot S \cdot \dot{Q}$
Amount expired = $P_{ex} \cdot \dot{V}$

Where S = solubility of the gas.

Thus, ventilation and perfusion can be calculated giving a ventilation:perfusion distribution.

Radioactive gases

Both blood flow and ventilation can be assessed by the use of radioactive gases and counters placed around the chest. This can give a general distribution; however, large differences in ventilation:perfusion ratios in adjacent lungs units cannot be detected.

- **What affects the concentration of oxygen in the alveolar compartment?**
- **Describe what is meant by the ventilation:perfusion ratio.**
- **State the two extremes of ventilation:perfusion ratio.**
- **Define venous admixture.**
- **Draw a graph of how the ventilation:perfusion ratio varies from lung apex to lung base.**
- **Outline how posture affects ventilation:perfusion ratio.**
- **Describe with the aid of a diagram how disease might affect the ventilation:perfusion ratio distribution.**

GAS TRANSPORT IN THE BLOOD

Oxygen transport

Dissolved oxygen

To meet the metabolic demands of the body, large amounts of oxygen must be carried in the blood. The solubility of oxygen in the blood is low:

The solubility of oxygen in blood is 0.000225 mL of oxygen per kilopascal per millilitre of blood. With normal arterial P_aO_2 (100 mmHg; 13.3 kPa), the dissolved oxygen is:

$13.3 \times 0.000225 = 0.003$ mL of oxygen per millilitre of blood

Normal cardiac output is 5.0 L/min; it is therefore capable of supplying:

$5 \times 1000 \times 0.003 = 15$ mL of oxygen per minute

At rest, the body requires approximately 250 mL of oxygen per minute. Thus, if all the oxygen in the blood was carried in the dissolved form, cardiac output would meet only 6% of the demand. There must, therefore, be an alternative mechanism for oxygen carriage.

In fact, the oxygen content of blood is approximately 200 mL of oxygen per litre of arterial blood. Therefore, most of the oxygen must be carried in chemical combination, not in simple solution. Oxygen is combined with haemoglobin.

Haemoglobin

Haemoglobin (Hb) is found in red blood cells and is a conjugate protein molecule, containing iron within its structure. The molecule consists of four polypeptide subunits, two α and two β. Associated with each polypeptide chain is a haem group that acts as a binding site for oxygen (Fig. 4.20).

The haem group consists of a porphyrin ring containing iron and is responsible for binding of oxygen:

- Haemoglobin contains iron in a ferrous (Fe^{2+}) or ferric (Fe^{3+}) state.
- Only haemoglobin in the ferrous form can bind oxygen.

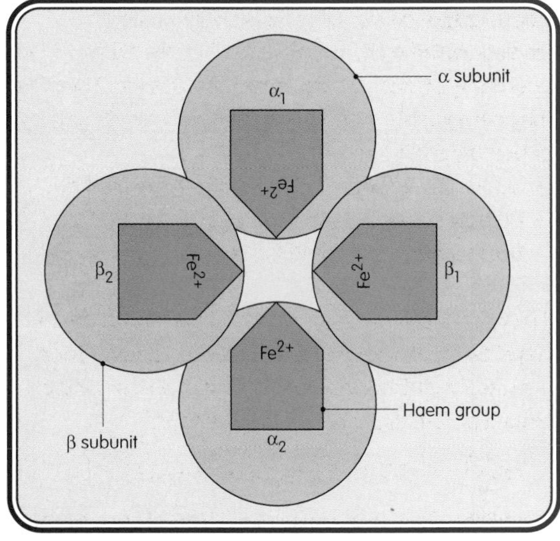

Fig. 4.20 Schematic diagram of Haemoglobin. α subunit consists of a polypeptide chain of 141 amino acids and one haem group. β subunit consists of a polypeptide chain of 146 amino acids and one haem group.

- Methaemoglobin (containing iron in a ferric state) cannot bind oxygen.

The quarternary structure of haemoglobin determines its ability to bind oxygen.

In its deoxygenated state, haemoglobin (known as reduced haemoglobin) has a low affinity for oxygen. The binding of one oxygen molecule to haemoglobin causes a conformational change in its protein structure; this positive cooperativity allows easier access to the other oxygen-binding sites, thus increasing haemoglobin's affinity for further binding of oxygen. Haemoglobin is capable of binding up to four molecules of oxygen.

$$Hb + 4O_2 \rightarrow Hb(O_2)_4$$

It should be noted that during this reaction the iron atom of the haem group remains in the ferrous Fe^{2+} form. It is not oxidized to the ferric Fe^{3+} form. The interaction of oxygen with haemoglobin is oxygenation *not* oxidation.

The main function of haemoglobin is to take up oxygen in the blood at the alveolar capillary membrane and to transport oxygen within the blood and release it into the tissues. However, haemoglobin also has other functions:

- Buffering of H^+ ions.
- Transport of CO_2 as carbamino compounds.

Haemoglobin binding and oxyhaemoglobin dissociation curve

Haemoglobin has four binding sites; the amount of oxygen carried by haemoglobin in the blood depends on how many of these binding sites are occupied. Therefore, the haemoglobin molecule can be said to be saturated or partially saturated:

- Saturated—all four binding sites are occupied by O_2.
- Partially saturated—some oxygen has bound to haemoglobin, but not all four sites are occupied.

If completely saturated, each gram of haemoglobin can carry 1.34 mL of oxygen. There are 150 g of haemoglobin per litre of the blood; therefore, the maximum binding of oxygen to haemoglobin we could expect is:

$$150 \times 1.34 = 201 \text{ mL of oxygen per litre of blood}$$

In addition, there is approximately 10 mL of O_2 in solution. The total (211 mL) is called the oxygen capacity; the haemoglobin is said to be 100% saturated ($SO_2 = 100\%$). The actual amount of oxygen bonded to haemoglobin and dissolved in the blood at any one time is called the oxygen content.

The oxygen saturation (SO_2) of the blood is defined as the amount of oxygen carried in the blood, expressed as a percentage of oxygen capacity:

$$SO_2 = O_2 \text{ content} \div O_2 \text{ capacity} \times 100$$

Cyanosis

Haemoglobin absorbs light of different wavelengths depending on whether it is in the reduced or oxygenated form. Oxyhaemoglobin appears bright red, whereas reduced haemoglobin appears purplish, giving a bluish pallour to skin. This is called cyanosis, which can be described as either central or peripheral. Cyanosis depends on the absolute amount of deoxygenated haemoglobin in the vessels, not the proportion of deoxgenated:oxygenated haemoglobin. In central cyanosis, there is more than 5 g/dL deoxygenated haemoglobin in the blood and this can be seen in the peripheral tissues (e.g lips, tongue). Peripheral cyanosis is due to a local cause (e.g. vascular obstruction of a limb).

It follows that an anaemic patient with low haemoglobin may become dangerously desaturated without appearing cyanosed!

How much oxygen binds to haemoglobin is dependent upon the partial pressure of oxygen in the blood. This relationship is represented by the oxyhaemoglobin dissociation curve (Fig. 4.21A); this is an equilibrium curve at specific conditions:

- 150 g of haemoglobin per litre of blood
- pH 7.4
- Temperature 37°C

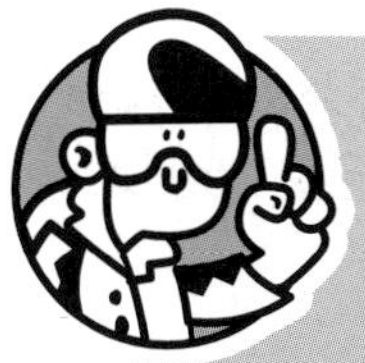

You will need to be able to reproduce this curve in your exams. The easiest way to remember it is by using four points. 25%, 50%, 75%, and 100% values are useful markers and the curve is easily drawn from the origin through these points. You will also need to remember arterial and mixed venous blood partial pressures of oxygen.

Factors affecting the oxygen dissociation curve

Various factors shift the oxygen dissociation curve to the right or to the left:

- A shift to the right allows easier dissociation of oxygen (i.e. lower oxygen saturation at any particular PO_2) and increases the oxygen release from oxyhaemoglobin.
- A shift to the left makes oxygen binding easier (i.e. higher oxygen saturation at any particular PO_2) and increases the oxygen uptake by haemoglobin.

The following factors shift the curve to the right (Fig. 4.21B):

- Increased PCO_2 and decreased pH (increased hydrogen ion concentration), known as the Bohr shift.
- Increased temperature.
- Increase in 2,3-diphosphoglycerate (2,3-DPG), which binds to the β chains.

2,3-Diphosphoglycerate is a product of anaerobic metabolism. Red blood cells possess no mitochondria

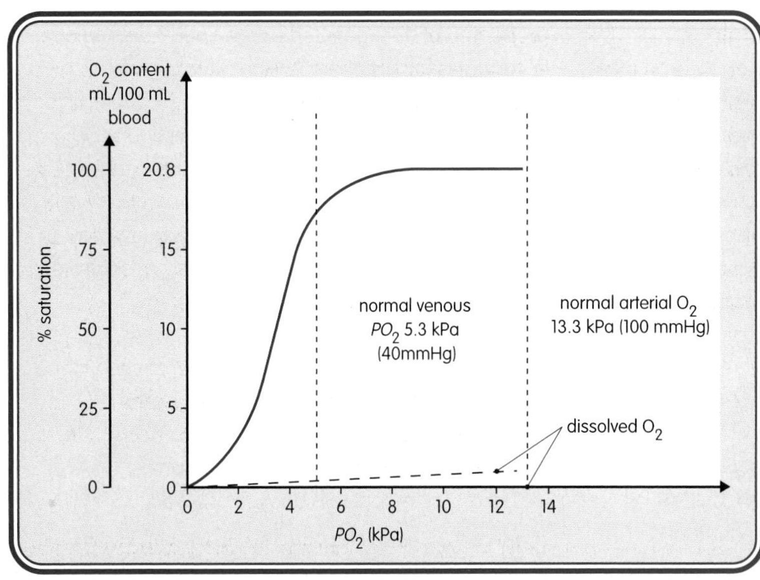

Fig. 4.21A Oxyhaemoglobin dissociation curve.

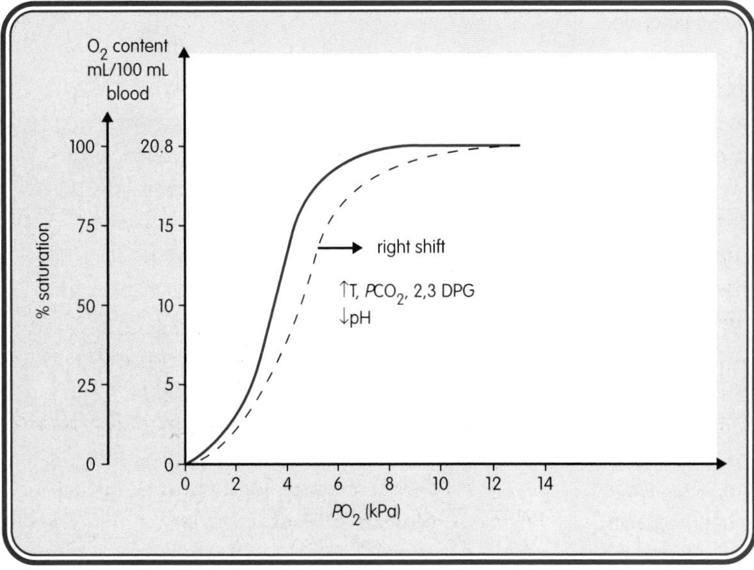

Fig. 4.21B The effect of temperature, PCO_2, pH and 2,3-DPG on the oxyhaemoglobin dissociation curve.

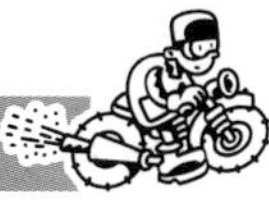

and therefore carry out anaerobic metabolism to produce energy. 2,3-DPG binds more strongly to reduced haemoglobin than to oxyhaemoglobin.

If you cannot remember how the above factors affect the oxygen dissociation curve, it is helpful to think of exercising muscle. It would be useful if its blood supply gave up oxygen more easily (right shift of the curve). An exercising muscle produces carbon dioxide (increased carbon dioxide), which forms carbonic acid in the blood, which in turn dissociates to form hydrogen ions (lowers the pH). Exercising muscle is hot (increased temperature) and uses up oxygen forming more reduced haemoglobin in red blood cells (increased 2,3-DPG concentration).

Other forms of haemoglobin

Myoglobin

Myoglobin is an iron-containing molecule found within skeletal muscle and cardiac muscle. It consists of a single polypeptide chain with a haem group:

- Myoglobin is capable of binding oxygen.
- It acts as a temporary storage of oxygen within skeletal muscle.
- Myoglobin has a higher affinity for oxygen than does normal adult haemoglobin (HbA), seen as a shift to the left of the dissociation curve (Fig. 4.22).
- Myoglobin is unsuitable for oxygen transport, because it binds oxygen at partial pressures below those of mixed venous blood (<40 mmHg) and so could not readily release O_2 to the tissues.

Sickle cell anaemia (HbS)

Sickle cell anaemia is an autosomal recessive disorder in which there is a defect in the β-globulin chain of the haemoglobin molecule.

There is a substitution of the amino acid valine for glutamine at position 6 of the β chain, forming HbS. The heterozygote has sickle cell trait and the homozygote sickle cell anaemia. The abnormal HbS molecules polymerise when de-oxygenated and cause the red blood cells containing the abnormal haemoglobin to sickle. The fragile sickle cells haemolyse and may block vessels leading to ischaemia and infarction.

The heterozygous patient may have painful crises with bone and abdominal pain; there may also be intrapulmonary shunting.

Thalassaemia

The thalassaemias are autosomal recessive disorders due to decreased production of either the α or the β chain of haemoglobin.

There are two genes for the β chain and, depending on the number of normal genes, the thalassaemia is quoted as major or minor. There are four genes which code for the α chain, leading to various clinical disorders depending on the genetic defect.

HbA_2

This is present in a small amount in the normal population and consists of 2 α and 2 δ chains. It is markedly raised in β thalassemia minor.

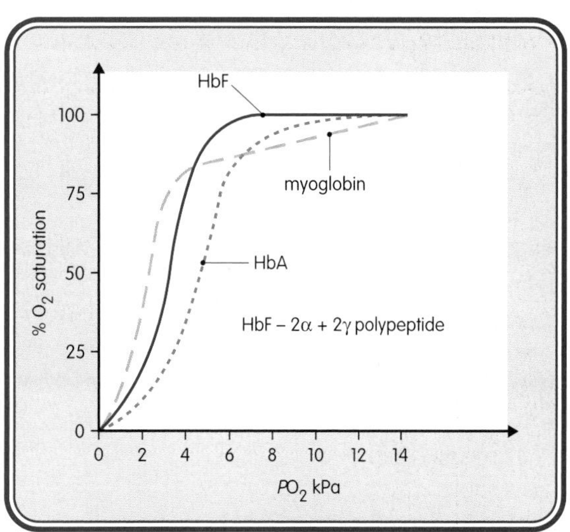

Fig. 4.22 Comparison of oxygen dissociation curves for myoglobin, fetal haemoglobin (HbF), and adult haemoglobin (HbA). (Adapted with permission from *Physiology* 3e, by R.M. Berne and M.N. Levy. Mosby Year Book, 1993.)

Fetal haemoglobin (HbF)

Fetal haemoglobin differs from adult haemoglobin by having two γ chains instead of two β chains (Fig. 4.22).

Fetal haemoglobin has a higher affinity for oxygen because its γ chains bind 2,3-DPG less avidly than the β chains of adult haemoglobin and are therefore able to bind oxygen at lower partial pressures (maternal venous P_vO_2 is low: <40 mmHg).

The double Bohr shift

Release of carbon dioxide from fetal haemoglobin causes a shift to the left of the fetal oxyhaemoglobin dissociation curve, thus increasing its affinity for oxygen. This released carbon dioxide binds to maternal haemoglobin, causing a shift to the right of maternal haemoglobin, thus reducing the affinity of the latter for oxygen. Oxygen is therefore released by maternal haemoglobin and bound by fetal haemoglobin.

Carbon monoxide poisoning

Carbon monoxide (CO) displaces oxygen from oxyhaemoglobin because the affinity of haemoglobin for carbon monoxide is more than 200 times that for oxygen. This changes the shape of the oxyhaemoglobin dissociation curve. Note that in Fig. 4.23, showing the effects of carbon monoxide poisoning:

- In this instance, oxygen capacity is 50% of normal (i.e. 50% HbO_2 and 50% HbCO). The actual value will depend on the partial pressure of CO (e.g. with a *P*CO of 16 mmHg, 75% of Hb will be in the form of HbCO).
- Saturation is achieved at a PO_2 of <40 mmHg (below venous PO_2).
- HbCO causes a shift to the left for the oxygen dissociation curve (i.e. HbCO has a higher affinity for oxygen than normal HbO_2).
- Carbon monoxide binds to two of the four available haem groups.
- Carbon monoxide takes a long time to be cleared, but this can be speeded up by ventilation with 100% oxygen.
- The patient is not cyanosed, because HbCO is cherry-red.

Carbon dioxide transport

There are three ways in which carbon dioxide can be transported in the blood:

- Dissolved in plasma.
- As bicarbonate ions.
- As carbamino compounds.

Dissolved carbon dioxide

The solubility of carbon dioxide in the blood is much greater than that of oxygen (20 times greater); so, unlike oxygen, a significant amount (approximately 10%) of carbon dioxide is carried in solution.

The solubility of carbon dioxide = 5.2 mL of carbon dioxide per kilopascal per litre of blood.

Normal P_aCO_2 = 5.3 kPa.

So, the normal dissolved carbon dioxide = 27.4 mL of carbon dioxide per litre of blood.

Bicarbonate ions

Approximately 60% of carbon dioxide is transported as bicarbonate ions. Dissolved carbon dioxide interacts with water to form carbonic acid as follows:

$$CO_2 + H_2O \leftrightarrow H_2CO_3 \qquad (1)$$

Carbonic acid rapidly dissociates into ions:

$$H_2CO_3 \leftrightarrow H^+ + HCO_3^- \qquad (2)$$

The total reaction being:

$$CO_2 + H_2O \leftrightarrow H_2CO_3 \leftrightarrow H^+ + HCO_3^-$$

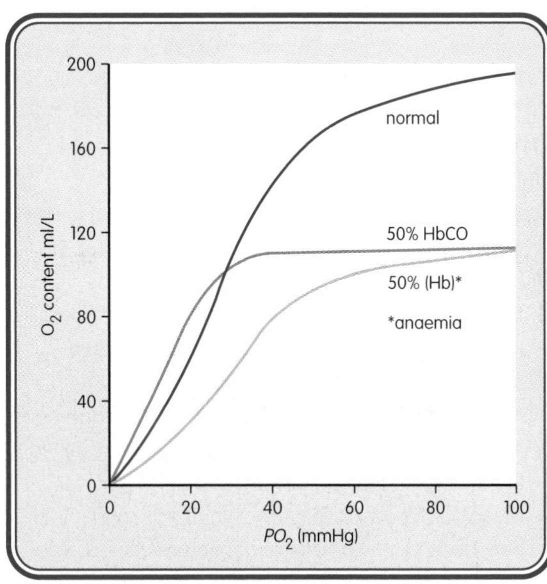

Fig. 4.23 Oxyhaemoglobin curve showing effects of anaemia and carbon monoxide poisoning (50% HbCO and anaemia compared with normal haemoglobin). (Adapted with permission from *Physiology* 3e, by R.M. Berne and M.N. Levy. Mosby Year Book, 1993.)

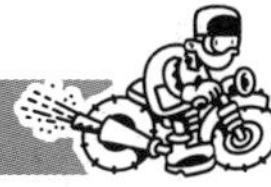

The first reaction is very slow in plasma, but within the red blood cell is dramatically speeded up by the enzyme, carbonic anhydrase. Reaction (2) is very fast, but if allowed to proceed alone, a large amount of H^+ ions would be formed, slowing down or halting the reaction. Haemoglobin has the property that it can bind H^+ ions and act as a buffer, thus allowing the reaction to proceed rapidly.

$$H^+ + HbO_2^- \leftrightarrow HHb + O_2$$

$$H^+ + Hb^- \leftrightarrow HHb$$

Reduced Hb can bind H^+ more actively; this is because reduced Hb is less acidic.

The buffering capacities of haemoglobin and oxyhaemoglobin are conferred by the imidazole groups of the 36 histidine residues in the haemoglobin molecule. The imidazole groups dissociate less readily in the deoxygenated form of haemoglobin, which is therefore a weaker acid and so a better buffer. This action reduces H^+ ions in the plasma and also pulls the second reaction to the right.

The bicarbonate produced in the red blood cells diffuses down its concentration gradient into the plasma in exchange for chloride ions (Cl^-). This process is known as the chloride shift (see Fig. 4.24).

Carbamino compounds

Carbon dioxide is capable of combining with proteins, interacting with their terminal amine groups to form carbamino compounds (Fig. 4.24).

$$RNH_2 + CO_2 \leftrightarrow RNHCOOH \leftrightarrow RNHCOO^- + H^+$$

The most important protein involved is haemoglobin, as it is the most abundant in the blood. It is also important to note that:

- The interaction of carbon dioxide and haemoglobin is rapid.
- No enzyme is involved.
- Haemoglobin binds carbon dioxide in its deoxygenated state (reduced haemoglobin).
- Approximately 30% of carbon dioxide is carried as carbamino compounds.

Haldane effect

Carriage of carbon dioxide is increased in deoxygenated blood because of two factors:

- Reduced haemoglobin has a greater affinity for carbon dioxide than oxyhaemoglobin.
- Reduced haemoglobin is less acidic (i.e. a better proton acceptor: H^+ buffer) than oxyhaemoglobin.

The haldane effect minimizes changes in pH of the blood when gaseous exchange occurs. The decrease in pH due to the oxygenation of Hb is offset by the increase that results from the loss of CO_2 to the alveolar air. The reverse occurs in the tissues.

This is an important effect because:

- In peripheral capillaries, the unloading of oxygen from haemoglobin aids the binding of carbon dioxide to haemoglobin.
- In pulmonary capillaries, the loading of oxygen on

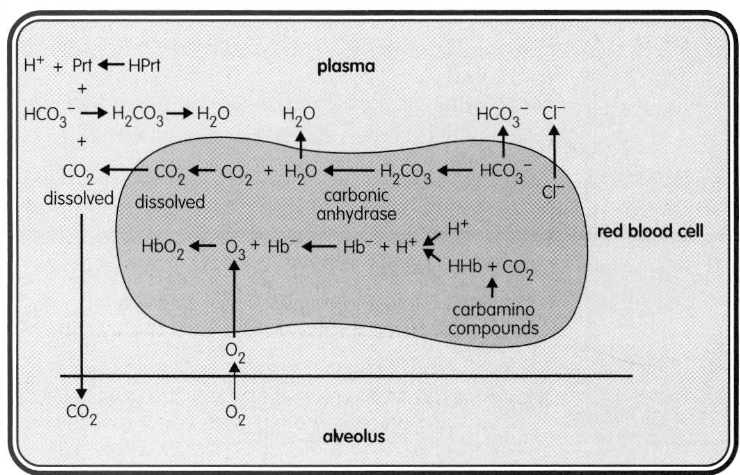

Fig. 4.24 Binding of CO_2. Bicarbonate produce in the red blood cell diffused out into the plasma down its concentration gradient. Chloride diffuses into the red blood cell to maintain electrical equilibrium pulling water with it. (Adapted with permission from *Physiology* 3e, by R.M. Berne and M.N. Levy. Mosby Year Book, 1993.)

haemoglobin reduces the binding of carbon dioxide to haemoglobin.

This allows efficient gaseous exchange of carbon dioxide in the tissues and the lungs.

Carbon dioxide dissociation curve

The carriage of carbon dioxide is dependent upon the partial pressure of carbon dioxide in the blood. This relationship is described by the carbon dioxide dissociation curve (Fig. 4.25). Compared with the oxygen dissociation curve:

- The carbon dioxide curve is more linear.
- The carbon dioxide curve is much steeper than the oxygen curve (between venous and arterial partial pressure of respiratory gases).
- The carbon dioxide curve varies according to oxygen saturation of haemoglobin.

The two main carbon dioxide dissociation curves, for mixed venous and arterial blood, can be drawn.

Stores of oxygen and carbon dioxide

There are only small stores (approximately 1550 mL) of oxygen in body tissues as follows:

- Lungs—450 mL.
- Blood—850 mL.
- Myoglobin—200 mL.
- Tissue fluids—50 mL.

On the other hand, carbon dioxide has vast stores (approximately 120 L):

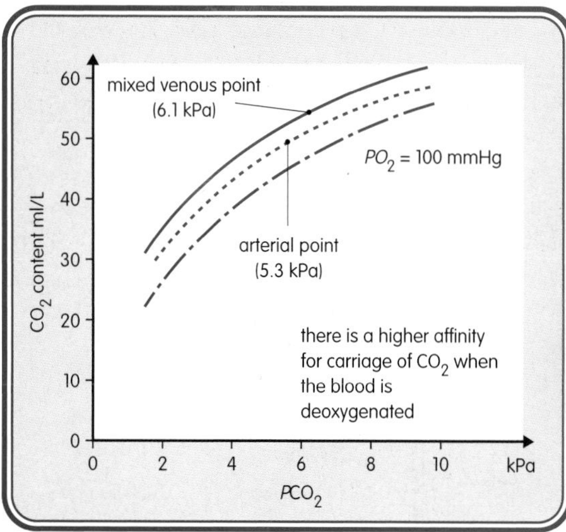

Fig. 4.25 Ventilation effects on oxygen and carbon dioxide levels in the blood.

- Blood carbonates.
- Bone carbonates.
- Tissue carbonates (including fat tissue).

A change in ventilation will affect both P_aO_2 and P_aCO_2. Because oxygen stores are small in comparison to those of carbon dioxide, a short-term variation in ventilation will affect P_aO_2. A persistent change in ventilation will be shown by a change in P_aCO_2. Clinically, ventilation is assessed by measurement of P_aCO_2.

Hypoventilation and hyperventilation

For the body to function normally, ventilation must meet the metabolic demand of the tissues (Fig. 4.26).

Thus, metabolic tissue consumption of oxygen must be equal to the oxygen taken up in the blood from alveolar gas. Or, metabolic tissue production of carbon dioxide must be equal to the amount of carbon dioxide blown off at the alveoli.

Hypoventilation

The term hypoventilation refers to a situation when ventilation is insufficient to meet metabolic demand.

Hyperventilation

The term hyperventilation refers to a situation where ventilation is excessive to metabolic demand. If we consider a component balance for carbon dioxide under steady-state resting conditions, the carbon dioxide exhaled ($\dot{V}CO_2$) will be equal to the minute ventilation ($\dot{V}_E$) multiplied by the fractional concentration of carbon dioxide in the expired air (F_ECO_2).

Carbon dioxide produced in the tissues = exhaled carbon dioxide

$$\dot{V}CO_2 = \dot{V}_E \cdot F_ECO_2$$

Because the amount of carbon dioxide expired equals the amount of carbon dioxide released at the alveoli, we can say

$$\dot{V}CO_2 = \dot{V}_A \cdot F_ACO_2$$

where $\dot{V}_A$ = alveolar ventilation; F_ACO_2 = fractional concentration of carbon dioxide at the alveoli.

$$F_ACO_2 = \dot{V}CO_2 / \dot{V}_A$$

Using Dalton's law, the partial pressure of a gas is related to its fractional concentration:

$$P_ACO_2 = F_ACO_2 \cdot P_{TOT}$$

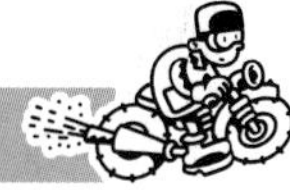

Comparison of hyperventilation and hypoventilation	
Hyperventilation	**Hypoventilation**
Causes anxiety brainstem lesion drugs	**Causes** obstruction: asthma chronic obstructive airways disease foreign body (e.g. peanut) brainstem lesion pneumothorax or lung collapse trauma (e.g. fractured rib) drugs, notably opioids
Consequences ventilation too great for metabolic demand too much CO_2 blown off from lungs P_aCO_2 <40 mmHg	**Consequences** ventilation is too small for metabolic demand not enough CO_2 is blown off at the lungs P_aCO_2 >40 mmHg

Fig. 4.26 Differences between hyperventilation and hypoventilation.

where P_ACO_2 = partial pressure of carbon dioxide in the alveoli; P_{TOT} = pressure of the gas in the alveoli.

Furthermore, we can say:

$$P_ACO_2 \propto \dot{V}CO_2/\dot{V}_A$$

Or:

$$P_ACO_2 = K \cdot \dot{V}CO_2/\dot{V}_A$$

where K is a constant.

Because alveolar gas is in equilibrium with the blood, P_ACO_2 can be estimated as P_aCO_2. Thus, it can be seen how ventilation will affect partial pressures of carbon dioxide and that hypoventilation and hyperventilation can be shown clinically by the partial pressure of carbon dioxide in the blood.

The alveolar gas equation shows the relationship between P_AO_2 and P_ACO_2 caused by hypoventilation:

$$P_AO_2 = P_IO_2 - (P_ACO_2/R) + K$$

where P_IO_2 = partial pressure of oxygen in inspired air and R = respiratory exchange ratio.

Mild or moderate exercise in a normal subject does not cause hyperventilation: the rate of breathing is increased (hypernoea) to balance the increased metabolic demand in exercise.

Hypercapnia and hypocapnia

Hypercapnia

A high partial pressure (concentration) of carbon dioxide in the blood (P_aCO_2 >45 mmHg) is termed hypercapnia (Fig. 4.27).

Hypocapnia

A low partial pressure of carbon dioxide in the blood (P_aCO_2 <40 mmHg) is termed hypocapnia.

Respiratory failure

Respiratory failure is defined as a P_aO_2 <8 kPa (60 mmHg). Respiratory failure is divided into type I and type II depending on the P_aCO_2.

In type I respiratory failure, P_aCO_2 <6.5 kPa. P_aO_2 is low (hypoxaemic), but P_aCO_2 may be normal or low; this represents a ventilation:perfusion mismatch.

In type II respiratory failure, P_aCO_2 >6.5 kPa. Both P_aO_2 and P_aCO_2 indicate that the lungs are not well ventilated.

The significance of this classification is that in type II respiratory failure the patient may have developed tolerance to increased levels of P_aCO_2; in other words, the drive for respiration no longer relies on hypercapnic drive (high P_aCO_2) but on hypoxic drive (low P_aO_2). Thus, if the patient is given high-concentration oxygen

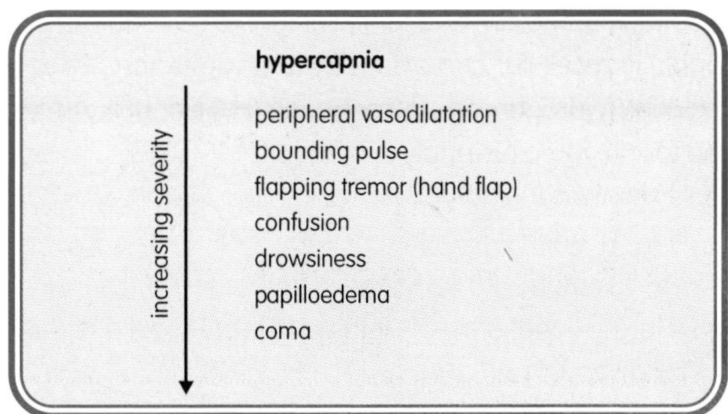

Fig. 4.27 Clinical signs of hypercapnia.

therapy the hypoxic drive for ventilation may decrease and the patient may stop breathing and die!

- **Explain with calculations why dissolved oxygen is insufficient for oxygen transport in the body.**
- **Describe the structure of haemoglobin and its ability to bind oxygen.**
- **Draw and explain the oxygen dissociation curve for haemoglobin. What factors affect the curve?**
- **Define the terms oxygen content, oxygen capacity, and saturation.**
- **Describe how fetal haemoglobin differs from adult haemoglobin and the double Bohr shift.**
- **List three ways in which haemoglobin can be transported in the blood.**
- **Explain the terms hypoventilation and hyperventilation.**

ACID–BASE BALANCE

Normal pH

Normal metabolism and functioning of cells requires a stable intracellular and extracellular environment. This includes hydrogen ion concentration [H^+] (i.e. pH). Also, the following points apply:

- Normal arterial pH = 7.4.
- Normal arterial pH range = 7.35–7.45 ([H^+] range, 45–35 nmol/L, 20% change in [H^+]).
- A larger variation in pH can be tolerated (pH 6.8–7.8) for a short time.
- If blood remains at pH 6.8 for long, recovery is often impossible.

Acids and bases

Remember from GCSE chemistry:

- Acids donate protons (H^+)
- Bases accept protons (H^+)

$$H_2SO_4 \leftrightarrow 2H^+ + SO_4^{2-} \text{ (acid} \leftrightarrow \text{protons + base)}$$

Strong acids dissociate to form protons easily. The reverse is true of strong bases; thus, by looking at the hydrogen ion concentration we can tell the strength of the acid. Because of the small numbers involved we use a logarithmic scale (pH).

$$pH = \log(1/[H^+]) = -\log[H^+]$$

Because pH is logarithmic, small variations in pH relate to large changes in H^+ ion concentration. The body is therefore relatively tolerant to a change in hydrogen ion concentration.

Metabolic production of acids

Products of metabolism (carbon dioxide, lactic acid, phosphate, sulphate etc.) form acidic solutions, thus increasing the hydrogen ion concentration and reducing pH. We also have an intake of acids in our diet (approximately 50–100 mmol H^+ per day).

We rely on three methods to control our internal hydrogen ion concentration:

- Dilution of body fluids.
- The physiological buffer system.
- Excretion of volatile and nonvolatile acids.

Buffers

A buffer is a substance that can either bind or release hydrogen ions, therefore keeping the pH relatively constant despite the addition of considerable quantities of acid or base.

Buffers are combinations of either:

- Weak acid and conjugate base
- Weak base and conjugate acid

$$\{1\}\ HA \leftrightarrow H^+ + A^- \text{ (acid} \leftrightarrow \text{protons + conjugate base)}$$
$$\{2\}\ B + H^+ \leftrightarrow BH^+ \text{ (base + proton} \leftrightarrow \text{conjugate acid)}$$

The equilibrium for reaction {1}:

$$K = [H^+]\cdot[A^-]/[HA]$$

pK is defined as log(1/K); therefore:

$$pK = \log([HA]/[A^-]) + \log(1/[H^+])$$
$$pH = \log(1/[H^+])$$

Thus, we can deduce the equation below:

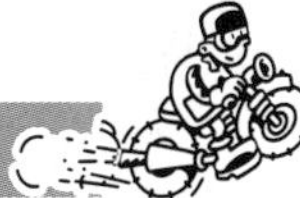

$$pH = pK + \log([base]/[acid])$$

Why do we need to know pK? The buffering capacity of a system is greatest when pK = pH (i.e. [base]/[acid] = 1, and the buffer is 50% dissociated) (Fig. 4.28). Therefore, different buffers in the body will be more or less effective depending on their concentration and pK value.

Buffers of the blood

There are four buffers of the blood:

- Haemoglobin.
- Plasma proteins.
- Phosphate.
- Bicarbonate.

Haemoglobin

As mentioned before, haemoglobin is a very good buffer, especially in its reduced form, although it can also act as a buffer as oxyhaemoglobin.

$$Hb^- + H^+ \leftrightarrow HHb$$
$$HbO_2^- + H^+ \leftrightarrow HHbO_2$$

Plasma proteins

Haemoglobin has six times the buffering capacity of plasma proteins.

$$Pr_p^- + H^+ \leftrightarrow HPr_p$$

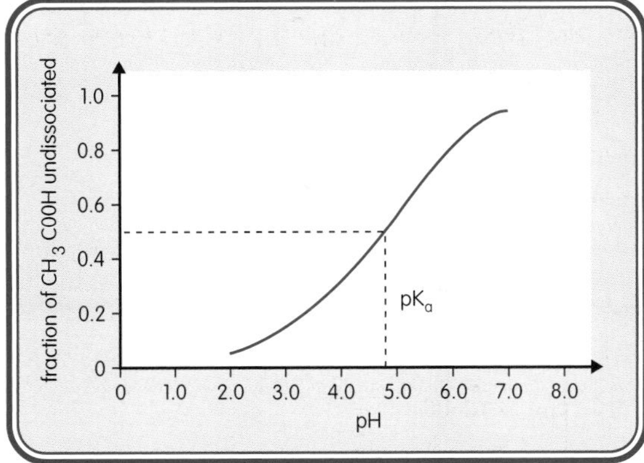

Fig. 4.28 pK_a Buffer. The pK_a of a buffer is the pH at which one-half of the molecules are neutral and one-half are dissociated. From Darnel, Lodish. (Adapted with permission from *Molecular Cell Biology* 2e, by J. Darnell, H. Lodish and D. Baltimore. Scientific American Books, 1990.)

Phosphate

There are two phosphate buffers: NaH_2PO_4 and Na_2HPO_4.

$$H^+ + HPO_4^{2-} \leftrightarrow H_2PO_4^-$$
$$pK = 6.8$$

Theoretically, this would be a good buffer; however, plasma concentrations are too low for it to be quantitatively important extracellularly; however, it is important intracellularly.

Bicarbonate

Bicarbonate is an important buffer because the lung regulates carbon dioxide concentration and the kidney regulates the bicarbonate concentration in the blood.

$$CO_2 + H_2O \leftrightarrow H_2CO_3 \leftrightarrow H^+ + HCO_3^-$$

Looking at the right-hand side of the equation, the equilibrium constant:

$$K = [H^+]\cdot[HCO_3^-]/[H_2CO_3]$$

Remember,

$$pH = pK + \log([base]/[acid])$$

Thus,

$$pH = pK + \log([HCO_3^-]/[H_2CO_3])$$

We know that, in the body, $[H_2CO_3]$ is proportional to $[CO_2]$.

$$[CO_2] = PCO_2 \cdot S$$

(Solubility, S = 0.03 mmol/mmHg·L)

$$pH = pK + \log([HCO_3^-]/(0.03 \times PCO_2))$$

This is known as the Henderson–Hassleblack equation. For this reaction, pK = 6.1 (at body conditions); arterial PCO_2 = 40 mmHg; $[HCO_3^-]$ = 24 mmol/L. Thus:

$$pH = 6.1 + \log(24/(0.03 \times 40)) = 6.1 + 1.3 = 7.4$$
Thus, we can say $pH \propto [HCO_3^-]/PCO_2$

Throughout the following text, it is easiest to follow the principles of acid–base by using the Davenport diagram.

Although the pK system is low relative to the pH of the blood, it is one of the most effective buffer systems of the body. This is because PCO_2 is readily controlled by respiration and [HCO_3^-] regulated by the kidney.

Regulation of plasma bicarbonate by the kidneys

Hydrogen ions, either formed by metabolism or consumed, react with bicarbonate in the plasma to form carbon dioxide, which is blown off at the lungs. The kidneys must try to maintain the remaining bicarbonate and if necessary produce additional bicarbonate (Fig. 4.29).

Normally, all the bicarbonate filtered at the glomerulus is converted into carbon dioxide and water by an interaction with hydrogen ions produced by the renal tubular cells and secreted into the tubular fluid. This reaction is catalysed by carbonic anhydrase (Ca). The process that generates hydrogen ions in the kidney is the same as that in the red blood cell. Carbonic anhydrase catalyses the conversion of carbon dioxide and water to hydrogen carbonate, which then dissociates to form hydrogen and bicarbonate. Bicarbonate passes preferentially into the plasma, replacing the bicarbonate lost in the tubular fluid. Thus, although bicarbonate is added to the plasma, it is not the same bicarbonate that was filtered at the glomerulus. The amount of hydrogen ions and bicarbonate produced depends on PCO_2. Increased PCO_2 will increase production, lowered PCO_2 will reduce production (Fig. 4.30).

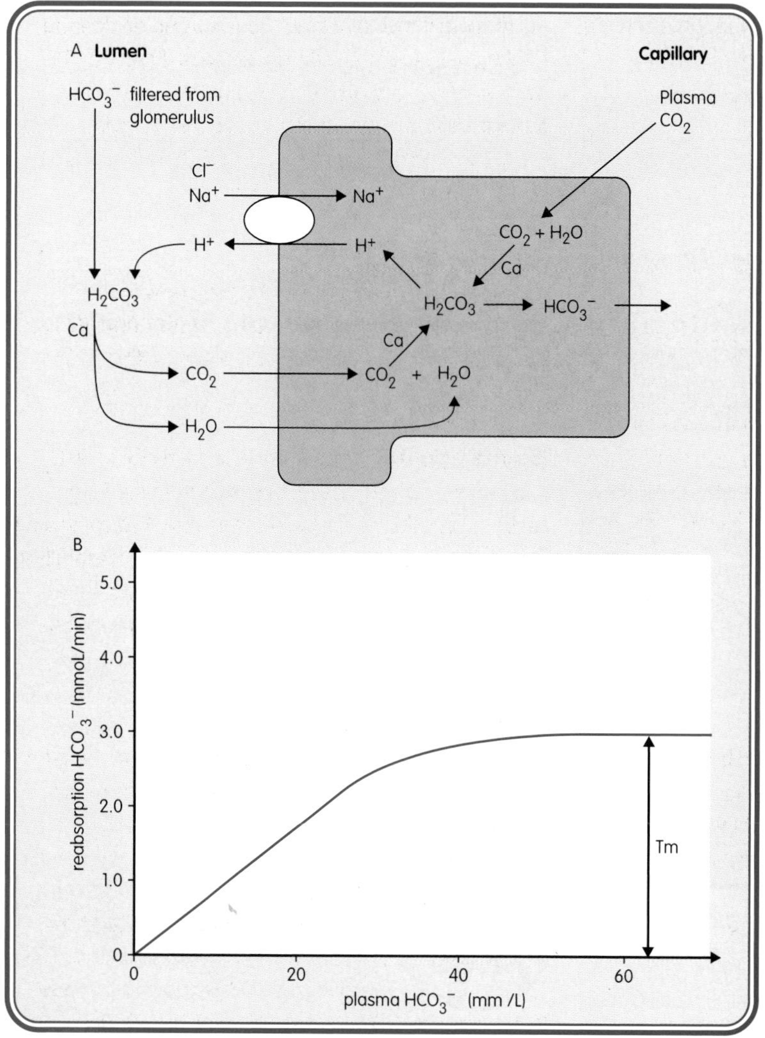

Fig. 4.29 Regulation of plasma blood bicarbonate in the kidneys. (A) Mechanism of reabsorption via carbonic anhydrase (Ca). (B) Saturation kinetics shown by reabsorption of plasma HCO_3^-. T_m is the maximum reabsorption rate of HCO_3^-.

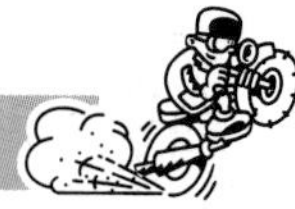

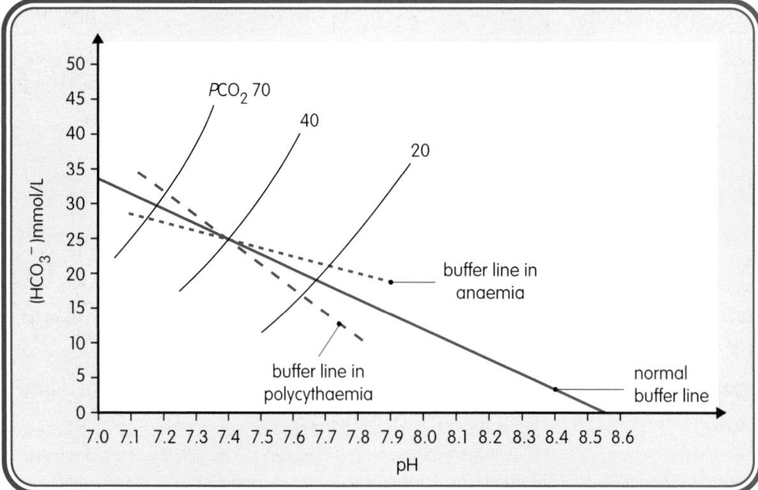

Fig. 4.30 The relationship between plasma [HCO_3^-], pH, and PCO_2. A buffer line runs from points A to B. Any change in PCO_2 will have an equivalent rise or fall in [HCO_3^-] because of bicarbonate buffering of hydrogen ions; this can be shown by moving up and down the buffer line. Point N shows the normal plasma pH and [HCO_3^-]. Lines running perpendicular to the buffer line are of constant PCO_2.

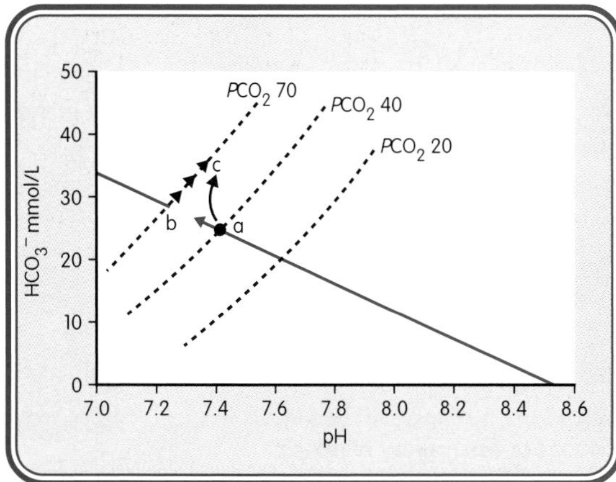

Fig. 4.31 Respiratory acidosis causes increases in PCO_2, HCO_3^- and reduction in pH shown as a moved from a to b. The kidneys compensate by increasing HCO_3^- reabsorption and production shown from point b to point c. Arrows a–c shows a real-life situation. (Adapted with permission from *Principles of Renal Physiology* 2e, by C. Lote. Chapman & Hall, 1994.)

Acid–base disturbances

Acid–base disturbances may be caused by either respiratory or metabolic disturbances. Blood pH disturbance can be tending either to a high pH (alkalosis) or a low pH (acidosis). This allows us to classify four types of disturbance:

- Respiratory alkalosis.
- Respiratory acidosis.
- Metabolic alkalosis.
- Metabolic acidosis.

Clinically, a pH level below 7.35 is termed acidaemia and a pH level above 7.45 is termed alkalaemia. The kidneys and lungs may try to return the acid–base disturbance towards normal values; this is called compensation. Return of PCO_2, [HCO_3^-], and pH to normal values is called correction.

Davenport diagram

A Davenport diagram (Fig. 4.30) can show the relationship between plasma [HCO_3^-], pH, and PCO_2. Remember: $CO_2 + H_2O \leftrightarrow H_2CO_3 \leftrightarrow H^+ \ HCO_3^-$

Respiratory acidosis

Respiratory acidosis results from an increase in PCO_2 caused by reduced gaseous exchange in the lungs (less carbon dioxide is blown off). In turn, this causes an increase in hydrogen ion concentration and a reduction in pH. Thus, plasma bicarbonate concentration increases to compensate for the increased hydrogen ion concentration (Fig. 4.31).

Renal compensation

The increase in hydrogen ion concentration in the blood results in increased filtration of hydrogen ions at the glomeruli, thus:

- Increasing HCO_3^- reabsorption.
- Increasing HCO_3^- production.
- Thus, plasma HCO_3^- rises compensating for the increased [H^+].

Renal compensation raises pH towards normal.

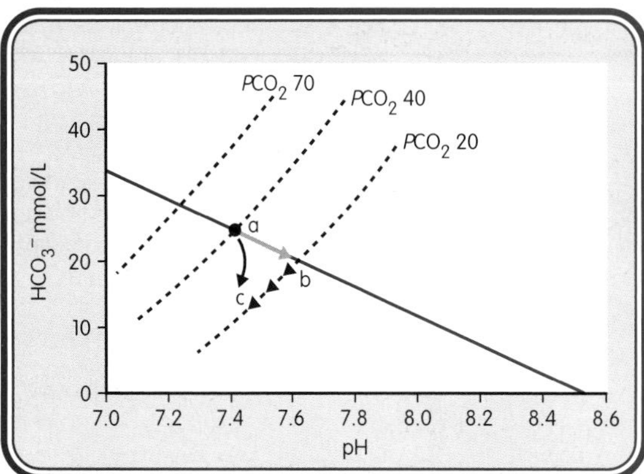

Fig. 4.32 Respiratory alkalosis causes reduced PCO_2, HCO_3^- and increases the pH. Shown as a move from point a to point b. The kidneys compensate by reducing the rate of renal excretion of H^+ so that less HCO_3^- is reabsorbed or produced by the kidney. This is shown as a move from point b to point c. The real-life situation is shown from point a–c. (Adapted with permission from *Principles of Renal Physiology* 2e, by C. Lote. Chapman & Hall, 1994.)

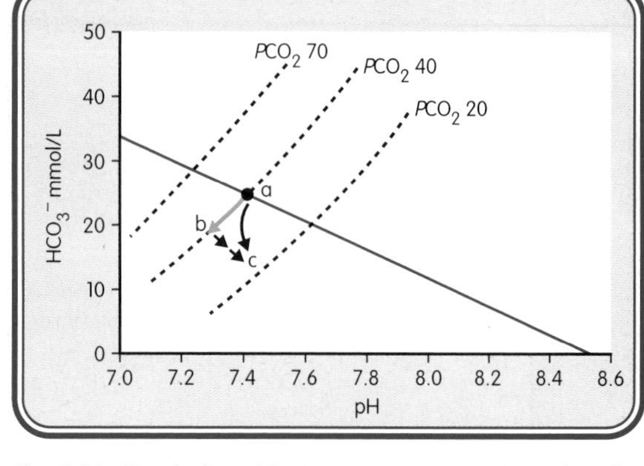

Fig. 4.33 Metabolic acidosis causes a rise in H^+, reduced HCO_3^- and reduced pH. Shown as a move from point a to point b. The lungs compensate by blowing off CO_2 and therefore increasing the pH shown as a move from point b to point c. The arrows a–c show the real-life situation. (Adapted with permission from *Principles of Renal Physiology* 2e, by C. Lote. Chapman & Hall, 1994.)

Causes of respiratory acidosis

The causes of respiratory acidosis are:

Decreased diffusion (has more effect on PO_2 than on PCO_2):

- Chronic obstructive pulmonary disease (chronic bronchitis, emphysema).
- Asthma.
- Blocked airway (by tumour or foreign body).
- Spontaneous lung collapse, brainstem lesion.
- Injury to the chest wall may also cause reduced ventilation.

Decreased diffusion (has more effect on PO_2 than on PCO_2):

- Emphysema.
- Fibrotic lung disease.

Drugs that reduce respiratory drive (ventilation):

- Morphine.
- Barbiturates.
- General anaesthetics.

Respiratory alkalosis

Respiratory alkalosis results from a decrease in PCO_2 caused by increased gaseous exchange in the lungs (more carbon dioxide is blown off). This causes a decrease in hydrogen ion concentration and thus an increase in pH (Fig. 4.32).

Renal compensation

The reduction in hydrogen ion concentration in the blood results in decreased hydrogen ion filtration at the glomeruli, thus:

- Reducing HCO_3^- reabsorption.
- Reducing HCO_3^- production.
- Thus, plasma HCO_3^- falls, compensating for the reduced [H^+].

Renal compensation reduces pH towards normal.

Causes of respiratory alkalosis

The causes of respiratory alkalosis are:

- Increased ventilation—caused by hypoxic drive in chronic obstructive pulmonary disease (chronic bronchitis, emphysema), high altitude.
- Hyperventilation—brainstem damage, infection causing fever, hysterical overbreathing.

Metabolic acidosis

Metabolic acidosis results from an excess of hydrogen ions in the body, which reduces bicarbonate concentration (shifting the equation below to the left). Respiration is unaffected; therefore, PCO_2 is normal (Fig. 4.33).

Respiratory compensation

$$CO_2 + H_2O \leftrightarrow H_2CO_3 \leftrightarrow H^+ + HCO_3^-$$

The reduction in pH is detected by the peripheral chemoreceptors. This causes an increase in ventilation, which lowers PCO_2. Also:

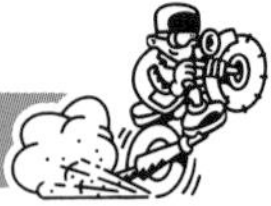

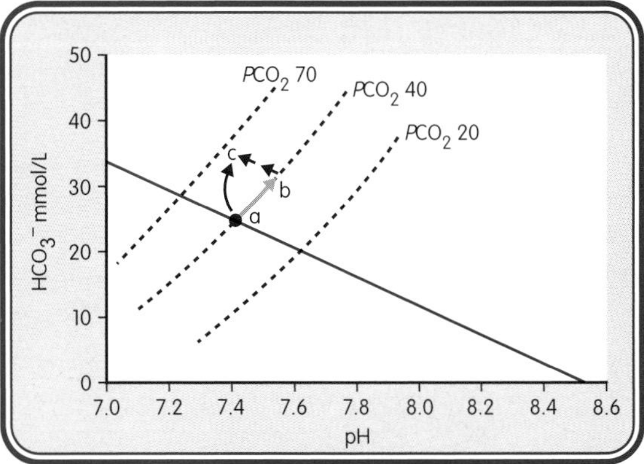

Fig. 4.34 Metabolic alkalosis due to loss of H^+ ions and increase in HCO_3^- with increase in pH shown as a move from point a to point b. The lungs compensate by reducing ventilation and increase PCO_2 shown as a move from point b to point c. The arrow from point a to point c shows the real situation. (Adapted with permission from *Principles of Renal Physiology* 2e, by C. Lote. Chapman & Hall, 1994.)

- The above equation is driven further to the left, reducing hydrogen ion concentration and bicarbonate.
- The decrease in hydrogen ion concentration raises pH towards normal.
- Respiratory compensation hinders renal correction of the fault.

Respiratory compensation cannot correct the values of PCO_2, $[HCO_3^-]$, and $[H^+]$. This can be carried out only by removing the excess hydrogen ions from the body or restoring the lost bicarbonate (i.e. correcting the metabolic fault).

Causes of metabolic acidosis

Causes of metabolic acidosis are:

- Ingestion of acid.
- Loss of HCO_3^- from the kidneys.
- Metabolic production of hydrogen ions. The kidneys may not be able to excrete the excess hydrogen ions immediately, or at all (as in renal failure).

Metabolic alkalosis

Metabolic alkalosis results from an increase in bicarbonate concentration or a fall in hydrogen ion concentration. Removing hydrogen ions from the right of the equation (below) drives the reaction to the right, increasing bicarbonate concentration. Decrease in hydrogen ion concentration raises pH; initially, PCO_2 is normal (Fig. 4.34).

Respiratory compensation

$$CO_2 + H_2O \leftrightarrow H_2CO_3 \leftrightarrow H^+ + HCO_3^-$$

The increase in pH is detected by the peripheral chemoreceptors. This causes a decrease in ventilation which raises PCO_2. Also:

- The above equation is driven further to the right, increasing hydrogen ion and bicarbonate concentrations.
- The decrease in hydrogen ion concentration raises pH towards normal.
- Respiratory compensation hinders renal correction of the fault.

Respiratory compensation cannot correct the values of PCO_2, $[HCO_3^-]$, and $[H^+]$. This can only be carried out by removing the problem either of reduced hydrogen ion concentration or increased bicarbonate concentration. This is done by reducing renal hydrogen ion secretion.

More bicarbonate is excreted because more is filtered at the glomerulus and less is reabsorbed in combination with hydrogen ions.

Causes of metabolic alkalosis

The causes of metabolic alkalosis are:

- Vomiting (hydrochloric acid loss from the stomach).
- Ingestion of alkaline substances.
- Increased plasma bicarbonate.

- **State the normal blood pH range.**
- **What is a buffer? Give four examples of buffers in the blood and their relative importance.**
- **Draw a Davenport diagram.**
- **Explain what is meant by an acid–base disturbance. Explain the four deviations.**
- **List the causes for respiratory acidosis and alkalosis.**
- **List the causes for metabolic acidosis and alkalosis.**

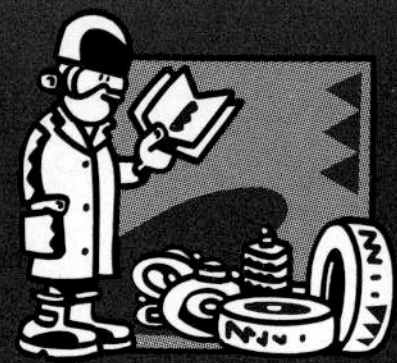

5. Control of Respiratory Function

CONTROL OF VENTILATION

Basics of control

Every control system (including respiratory control) needs various individual parts for it to function correctly:

- A control variable—a variable to be kept within certain limits (e.g. P_aCO_2 or P_aO_2).
- A desired value for that control variable, often quoted as normal physiological range (e.g. P_aCO_2 of around 40 mmHg).
- A measured value for the control variable (e.g. actual $P_aCO_2 = 46$ mmHg, 35 mmHg, etc.).
- Sensors to detect the measured value or a difference from the desired value (e.g. muscle spindle stretch receptors or chemoreceptors).
- Effectors (e.g. respiratory muscles, which alter ventilation and thus change P_aCO_2).
- A controller that relates the measured value to the desired value and changes output to the effectors (respiratory muscles), altering ventilation.

Types of control within the respiratory system

There are two types of control: feedback and feed-forward:

- Feedback control—the system detailed below (Fig. 5.1), in which the controller looks at the measured value of the control variable (e.g. P_aCO_2) and relates this to the desired value. Adjustments to the system are then made.
- Feed-forward control—the system detailed below (Fig. 5.2), which anticipates the effects of external factors to the system and makes adjustments to the system in an attempt to control their effect. An example of this is behavioural control of breathing when we sing.
- Control of breathing—when considering control of the breathing, the main control variable is P_aCO_2 (we try to control this value near to 40 mmHg). This can be carried out by adjusting the respiratory rate, the tidal volume, or both.

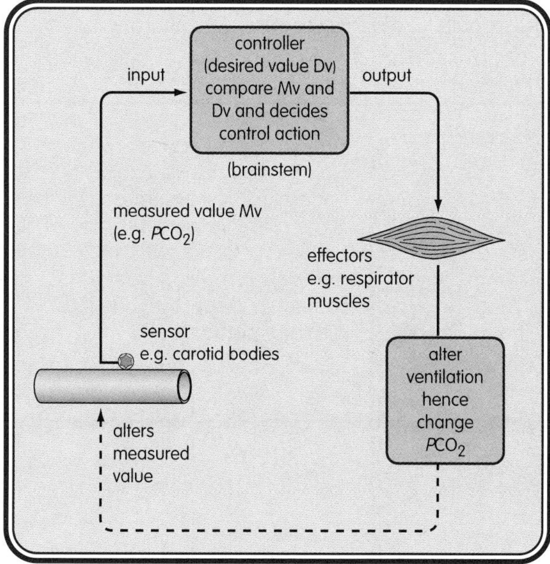

Fig. 5.1 Example of feedback control in the respiratory system. P_aCO_2 is used as the control variable.

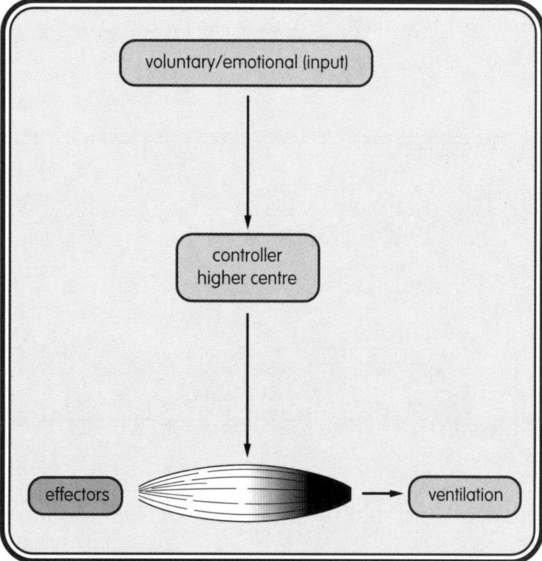

Fig. 5.2 Example of feed-forward control in the respiratory system. Higher centres predict the effect of external changes (e.g. emotion or singing) and alter the output to the effectors (respiratory muscles) to achieve the required ventilation.

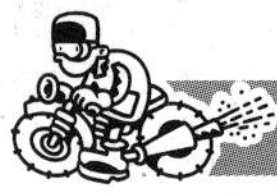

By controlling P_aCO_2 we are effectively controlling alveolar ventilation (see Chapter 3) and thus P_ACO_2.

Although P_aCO_2 is the main control variable, P_aO_2 is also controlled, but normally to a much lesser extent than P_aCO_2. However, the P_aO_2 control system can take over and become the main controlling system when the P_aO_2 drops below 50 mmHg.

Control can seem to be brought about by:

- Metabolic demands of the body (*metabolic control*)—tissue oxygen demand and acid–base balance.
- Behavioural demands of the body (*behavioural control*)—singing, coughing, laughing (i.e. control is voluntary).

These are essentially feedback and feed-forward control systems, respectively. The behavioural control of breathing overlays the metabolic control. Its control is derived from higher centres of the brain. The axons of neurons whose cell bodies are situated in the cerebral cortex bypass the respiratory centres in the brainstem and synapse directly with lower motor neurons that control respiratory muscles. This system will not be dealt with within this text; we shall deal only with the metabolic control of respiration.

Metabolic control of breathing

Metabolic control of breathing is a function of the brainstem (pons and medulla). The controller can be considered as specific groups of neurons (previously called respiratory centres).

Pontine neurons

Those located in the pons are the pontine respiratory group and consist of two groups of neurons:

- Expiratory neurons in the nucleus parabrachialis medialis.
- Inspiratory neurons in the lateral parabrachial nucleus and Kölliker's fuse nucleus.

The role of the pontine respiratory group (PRG) is to regulate (i.e. affect the activity of) the dorsal respiratory group (DRG) and possibly the ventral respiratory group (VRG, neuron groups in the medulla).

Medullary neurons

Three groups of neurons associated with respiratory control have been identified in the medulla:

- The dorsal respiratory group, situated in the nucleus of tractus solitarius.
- The ventral respiratory group, situated in the nucleus ambiguus and the nucleus retroambigualis.
- The Bötzinger complex, situated rostral to the nucleus ambiguus.

These groups receive sensory information, which is compared with the desired value of control; adjustments are made to respiratory muscles to rectify any deviation from ideal.

The dorsal respiratory group (Fig. 5.3) contains neuron bodies of inspiratory upper motor neurons. These inhibit the activity of expiratory neurons in the ventral respiratory group and have an excitatory effect

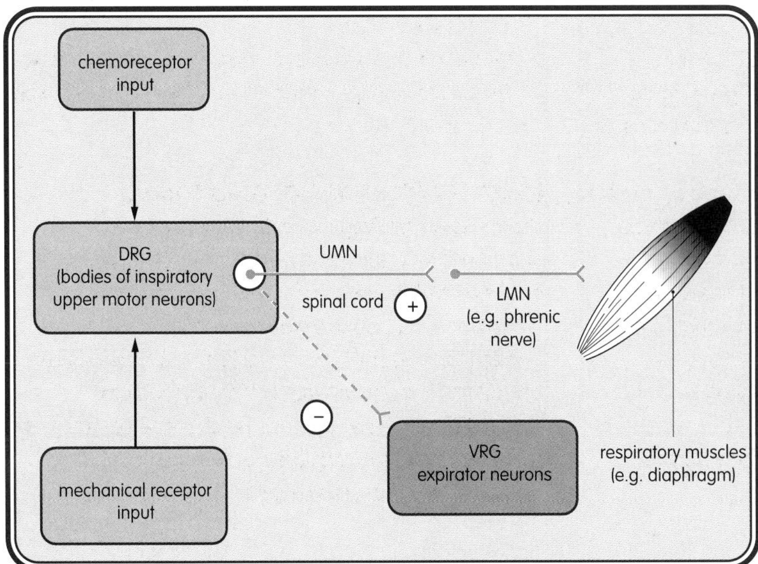

Fig. 5.3 Dorsal respiratory group. Note the output to respiratory muscle and inhibition of expiratory neurons in the ventral respiratory group. UMN = upper motor neuron; LMN = lower motor neuron; VRG = ventral respiratory group; DRG = dorsal respiratory group.

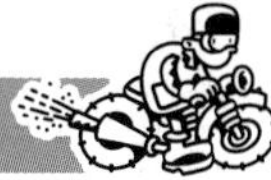

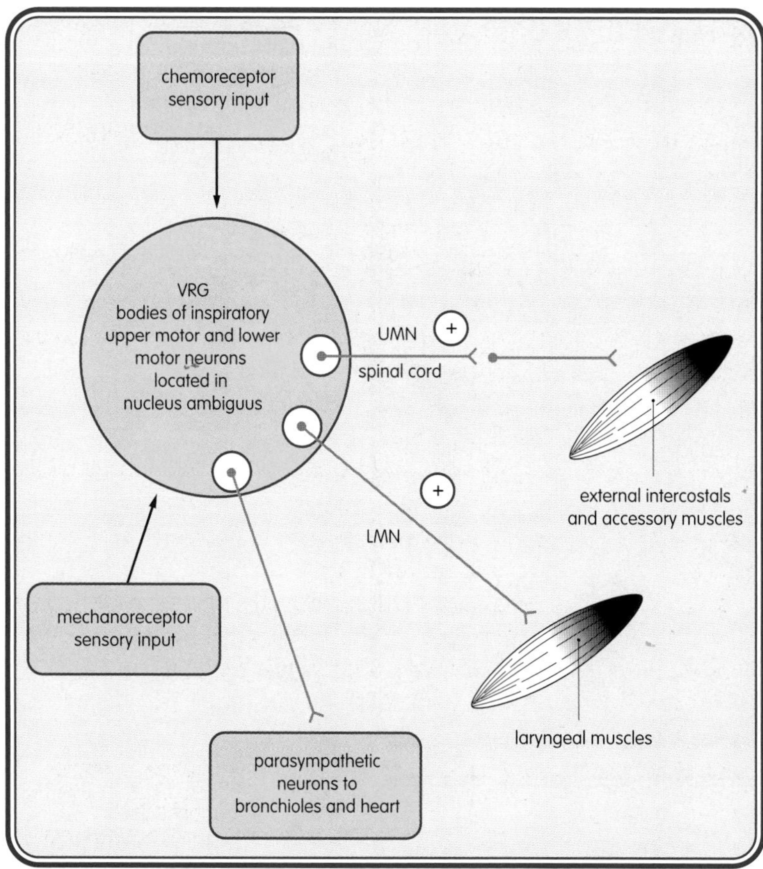

Fig. 5.4 Ventral respiratory group in the nucleus ambiguus. LMN = lower motor neuron; UMN = upper motor neuron; VRG = ventral respiratory group.

on lower motor neurons to the respiratory muscles, increasing ventilation.

Ventral respiratory group neurons in the nucleus ambiguus (Fig. 5.4) are again inspiratory upper motor neurons.

Ventral respiratory group neurons in the rostral part of the nucleus retroambigualis (Fig. 5.5) contain inspiratory upper motor neurons which go on to supply through their lower motor neurons external intercostal muscles and accessory muscles.

Ventral respiratory group neurons in the caudal part of the nucleus retroambigualis (Fig. 5.6) are expiratory upper motor neurons.

The Bötzinger complex (Fig. 5.7) contains only expiratory neurons. Its sensory input is through the nucleus tractus solitarius. It has two functions:

- Inhibition of inspiratory neurons of the dorsal and ventral respiratory groups.
- Excitation of expiratory neurons in the ventral respiratory group.

It is believed that the medulla is responsible for the respiratory rhythm (Fig. 5.8); two main theories exist as to how this is brought about:

- Dorsal respiratory group inspiratory pacemaker—neurons discharge in a phasic manner, inhibiting expiratory neurons.
- Neural networks—local re-excitation causes phasic firing in both inspiratory and expiratory neurons with reciprocal inhibition.

Effectors (muscles of respiration)

The muscles involved in respiration have been described in Chapter 3. The major muscle groups involved are the diaphragm, internal and external intercostals, and abdominal muscles.

Effectors carry out the control action for the central controller. Thus, the strength of contraction and coordination of these muscles is set by the central controller. If the muscles are not coordinated, this will result in abnormal breathing patterns.

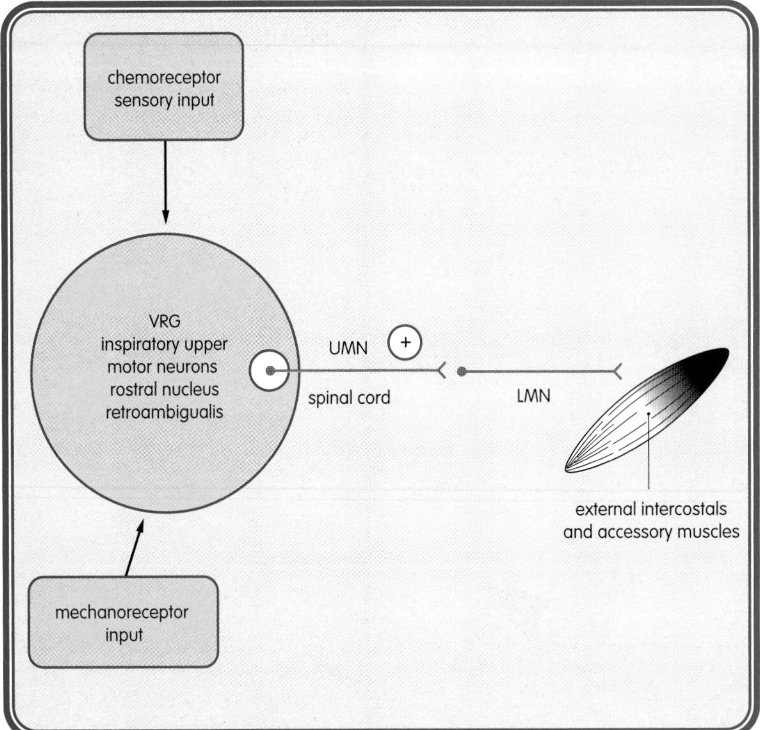

Fig. 5.5 Ventral respiratory group located in rostral nucleus retroambigualis. UMN = upper motor neuron; LMN = lower motor neuron; VRG = ventral respiratory group.

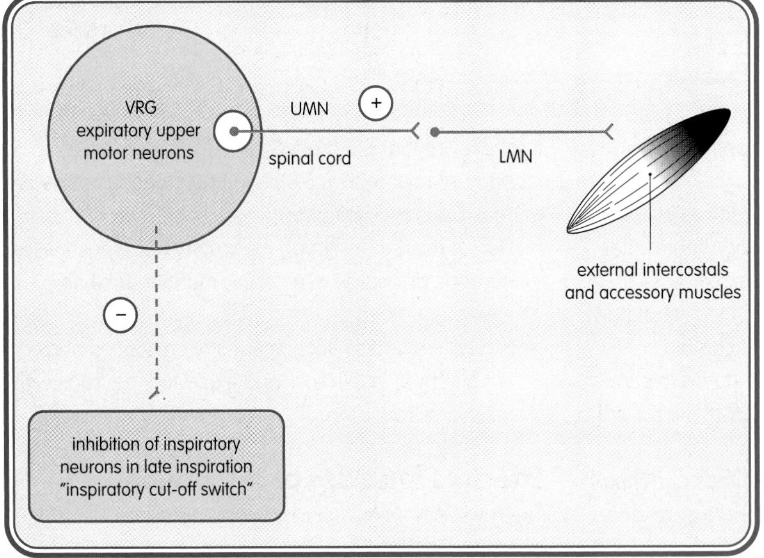

Fig. 5.6 Ventral respiratory group located in caudal nucleus retroambigualis (expiratory neurones). (Adapted with permission from *Consultation in Diagnostic Imaging* by W.W. Scott and P.P. Scott. BC Decker, 1985.)

Sensors (receptors)

Sensors report current values or discrepancies from ideal values for the various variables being controlled (e.g. P_aCO_2, P_aO_2, and pH) to the central controller.

There are many types of sensors and receptors involved with respiratory control:

- Chemoreceptors—central and peripheral.
- Lung receptors—irritant, pulmonary stretch, and juxtapulmonary.
- Receptors in the chest wall—muscle spindles and Golgi tendon organs.
- Other receptors—nasal, tracheal, and laryngeal receptors, arterial baroreceptors, pain receptors.

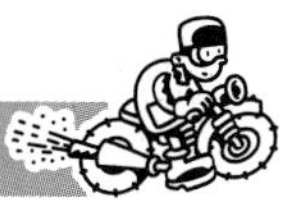

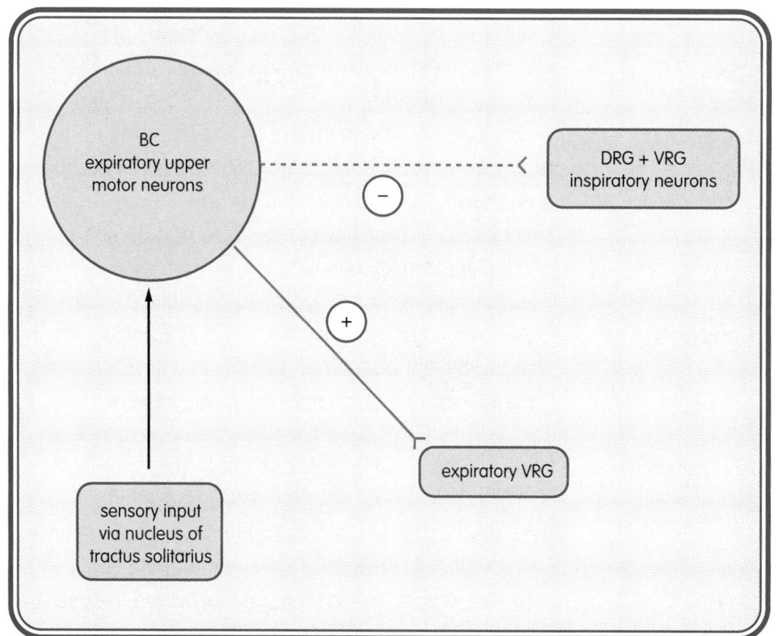

Fig. 5.7 Bötzinger complex (BC); located first rostral to nucleus ambiguus and comprised entirely of expiratory neurons. PRG = pontine respiratory group; DRG = dorsal respiratory group. (Adapted with permission from *Decision making in medicine*, by H.L. Green and W.P. Johnson. Mosby Year Book, 1993.)

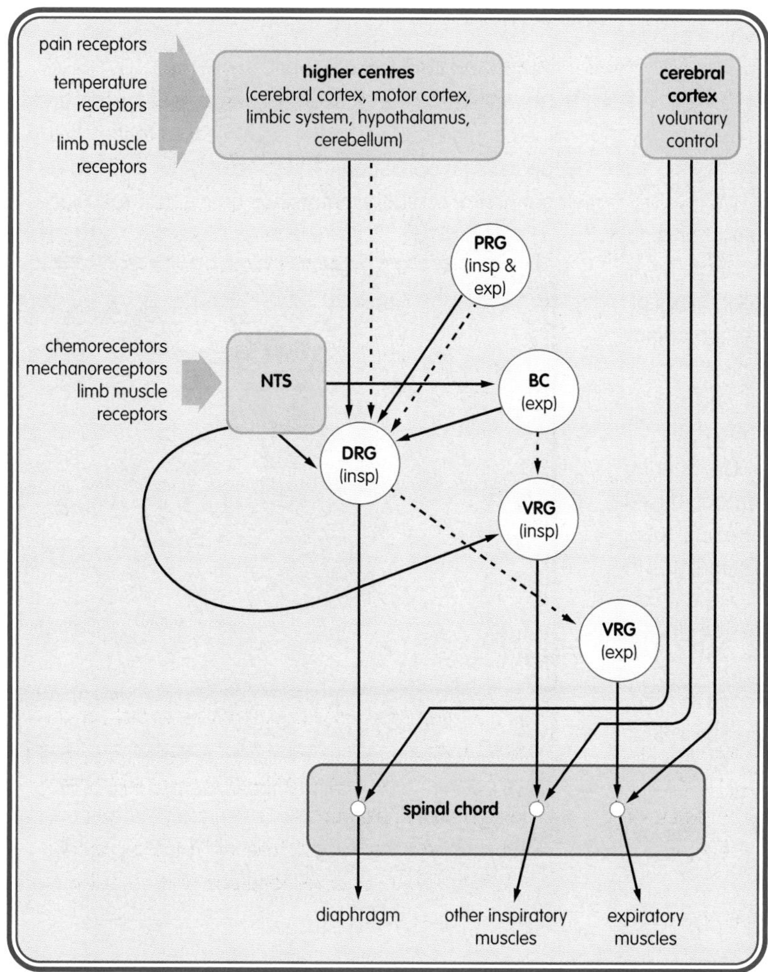

Fig. 5.8 Summary of the control pathways of ventilation. BC = Bötzinger complex; NTS = nucleus tractus solitarius; PRG = pontine respiratory group; DRG = dorsal respiratory group; VRG = ventral respiratory group. Dotted line = inhibitory, full line = excitatory.

Chemoreceptors

Chemoreceptors monitor blood gas tensions, P_aCO_2, P_aO_2, and pH, and help keep $\dot{V}_E$ appropriate to metabolic demands of the body. Therefore, chemoreceptors respond to:

- Hypercapnia.
- Hypoxia.
- Acidosis.

Chemoreceptors are divided into central and peripheral chemoreceptors.

Central chemoreceptors

Central chemoreceptors are located in the brainstem on the ventrolateral surface of the medulla, close to the exit of cranial nerves IX and X.

Chemoreceptor neurons are anatomically separate from the medullary respiratory control centre.

Central chemoreceptors respond to hydrogen ion concentration within the surrounding brain tissue and cerebrospinal fluid.

- Raised hydrogen ion concentration increases ventilation.
- Lowered hydrogen ion concentration decreases ventilation.

Diffusion of ions across the blood–brain barrier is poor. Blood levels of hydrogen ions and bicarbonate have little effect in the short term on the concentrations of hydrogen ions and bicarbonate in the cerebrospinal fluid and thus have little effect on the central chemoreceptors.

Carbon dioxide, however, can pass freely by diffusion across the blood–brain barrier. On entering the cerebrospinal fluid, the increase in carbon dioxide increases the free hydrogen ion concentration. This increase in hydrogen ion concentration stimulates the central chemoreceptors. Thus:

- Central chemoreceptors are sensitive to P_aCO_2 not arterial hydrogen ion concentration.
- Central chemoreceptors are not sensitive to P_aO_2.
- Because there is less protein in the cerebrospinal fluid (<0.4 g/L) than in the plasma (60–80 g/L), a rise in P_aCO_2 has a larger effect on pH in the cerebrospinal fluid than in the blood (CSF has lower buffering capacity).

Long-standing raised P_aCO_2 causes the pH of the cerebrospinal fluid to return towards normal—this is explained below.

The carbon dioxide in glial cells is hydrated to hydrogen ions and bicarbonate (catalysed by carbonic anhydrase). The hydrogen ions produced are buffered by intracellular proteins, but the bicarbonate diffuses into the cerebrospinal fluid.

Hypercapnia causes glial cells to reduce anerobic metabolism and hence production of lactic acid, allowing bicarbonate to diffuse freely into the cerebrospinal fluid. Diffusion of bicarbonate from the blood into the cerebrospinal fluid causes central chemoreceptors to become insensitive to high levels of P_aCO_2.

The receptors are tonically active and vital for maintenance of respiration. Eighty per cent of the drive for ventilation is a result of stimulation of the central chemoreceptors. When they are inactivated, respiration ceases. These receptors are readily depressed by drugs (e.g. opiates and barbiturates).

Peripheral chemoreceptors

Fig. 5.9 shows the location of chemoreceptors around the carotid sinus and aortic arch. These are the carotid bodies and aortic bodies, respectively. Stimulation of peripheral chemoreceptors has both cardiovascular

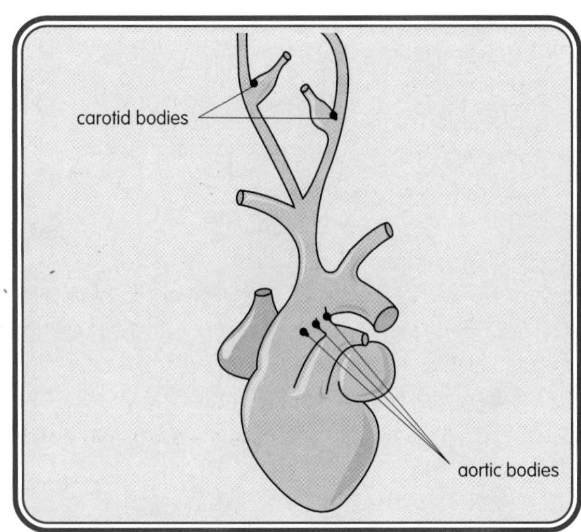

Fig. 5.9 Peripheral chemoreceptors. Carotid bodies are situated around the carotid sinus and are sensitive both to P_aCO_2 and P_aO_2. Aortic bodies are situated around the aortic arch and are sensitive only to P_aCO_2.

and respiratory effects. Of the two receptor groups, the carotid bodies have the greatest effect on respiration.

Carotid bodies

The carotid bodies contains two different types of cells: type I (glomus) cells and type II (sustentacular) cells. Type I cells are stimulated by hypoxia; they connect with afferent nerves to the brainstem. Type II cells are supportive (structural and metabolic), similar to glial cells of the central nervous system.

There is a rich blood supply to the carotid bodies (blood flow per mass of tissue far exceeds that to the brain); venous blood flow, therefore, remains saturated with oxygen.

The exact mechanism of action of the carotid bodies is not known. It is believed that type I (glomus) cells are activated by hypoxia and release transmitter substances that stimulate afferents to the brainstem.

Peripheral chemoreceptors are sensitive to:

- P_aO_2.
- P_aCO_2.
- pH.
- Blood flow.
- Temperature.

The carotid bodies are supplied by the autonomic nervous system, which appears to alter their sensitivity to hypoxia by regulating blood flow to the chemoreceptor:

- Sympathetic action vasoconstricts, increasing sensitivity to hypoxia.
- Parasympathetic action vasodilates, reducing sensitivity to hypoxia.

At a low P_aO_2 (<50 mmHg), a further decrease in arterial oxygen tension significantly increases ventilation (Fig. 5.10). However, at levels of oxygen tension close to 100 mmHg, changes have little effect on ventilation. If P_aO_2 increases above 100 mmHg (achieved when breathing high-concentration oxygen), ventilation is only slightly reduced.

Unlike central chemoreceptors, peripheral chemoreceptors are directly stimulated by blood pH. Although peripheral chemoreceptors are stimulated by P_aCO_2, their response is much less than that of central chemoreceptors (less than 10% of the effect).

In summary:

- Lowered P_aO_2 (especially below 50 mmHg) increases ventilation.
- Increased P_aCO_2 increases ventilation (<10% of the effect of central receptors).
- Raised hydrogen ion concentration increases ventilation (however, aortic bodies do not respond).
- The response of these receptors is very fast and can oscillate within a respiratory cycle.
- The receptors are very rugged.

Receptors in the lung

The receptors in the lung monitor mechanical activity. There are three types of receptors in the lung:

- Pulmonary stretch receptors—slowly and rapidly adapting.
- Pulmonary and bronchial C fibre receptors—formerly juxtapulmonary, J receptors.
- Irritant receptors.

Stretch receptors

These receptors are situated in the smooth muscle of the bronchial walls and respond to changes in transmural pressure. They are classified into two types: slowly adapting, which produce maintained response to a maintained stimulus; and rapidly adapting, which produce a transient response to a maintained stimulus.

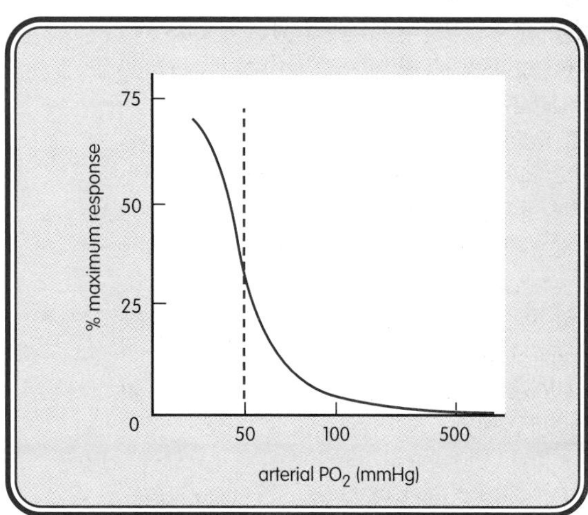

Fig. 5.10 Response of ventilation to P_aO_2. The response to a lowered P_aO_2 is small until the P_aO_2 falls below a value of 50 mmHg, after which point the response increases dramatically.

Slowly adapting

With slowly adapting stretch receptors, a maintained stimulus leads to a maintained response. Primarily, these receptors are concerned with physiological control and regulatory reflexes. They are stimulated by inflation (which stretches the lungs):

- Inflation leads to decreased respiration (inflation reflex or Hering–Breuer reflex).
- Deflation leads to increased respiration (deflation reflex).

These reflexes are active in the first year of life, but are weak in adults. Therefore, they are not thought to determine the rate and depth of breathing in adults. However, these reflexes are seen to be more active if the tidal volume increases above 1.0 L and therefore might have a role in exercise.

Afferent fibres travel to the respiratory centres through the vagus nerve.

The functions of these receptors are:

- The termination of inspiration.
- Regulation of the work of breathing.
- Reinforcement of respiratory rhythm in the first year of life.

However, if the nerve is blocked by anaesthesia there is no change seen in the rate and depth of breathing.

Pulmonary and bronchial C fibre receptors

These receptors are stimulated by:

- Large inflation.
- Forced deflation.
- Pulmonary vascular congestion.
- Oedema—interstitial fluid in the alveolar wall.
- Chemical mediators—histamine and capsacin.

The receptors are thought to be situated in the alveolar wall close to pulmonary capillaries. Afferent fibres travel to respiratory centres through the vagus nerve (nonmyelinated C fibres).

When stimulated they cause:

- Closure of the larynx.
- Rapid, shallow breathing.
- Bradycardia.
- Hypotension.

They also contribute to the breathlessness in heart failure.

Irritant receptors

These receptors are scattered through the airways and lie between epithelial cells. They are stimulated by inhaled particles, noxious gases, increased airflow, pulmonary congestion, and mechanical deformation. Chemical mediators of allergic reactions also stimulate these receptors which in part account for an increase in ventilation in asthma.

Stimulation of these receptors in the trachea causes a cough reflex, thereby eliminating the particles from the airways. Receptors in lower areas cause bronchoconstriction, laryngeal constriction, and rapid, shallow breathing. This is an attempt to limit how far a particle is inhaled.

In the nose and upper airways, there are irritant receptors (Chapter 2), which act to protect the lower airway.

Receptors in the chest wall

Receptors in the chest wall consist of:

- Joint receptors—measure the velocity of rib movement.
- Golgi tendon organs—found within the muscles of respiration (e.g. diaphragm and intercostals) and detect the strength of muscle contraction.
- Muscle spindles—monitor the length of muscle fibres both statically and dynamically (i.e. detect muscle length and velocity).

These receptors help to minimize changes to ventilation imposed by an external load (e.g. lateral flexion of the trunk). They achieve this by modifying motor neuron output to the respiratory muscles. The aim is to achieve the most efficient respiration in terms of tidal volume and frequency. Thus, reflexes from muscles and joints stabilize ventilation in the face of changing mechanical conditions.

Arterial baroreceptors

Hypertension stimulates arterial baroreceptors, which inhibit ventilation. Hypotension has the opposite effect.

Pain receptors

Stimulation of pain receptors causes a brief apnoea, followed by a period of hyperventilation.

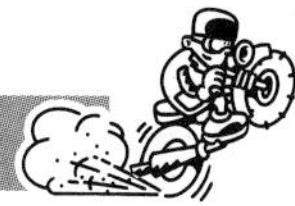

Coordinated responses of the respiratory system

Response to carbon dioxide

Carbon dioxide is the most important factor in the control of ventilation. Under normal conditions P_aCO_2 is held within very tight limits and ventilatory response is very sensitive to small changes in P_aCO_2.

The response of ventilation to carbon dioxide has been measured by inhalation of mixtures of carbon dioxide, raising the P_aCO_2 and observing the increase in ventilation (Fig.5.11).

Note that a small increase in P_ACO_2 causes a significant increase in ventilation. The response to P_aCO_2 is also dependent upon the arterial oxygen tension. At lower values of P_aO_2 the ventilatory response is more sensitive to changes in P_aCO_2 (steeper slope) and ventilation is greater for a given P_aCO_2. If the P_aCO_2 is reduced, this causes a significant reduction in ventilation.

Factors that affect ventilatory response to P_aCO_2 are:

- P_aO_2.
- Blood pH.
- Genetics.
- Age.
- Personality.
- Fitness.
- Drugs (e.g. opiates, such as morphine and diamorphine, reduce respiratory and cardiovascular drive).

Response to oxygen

As mentioned above, the response to reduced P_aO_2 is by stimulation of the peripheral chemoreceptors. This response, however, is not significant until the P_aO_2 drops to around 50 mmHg. The relationship between P_aO_2 and ventilation has been studied by measuring changes in ventilation while a subject breathes hypoxic mixtures (Fig. 5.12). It is assumed that end expiratory P_AO_2 and P_ACO_2 are equivalent to arterial gas tensions.

The response to P_AO_2 is also seen to change with different levels of P_ACO_2.

- The greater the carbon dioxide tension, the earlier the response to low oxygen tension.
- Therefore, at high P_ACO_2, a decrease in oxygen tension below 100 mmHg causes an increase in ventilation.

Under normal conditions, P_aO_2 does not fall to values of around 50 mmHg and, therefore, daily control of ventilation does not rely on hypoxic drive. However, under conditions of severe lung disease, hypoxic drive becomes increasingly important. The patient may rely almost entirely on hypoxic drive alone, having lost ventilatory response to carbon dioxide (described above). Central chemoreceptors have become unresponsive to carbon dioxide; in addition, ventilatory drive from the effects of reduced pH on peripheral chemoreceptors is also lessened by renal compensation for the acid–base abnormality. Administration of high-concentration oxygen therapy

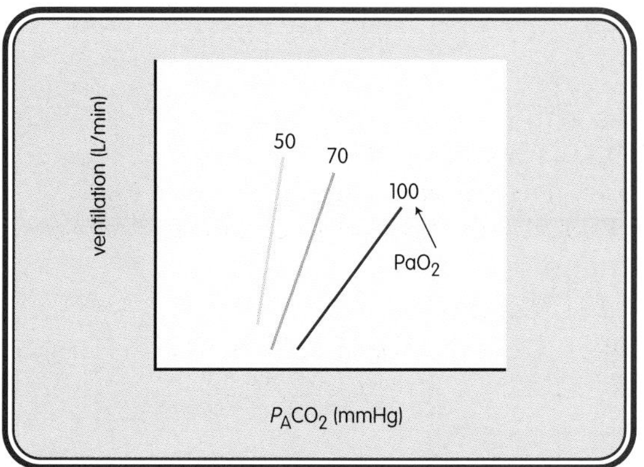

Fig. 5.11 The response of ventilation to CO_2.

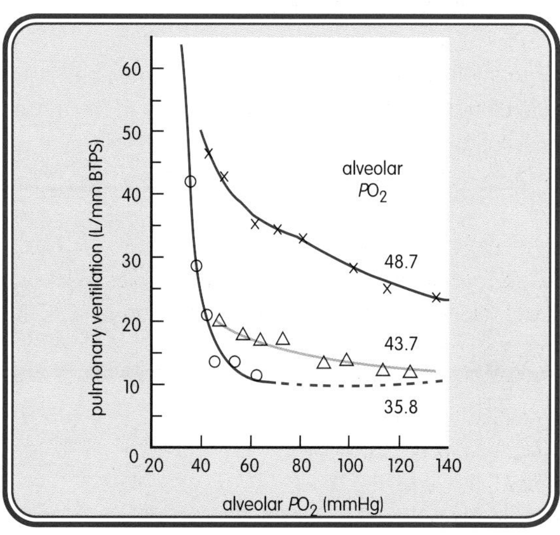

Fig. 5.12 The response of ventilation to P_AO_2 at three values of P_ACO_2. Lowered P_AO_2 has a much greater effect on ventilation when increased values of P_ACO_2 are present.

(e.g. 100% O_2) may abolish any hypoxic drive the patient was previously relying upon, depressing ventilation and worsening the patient's condition.

Response to pH

From earlier in the chapter you should remember that hydrogen ions do not cross the blood–brain barrier and therefore affect only peripheral chemoreceptors. It is difficult to separate the response from increased P_aCO_2 and decreased pH. Any change in pH may be compensated in the long term by the kidneys and therefore has less effect on ventilation than might be expected.

An example of how pH may drive ventilation is seen in the case of metabolic acidosis. The patient will try to achieve a reduction in hydrogen ion concentration by blowing off more carbon dioxide from the lungs. This is achieved by increasing ventilation.

Response to exercise

As human beings, we are capable of a huge increase in ventilation in response to exercise: approximately 15 times the resting level. In moderate exercise, the carbon dioxide output and oxygen uptake are well matched. The increase in respiratory rate and tidal volume do not cause hyperventilation, and the subject is said to be hyperpnoeic:

- P_aCO_2 does not increase, but may fall slightly.
- P_aO_2 does not decrease.
- In moderate exercise, arterial pH varies very little.

So where does the drive for ventilation come from? There have been many possible causes of the increase in ventilation seen during exercise, but none is completely satisfactory:

- Carbon dioxide load within venous blood returning to the lungs affects ventilation.
- Change in pattern of oscillations of P_aCO_2 (Fig. 5.13).
- Central control of P_aCO_2 is reset to a lower value and held constant during exercise.
- Movement of limbs activates joint receptors, which contribute to increase ventilation.
- Increase in body temperature during exercise may also stimulate ventilation.
- The motor cortex stimulates respiratory centres.
- Adrenaline released in exercise also stimulates respiration.

The possible role of oscillations of P_aCO_2

It is suggested that there are cyclical changes of P_aCO_2, with inspiration and expiration. Although mean P_aCO_2 does not change during moderate exercise, the amplitude of these oscillations may increase, providing the stimulus for ventilation.

In heavy exercise, there can be measurable changes in P_aO_2 and P_aCO_2, which stimulate respiration. In addition, the pH falls because anerobic metabolism leads to production of lactic acid (blood lactate levels increase 10-fold). This lactic acid is not oxidized because the oxygen supply cannot keep up with the demands of the exercising muscles (i.e. an 'oxygen debt' is incurred). Rises in potassium ion concentration and temperature may also contribute to the increase in ventilation.

When exercise stops, respiration does not immediately return to basal levels. It remains elevated

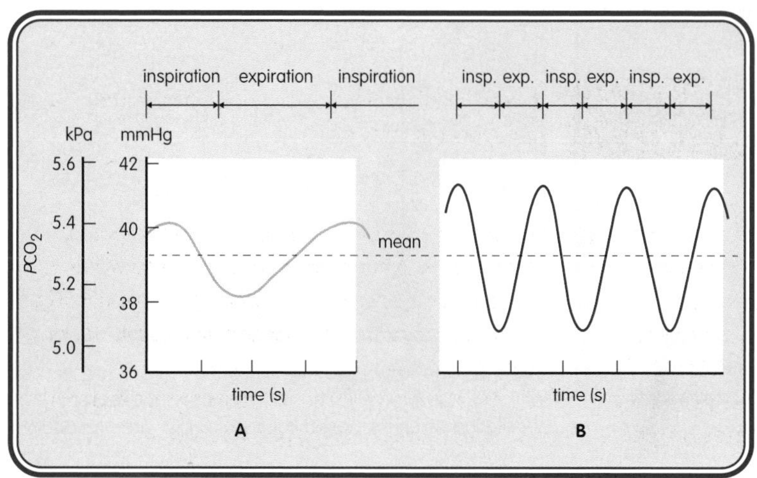

Fig. 5.13 Cyclical changes of P_aCO_2 with inspiration and expiration, (A) at rest, (B) during exercise. Larger oscillations are thought to alter ventilation.

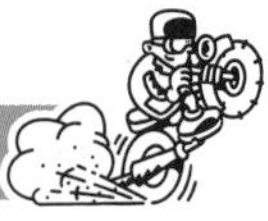

to provide an increased supply of oxygen to the tissues to oxidize the products of anerobic metabolism ('repaying the oxygen debt').

Abnormalities of ventilation control

Cheyne–Stokes respiration

In Cheyne–Stokes respiration, ventilation alternates between progressively deeper breathes and then progressively shallower breathes, in a cyclical manner. Ventilatory control is not achieved and the respiratory system appears to become unstable:

- Arterial carbon dioxide and oxygen tensions vary significantly.
- Tidal volumes wax and wane (Fig. 5.14).
- There are short periods of apnoea separated by periods of hyperventilation.

Cheyne–Stokes breathing is observed at various times:

- At altitude, often when asleep.
- During sleep.
- During periods of hypoxia.
- After voluntary hyperventilation.
- During disease, particularly with combined right and left heart failure and uraemia.
- Secondary to brainstem lesions or compression.

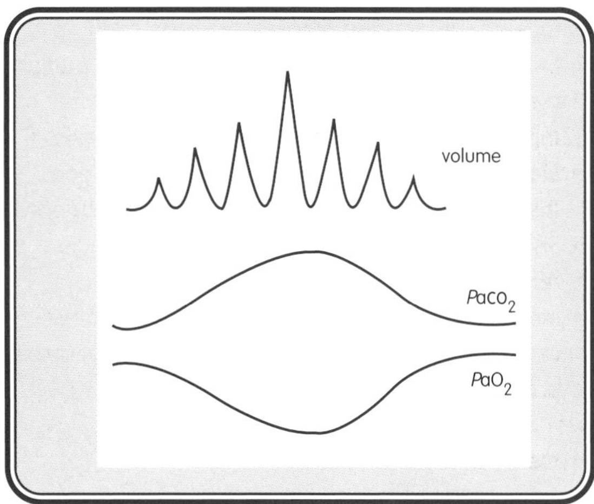

Fig. 5.14 Cheyne–Stokes respiration. (Adapted with permission from *Physiology* 3e, by R.M. Berne and M.N.Levy. Mosby Year Book, 1993.)

- **Describe what is meant by feedback and feed-forward control.**
- **Discuss the central control of breathing with reference to the pontine respiratory group, and the dorsal and ventral respiratory groups of the medulla.**
- **List the different types of receptors involved in control.**
- **What factors stimulate central and peripheral chemoreceptors?**
- **Outline the responses of the respiratory system to changes in carbon dioxide concentration, oxygen concentration, and pH.**
- **Discuss the mechanisms thought to influence the control of ventilation in exercise.**

RESPIRATORY RESPONSE TO EXTREME ENVIRONMENTS

Response to high altitude

At high altitude, the barometric pressure is much lower than at sea level; for example, at the top of Mount Everest (8848 m), the barometric pressure is only 250 mmHg compared with 760 mmHg at sea level. Hence, the partial pressure of oxygen is lower. Dalton's law of partial pressures states that 'The pressure exerted by a mixture of nonreacting gases is equal to the sum of the partial pressures of the separate components.' Thus:

$$P_{atm} = PO_2 + PN_2 + PCO_2 + PH_2O$$

In addition, the partial pressure of water vapour is constant, because inspired air is saturated at body temperature. Therefore, the partial pressure of oxygen in the alveoli (and in the blood) is significantly lower than at sea level.

The carriage of oxygen in the blood is dependent on:

- Partial pressure of oxygen in the blood.

- Haemoglobin concentration.
- The oxyhaemoglobin dissociation curve.

At altitude the partial pressure of oxygen in the blood is lowered. This would tend to limit the amount of oxygen carriage. To combat this problem the body can:

- Hyperventilate in an attempt to decrease the partial pressure of carbon dioxide in the alveoli and therefore increase the partial pressure of oxygen.
- Increase the amount of haemoglobin in the blood, thereby increasing oxygen carriage (oxygen capacity).
- Shift the oxygen dissociation curve.
- Alter the circulation.
- Increase anerobic metabolism in tissues, increase cytochrome oxidase activity, and increase myoglobin in muscle tissue.

Hyperventilation

It can be seen by looking at the alveolar gas equation that if we hyperventilate it is possible to bring the partial pressure of oxygen in the alveolar gas much closer to the partial pressure of inspired gas.

$$P_AO_2 = P_IO_2 - (P_ACO_2/R) + K$$

This is very advantageous at altitude—at 5000 ft, the partial pressure of oxygen is about 130 mmHg. Thus, for saturated air entering the lungs: $P_IO_2 = 130 - 47 = 93$ mmHg

If a subject's P_ACO_2 was 40 mmHg and R = 0.8, then from the alveolar gas equation:

$$P_AO_2 = 93 - (40/0.8) = 43 \text{ mmHg}$$

If the P_ACO_2 were reduced to 10 mmHg, then the P_AO_2 would be 80.5 mmHg.

At higher altitudes, because of the shape of the oxyhaemoglobin dissociation curve, the effect on oxygen carriage in the blood is more dramatic.

Hyperventilation is stimulated by the effect of hypoxia on peripheral chemoreceptors. The effect of this hypoxia is offset by the resultant hypocapnia (low PCO_2), which reduces central chemoreceptor drive. Eventually, the plasma bicarbonate levels fall because there is an increased loss of bicarbonate in the urine and a reduction in the amount of bicarbonate produced by the renal tubular cells and transferred into the blood (renal compensation).

Similar changes occur in the cerebrospinal fluid because of alterations in:

- Production of bicarbonate by the glial cells.
- Movement of bicarbonate across the blood–brain barrier.

The low PCO_2 is now matched by a decrease in bicarbonate concentration, so the pH of the cerebrospinal fluid rises back to normal (see Henderson–Hasselbach equation, Chapter 4). This results in further increase in ventilation as the central chemoreceptor drive returns to normal.

However, the system is now more sensitive to changes in PCO_2.

Polycythaemia

The function of the polycythaemia that is experienced by those living at altitude is not to give a rosy-cheeked complexion, but to increase the haemoglobin concentration and therefore the oxygen-carrying capacity of the blood. The P_aO_2 and oxygen saturation of the haemoglobin is unchanged, but the total amount of oxygen per unit volume of blood is increased towards normal levels.

Hypoxaemia stimulates the kidney to release the hormone erythropoietin, which increases red-cell production. This leads to a higher oxygen capacity, but has the adverse effect of increasing blood viscosity and therefore increasing the tendency for thrombus formation.

Shifting of the oxyhaemoglobin dissociation curve

It would be extremely advantageous if we as humans could significantly shift the oxyhaemoglobin dissociation curve to the left when loading haemoglobin with oxygen, and to the right when unloading oxygen. At altitude, there is a shift to the right, which aids unloading. This is caused by an increase in 2,3-diphosphoglycerate as a result of respiratory alkalosis. Other factors mentioned in Chapter 4 shift the oxygen dissociation curve.

Adverse effects of altitude

Low oxygen tensions in the alveoli cause vasoconstriction of the pulmonary vasculature. This leads to hydrodynamic pulmonary hypertension and increased work for the right heart. Because this alters the Starling forces affecting the pulmonary vessels, pulmonary oedema may occur (reducing gaseous exchange). The permeability of capillaries is increased and a high-protein transudate forms.

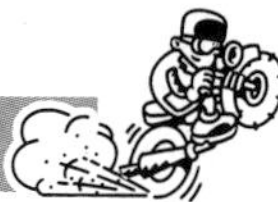

Oxygen intoxication

The use of high-concentration oxygen therapy can have deleterious effects on the respiratory system. This is especially evident after prolonged use.

Oxygen intoxication was first recognized by Paul Bert in 1878. He noticed that breathing oxygen at 1 atm for as little as 12 hours can lead to pulmonary congestion (reducing vital capacity), pulmonary oedema, exudation (reducing gaseous exchange), and damage to the pulmonary epithelium.

In the premature infant, administration of high-concentration oxygen can also cause retrolental fibroplasia. Fibrous tissue forms behind the lens and can lead to permanent blindness. This is thought to be caused by vasoconstriction, secondary to a high partial pressure of oxygen. This can be avoided by keeping a low PO_2.

Respiratory distress can occur because of absorption atelectasis.

Absorption atelectasis

Absorption atelectasis is the collapse of an alveolus due to blockage (Fig. 5.15). When breathing 100% O_2, the oxygen in the alveolus is quickly absorbed because there is a huge partial pressure difference between the alveolar gas (about 760 mmHg) and the partial pressure of gases in the venous blood. This results in collapse of the alveolus. It is then difficult to open the collapsed alveoli because of high surface tension effects.

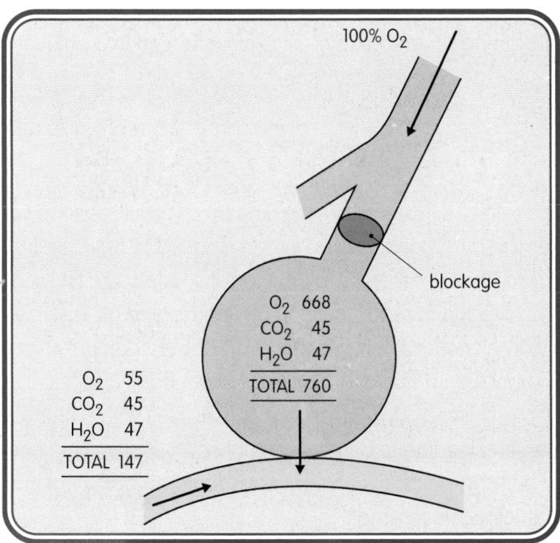

Fig. 5.15 Absorption atelectasis. The sum of the partial pressures (in mmHg) of alveolar gas far exceed those in the mixed venous blood. Oxygen is taken up rapidly by the blood causing collapse of the alveoli. (Adapted from *Respiratory Physiology* 3e by J. West. Williams & Wilkins, 1995.)

Absorption atelectasis also occurs when breathing a normal air mixture. The rate of absorption is much slower as driving force (the partial pressure difference between venous blood and alveolar gas) is much lower. There is still a partial pressure difference driving diffusion because the fall in oxygen tension from arterial to venous blood is greater than the rise in carbon dioxide tension. Nitrogen is poorly absorbed because of its poor solubility; this tends to prevent alveolar collapse.

Space flight

During space flight, the main changes to respiratory physiology are caused by gravitational effects. Blood and air distribution within the lungs is dependent on gravity (Chapter 4). In space flight, these gravitational effects are absent and the distribution is more uniform from apex to lung base. This results in a slight improvement to overall gaseous exchange.

Gravity also has an effect on inhaled particles entering the lung. Larger particles tend to impact on the upper respiratory tract because of their momentum and inability to turn corners. Medium-sized particles tend to sediment out. Sedimentation is a process dependent on gravity. Hence, in space flight, these particles will travel further down the respiratory tract.

Effects on other systems are:

- Cardiovascular system—reduced venous pooling in the legs; postural hypotension on return to earth.
- Muscular system—wasting of musculature; atrophy caused by reduced work performed by muscles.
- Skeletal system—bone demineralization because the skeleton is no longer supporting body weight.

Increased pressure

Increased pressure applies in underwater situations. When diving, pressure increases because of the weight of the column of water above. The pressure rises by 1 atm (760 mmHg) for every 10 m descended. Solids and liquids are incompressible, and any increased pressure has little effect on these. Gases, however, are compressible and gas contained within a cavity or in solution (Henry's law) is affected by pressure changes.

Thus, on descent, the pressure increases and a gas is:

- Compressed.
- Forced into solution.

On ascent gas may:

- Expand (which if enclosed in a cavity or sinus could rupture the surrounding structure).
- Come out of solution.

There are different types of dive. A dive may be:

- Short enough to be accomplished on the air inhaled at the surface—a single-breath dive.
- Carried out at a shallow depth, so that connection with the air can be maintained by a tube—a snorkel dive.
- Long enough and deep enough to demand a continual supply of air. This will be provided at the increased ambient pressure to which the diver is exposed—a conventional dive or SCUBA dive.

Single-breath dive

The diver holds his breath and submerges. The air in the diver's lung is subjected to increased pressure, increasing the PO_2 and PCO_2. Oxygen supply is increased, but so is carbon dioxide, stimulating the chemoreceptors: the diver soon must return to the surface. The dive can be prolonged by hyperventilation before submerging, but this can be dangerous on ascent because, as the ambient pressure falls, so the PO_2 falls to levels at which the diver may become unconscious. Standard advice is that four maximum breaths are allowed.

The ratio of total lung volume to residual volume limits the depth of the dive (6.0/1.5 = 4 atm—i.e. 40 m).

Snorkel dive

The maximum lung pressure that the inspiratory muscles can generate is about 100 mmHg, equivalent to a depth of about 1.2 m. This pressure cannot be maintained for more than a few minutes, thus the length of the snorkel is reduced to approximately 40 cm, reducing the dead space in the tube.

Conventional and SCUBA dives

Conventional dives involve being enclosed within a chamber while breathing compressed gases.

During SCUBA (self-contained underwater breathing apparatus) dives, gas is breathed through a regulated valve system from a pressure tank carried by the diver. The pressure of gas breathed is ambient, eliminating problems of lung mechanics. There are problems with conventional and SCUBA dives at depths over 50 m (5 atm) because of:

- Increased density of the inhaled gas, increasing the work of breathing.
- Nitrogen narcosis.
- Decompression sickness.

Nitrogen narcosis

Nitrogen has high solubility in fat and this solubility increases with increasing pressure. Nitrogen acts like a general anaesthetic, expanding the lipid components of cell membranes, leading to the destruction of membrane proteins, including ion channels that are responsible for neural signalling. It is believed this property leads to narcosis. Symptoms of nitrogen narcosis include:

- Euphoria.
- Mental confusion.
- Impaired neuromuscular coordination (clumsiness).
- Loss of consciousness.

Effects are detectable at 4 atm; serious impairment of performance occurs at 10 atm; full surgical anaesthesia occurs at 30 atm.

Decompression sickness

Under normal atmospheric pressure, the solubility of nitrogen is low and body tissues contain little nitrogen in solution: 9 mL nitrogen dissolved per litre of body water; 50 mL of nitrogen dissolved per litre of body fat. As we descend during a dive, ambient pressure increases, thus increasing the partial pressure of nitrogen. When breathing an air mixture, nitrogen is forced into solution (especially in adipose tissue) because of its high partial pressure (Henry's law).

On ascending, the nitrogen comes out of solution. Because the blood supply of adipose tissue is poor and the rate of diffusion slow, the time taken for nitrogen to be removed from the tissues and transported to the lung is great. Thus, if ascent is rapid, there is inadequate time for the nitrogen to reach the lungs and be blown off. Instead it comes out of solution and forms bubbles (like formation of bubbles on opening a bottle of lemonade). Bubbles obstruct the circulation, especially in tissues with a high fat content, leading to bends and chokes.

Symptoms and signs of bends (bubble formation in the joints etc.) include:

- Pain in the joints.
- Reduced skin temperature and blanched skin.
- Central nervous system effects—disorientation, visual disturbances, convulsions, and loss of conciousness, obstruction to blood flow and stroke.

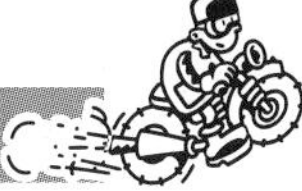

Symptoms and signs of chokes (bubble formation in the pulmonary blood vessels) include:

- Dyspnoea.
- Coughing.
- Substernal distress.
- Rapid shallow breathing (up to 100 breaths per minute)—little gas exchange.
- Bradycardia.
- Mental confusion.

Decompression sickness can be treated by returning the diver to a high-pressure chamber (a decompression chamber) which recompresses the bubbles and forces them back into solution. The pressure is then gradually increased in steps, allowing the nitrogen to come out of solution slowly. To prevent bends and chokes, divers can:

- Limit the depth of dives to about 40 m.
- Have scheduled decompression stops, giving time for nitrogen to come out of solution slowly, and preventing the formation of harmful large bubbles.
- Another way to prevent decompression sickness is to use an inert carrier gas with oxygen (e.g. Heliox) that is less soluble than nitrogen. The solubility of helium is about one-half that of nitrogen and less gas is forced into solution. In addition, the diffusivity of helium is much greater, allowing faster transport to the lungs and hence elimination.

Fatty tissues tend to have a lower blood flow than tissues with a high water content: 0.6 L/min and 5.2 L/min, respectively. Longer dives lead to increased build-up of nitrogen; thus, increased decompression limits effective working time underwater. Eventually, saturation of all body tissues with dissolved nitrogen occurs; decompression time will then be constant.

Saturation divers in the North Sea may spend 28 days underwater: 14 days diving or in high-pressure compression chambers and 14 days in decompression.

Oxygen toxicity

If the partial pressure of inhaled oxygen exceeds atmospheric pressure (usually, at pressures >2 atm), toxic effects on the central nervous system are observed:

- Convulsions (associated with reduction of GABA, an inhibitory transmitter in the brain).
- Nausea.

Predisposing factors to central nervous toxicity are:

- Partial pressure of oxygen.
- Duration of breathing high-partial-pressure oxygen.

For this reason, oxygen concentration in a diver's tanks is reduced for deeper dives.

Liquid breathing

Not something to be tried at home! If the concentration of dissolved oxygen in a carrier liquid (such as saline) is high enough, animals breathing this mixture can survive for some time. The high concentration of oxygen is achieved by saturating the saline with very high pressure 100% O_2. There are two problems with breathing liquids:

- The work of breathing is vastly increased.
- The rate of diffusion of gases in liquids is much slower than in gases. This leads to retention of carbon dioxide and acidosis.

- **Discuss the changes that occur in response to high altitude.**
- **Describe absorption atelectasis.**
- **Give two effects of space flight on respiratory systems.**
- **Describe decompression sickness and nitrogen narcosis.**
- **Outline the changes that occur in long-term oxygen therapy.**

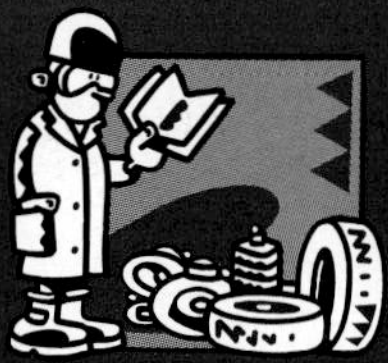

6. Pharmacology of the Respiratory System

DRUGS AND THE RESPIRATORY SYSTEM

Overview

Many drugs are used to treat diseases of the respiratory system.

These can be classified into the following types:

- Drugs used in asthma—bronchodilators, cromoglycate, and corticosteroids.
- Respiratory stimulants.
- Drugs used in allergies and anaphylaxis.
- Oxygen (see Chapter 5).
- Mucolytics.
- Cough preparations.

In addition, a number of drugs have side effects upon the respiratory system. This chapter deals with those drugs not dealt with in Chapter 11 as well as drugs that have the side effects of respiratory depression.

Drugs used in the treatment of asthma

Drugs used in the treatment of asthma can be split into three main categories:

- Bronchodilators.
- Preventors of mast-cell degranulation.
- Anti-inflammatory drugs.

The latter two categories can be used for prophylaxis, and if used correctly reduce the risk of having an attack.

Bronchodilators

Bronchodilators can be split into three groups:

- β_2 agonists.
- Xanthines.
- Antimuscarinics.

β_2 agonists

Bronchial smooth muscle contains numerous β_2 receptors, which act through an adenylate cyclase/cAMP second-messenger system to cause smooth muscle relaxation and hence bronchodilation (Fig. 6.1).

Examples of β_2 agonists are:

- Salbutamol.
- Terbutaline.
- Salmeterol.

These drugs are usually inhaled, either as an aerosol, a powder, or as a nebulized solution. They can also be given intravenously, intramuscularly, and subcutaneously. Salbutamol and terbutaline are used for acute symptoms and act within minutes, producing effects lasting 3–5 hours. Salmeterol has a slower onset than salbutamol and terbutaline, but its effects last much longer. For this reason, it is not used for acute attacks. In addition, salmeterol can also cause bronchoconstriction acutely.

The β_2 agonists are not completely specific and have some β_1 agonistic effects, especially in high doses.

Side effects of β_2 agonists include:

- Tachycardia.
- Fine tremor.
- Nervous tension.
- Headache.

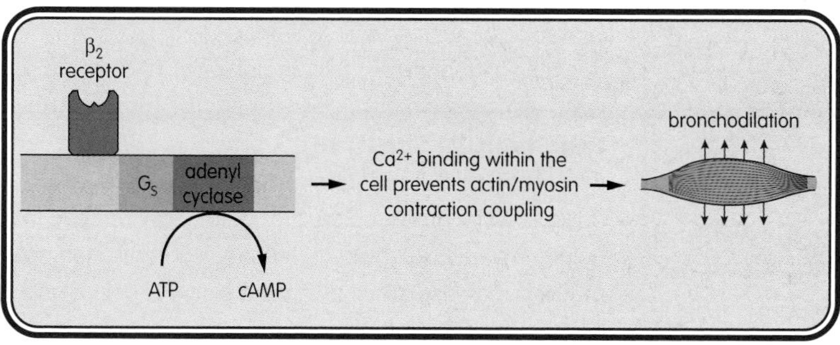

Fig. 6.1 Mechanisms of action of β_2 agonists—relaxation of bronchial muscle (which leads to bronchodilation) and inhibition of mast-cell degranulation (β receptors on mast cell).

At the doses given by aerosol, these side effects seldom occur. Tolerance may occur with high repeated doses.

Xanthines

Xanthines work by preventing the breakdown of cAMP (Fig. 6.2). The amount of cAMP within the bronchial smooth muscle cells is therefore increased, which causes bronchodilation in a similar way to β_2 agonists.

These drugs are metabolized in the liver and there is a considerable variation in half life between individuals. This has important implications because there is a small therapeutic window.

Theophylline can be given intravenously in the form of aminophylline (theophylline with ethylenediamine), but must be administered very slowly (over 20 minutes to administer dose). Aminophylline is given in cases of severe asthma attacks that do not respond to β_2 agonists and in acute asthma.

Antimuscarinics

Antimuscarinics block the vagal control of bronchial smooth muscle tone in response to irritants and therefore reduce the reflex bronchoconstriction. An example of a antimuscarinic is ipratropium bromide; it has two mechanisms of action:

- Reduction of reflex bronchoconstriction (e.g. from dust or pollen).
- Reduce mucous secretions.

These drugs have a slow onset (30–60 mins) and are poorly absorbed orally; they must, therefore, be given by aerosol. They are used for chronic bronchitis that does not respond to β_2 agonists.

Side effects are rare, but include:

- Dry mouth.
- Urinary retention.
- Constipation.

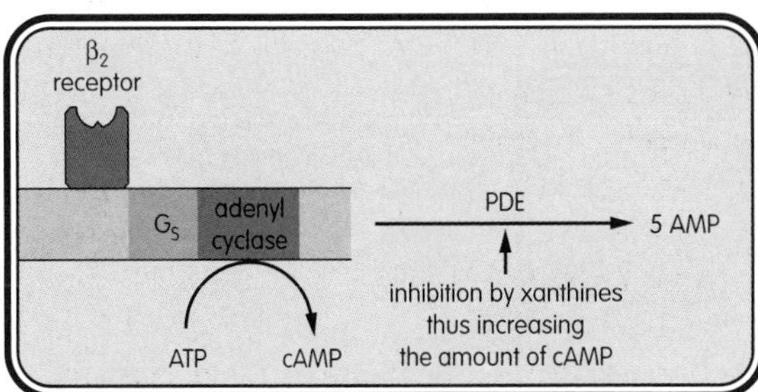

Fig. 6.2 Xanthines. The inhibition of phosphodiesterase (PDE) leads to an increase in cellular cyclic AMP which is believed to lead to bronchodilation as in Fig. 6.1

Preventors of mast-cell degranulation

The main drug in this class is sodium cromoglygate. It acts to stabilize mast cells and has no bronchodilator effect. It cannot be used to treat an acute attack, but is given for prophylaxis, especially in patients with atopy. The route of administration is by inhalation.

Its mechanism of action is to:

- Prevent mast-cell degranulation and hence mediator release.
- Reduce C fibre response to irritants therefore reducing bronchoconstriction.
- Inhibit platelet-activating factor (PAF) induced bronchoconstriction.

Sodium cromoglygate is effective in antigen-induced, exercise-induced asthma and continued use results in reduced bronchial hyperactivity. Best results are seen in children.

Anti-inflammatory drugs

Anti-inflammatory drugs act by reducing inflammation of the bronchial mucosa (Fig. 6.3). They inhibit phospholipase A_2 and thus block the production of inflammatory mediators.

Glucocorticoids can be given either by inhalation as prophylaxis or orally as a second-line drug. β_2 agonists have not been effective (oral prednisolone).

Drugs given by inhalation are:

- Beclomethasone.
- Betamethasone.
- Budesonide.

Prednisolone is an orally active steroid, which has value in acute asthma. It should be given for only a short period because long-term administration of oral steroids is associated with severe side effects (e.g. salt and water retention, osteoporosis, thinning of the skin, etc.).

Respiratory stimulants

Respiratory stimulants (analeptics) can be used for patients with chronic obstructive pulmonary disease in respiratory failure; however, mechanical ventilation has reduced their use. Most drugs are centrally acting and all must be given intravenously. These drugs are used specifically for ventilatory failure (type II) in acute

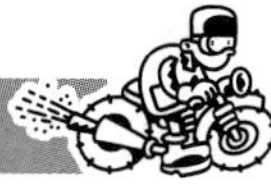

exacerbations of chronic bronchitis.

Examples of drugs used are:

- Doxapram: stimulates carotid chemoreceptors and the respiratory centre.
- Aminophylline.

Side effects of these drugs are:

- Tachycardia (doxapram and aminophylline).
- Palpitations (doxapram and aminophylline).
- Nausea (doxapram and aminophylline).
- Sweating (doxapram).
- Tremor (doxapram).
- Gastrointestinal upset (aminophylline).

Contraindications of doxapram are:

- Epilepsy.
- Hypertension.
- Hyperthyroidism.

Caffeine is a respiratory stimulant that may be used in premature infants.

Drugs used for allergies and anaphylaxis

H_1 Histamine antagonists

These drugs are used in the treatment of allergies, such as hayfever. Examples of these drugs are:

- Promethazine.
- Trimeprazine.

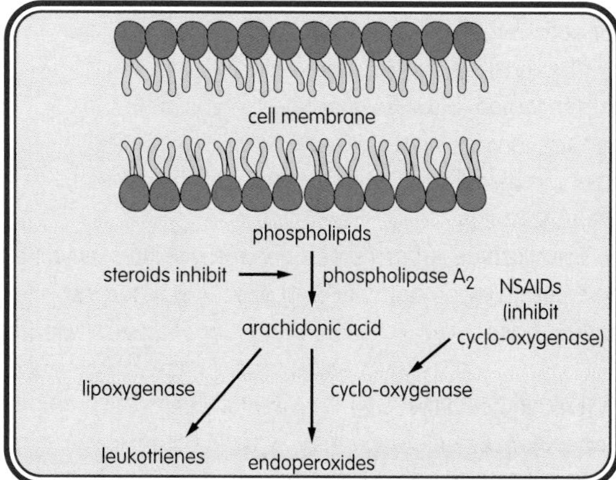

Fig. 6.3 Mechanism of action of the anti-inflammatory drugs. Steroid inhalers inhibit the action of phospholipase A_2 and therefore block the production of inflammatory mediators. Non-steroidal anti-inflammatory drugs (NSAIDs) inhibit cyclooxygenase and, it is believed, shunt the pathway to produce excess leukotrienes. It is for this reason that NSAIDs are believed to precipitate asthma.

The mechanism of action is to block H_1 receptors. These drugs cross the blood–brain barrier and have a general depressant action (sedative); in high doses, this action can cause respiratory depression.

Newer drugs such as terfenadine do not readily cross the blood–brain barrier and therefore do not cause respiratory depression.

Anaphylaxis

Anaphylactic shock is a systemic allergic reaction which is a life threatening condition. The features of anaphylactic shock are:

- Severe hypotension.
- Laryngeal spasm.
- Bronchoconstriction.

The treatment of anaphylaxis must therefore be rapid:

- Secure the airway.
- Maintain blood pressure by lying the patient flat and raising his or her legs.

Drug therapy is as follows:

- Intramuscular adrenaline (0.5–1.0 mg, 0.5–1.0 mL of adrenaline injection 1:1000), repeated at 10-minute intervals depending on the blood pressure.
- 100% oxygen.
- Chlorpheniramine (antihistamine) 10–20 mg intravenously, continued for 24–48 hours.
- Salbutamol can be given intravenously for those patients not responsive to adrenaline.
- Hydrocortisone 200–300 mg intravenously may be given as a second-line drug to reduce further deterioration.

Mucolytics

Mucolytics (e.g. carbocisteine and methyl cysteine hydrochloride) are designed to reduce the viscosity of sputum, thereby aiding expectoration. The indications for use have been in:

- Chronic bronchitis.
- Chronic asthma.
- Cystic fibrosis.
- Bronchiectasis.

There is little evidence that these drugs are effective.

Cough preparations

The cough reflex is a protective mechanism to eliminate

particulate matter and mucus from the respiratory tree. Inhibition of this reflex may have a deleterious effect, causing build up of secretions and the risk of infection, especially in patients with chronic bronchitis and bronchiectasis. They may have some use in a dry cough or a nonproductive cough found in bronchial carcinoma.

Typical drugs used are weak opioids, which suppress the cough reflex. Examples are:

- Codeine phosphate.
- Dextromethorphan.

Codeine phosphate inhibits the cough reflex centrally. A side effect is the inhibition of ciliary activity, which reduces the clearance of secretions. It also causes constipation.

Dextromethorphan is a synthetic, non-narcotic, nonanalgesic, and nonaddictive opioid. It has a similar efficacy to codeine but does not have the side effects. It should be noted that both drugs in large doses cause respiratory depression.

Drugs that have adverse effects on the respiratory system

If a drug has a depressant action on the central nervous system, large enough doses of it will cause respiratory depression. The most notable of the drugs which cause respiratory depression are the opioid analgesics.

Other drugs that may also cause respiratory depression are listed below:

- Barbiturates.
- Benzodiazepines.
- H_1 histamine antagonists.
- Alcohol.

Opioids and barbiturates depress central chemoreceptor activity and this contributes to the respiratory depression they cause.

Opioid analgesics

These drugs are in very common use in clinical medicine, and include:

- Morphine.
- Diamorphine (heroin).
- Pethidine.

In high doses, these drugs cause respiratory and cardiovascular depression, which can be lethal. These drugs bind to opioid receptors in the spinal cord, pons, and midbrain, and mimic the action of endogenous opioid.

Overdose is usually iatrogenic in origin or from illicit drug abuse (heroin). The effects of overdose can be reversed by administration of an opioid-receptor antagonist (e.g. naloxone).

Overdose may occur in the newborn if the mother has been given opioids during a caesarean section because the drug crosses the placenta. This can cause respiratory depression in the neonate. The infant is injected with naloxone and resuscitation commenced immediately.

Signs of overdose are varied state of consciousness, respiratory depression, and pin-point pupils.

Other main side effects of opioids are:

- Nausea and vomiting.
- Constipation.
- Difficulty in micturition.
- Drowsiness.

Contraindications to opioid analgesics are respiratory depression and acute alcoholism.

Barbiturates

All barbiturates have a depressant activity on the central nervous system. They are used as induction agents for general anaesthesia (thiopentone), for treatment of grand mal epilepsy (phenobarbitone), and for sedation.

The mechanism of action of barbiturates is enhancement of GABA-mediated inhibition of the central nervous system. These drugs prolong the opening of individual chloride channels by a given GABA stimulus.

Barbiturates cause respiratory and cardiovascular depression when administered at 10–100 times the clinical dose.

Benzodiazepines

Benzodiazepines are extensively used as anxiolytics, hypnotics, and for sedation. Their use has become unfashionable because of tolerance and withdrawal effects, which develop after about 2–4 weeks of use.

Their mechanism of action is the same as that of the barbiturates, although benzodiazepines bind to a different site on the $GABA_A$ receptor complex.

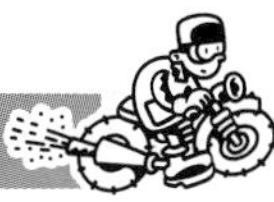

Normally, even high orally administered doses of benzodiazepines do not cause severe respiratory depression. However, intravenous administration or oral administration either to elderly patients or to patients with underlying pulmonary disease can cause respiratory depression.

- **Outline the treatment of a patient with an acute asthma attack.**
- **Explain the mechanism of action of the β_2 agonists.**
- **Outline the prophylaxis of asthma.**
- **List the classes of drugs used to treat diseases of the respiratory system.**
- **Give examples of two respiratory stimulants.**
- **List the treatment measures for management of anaphylaxis**
- **Describe the drugs that have an adverse effect on the respiratory system.**

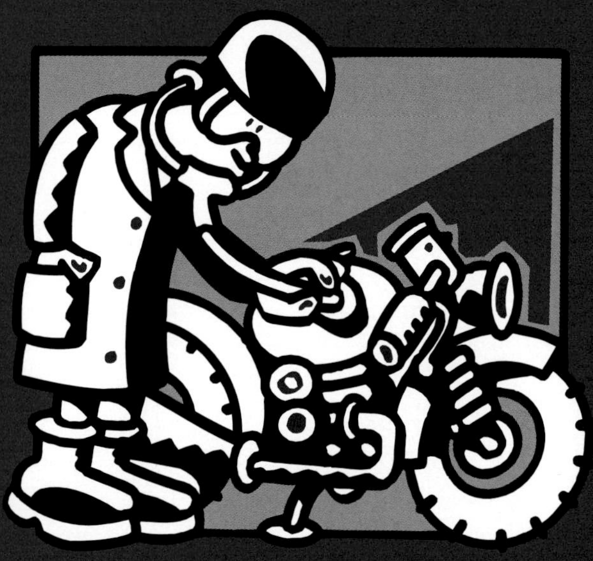

CLINICAL ASSESSMENT

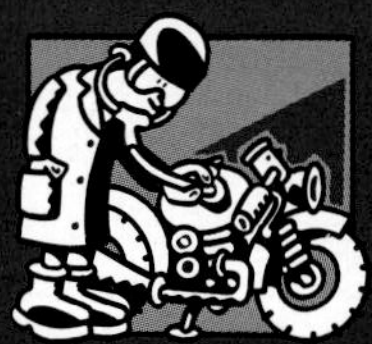

7. Taking a History

THE HISTORY

Things to remember when taking a history

A good history should tell you the diagnosis (Fig. 7.1). Take a few minutes before you begin to introduce yourself and to put the patient at ease.

Simple observation at the bedside can often give a good clue to the likely diagnosis:

- Inhalers and oxygen bottles.
- Sputum pots.
- Walking sticks or frames.

How does the patient appear during the interview? Agitated, distressed, or dyspnoeic? Is there a visible tremor? Simple observations now will save time later.

Structure of the history

Presenting complaint

The presenting complaint is the collection of symptoms felt by the patient. Use the patient's own words—this is not a diagnosis. For example, for shortness of breath the patient might use 'out of puff' or 'can't get any air in'.

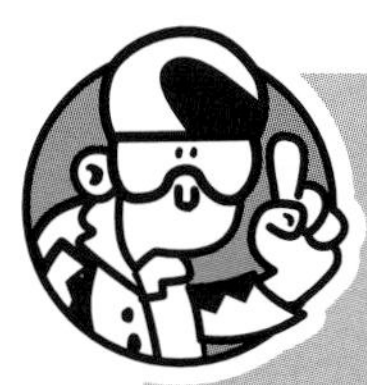

Allow yourself 25 minutes to take the history: 20 minutes to examine the patient and 5 minutes to plan the management of the case.

Systems review		
Body system	**Symptom**	**Relevance**
cardiovascular system	swollen legs or ankles	peripheral oedema caused by cor pulmonale
peripheral venous system	pain in calf	deep vein thrombosis; risk of pulmonary embolus
gastrointestinal tract	right upper quadrant pain	right lower lobe pneumonia
	difficulty in swallowing	laryngeal mass
locomotor system	arthralgia with wrist and ankle swelling	hypertrophic pulmonary osteoarthropathy
	shoulder pain	pathology involving diaphragm
skin	butterfly-shaped rash	systemic lupus erythematosus
	erythema nodosum; skin nodules	sarcoidosis
general	weight loss	chronic illness
	weight gain	can cause dyspnoea

Fig. 7.1 Systems review.

History of presenting complaint

It is vital that time is taken to find the history of the presenting complaint (HPC). Ascertain the nature of the complaint as follows:

- Onset: acute or gradual.
- Pattern: intermittent or continuous.
- Frequency: daily, weekly, or monthly.
- Duration: minutes or hours.
- Progression: better or worse than in the past.
- Severity: mild, moderate, or severe.
- Character: e.g. is the pain sharp, dull, or aching?
- Precipitating and relieving factors: e.g. are any medications used?
- Associated symptoms: e.g. cough, wheeze, haemoptysis, dyspnoea, chest pain, or orthopnoea.

Has the patient had the problem before? If so, what was the diagnosis, treatment, and outcome.

Ask the patient how disabling the problem is and how it affects daily life.

Past medical history

Find out any past medical history (PMH) that might contribute to the presenting complaint; for example:

- Chronic infection.
- Anaemia.
- Vitamin deficiencies.

Present the PMH in chronological order, listing any surgical operations that the patient may have had and the primary diagnosis. Note any foreign travel, especially recently. Has the patient received BCG immunization or experienced tuberculosis contact in the past? Is there a history of natural measles or pertussis? Has he or she ever had a chest radiograph: it may be useful for comparison.

Drug history

When taking the drug history (DH), list the patient's current intake of both prescribed and over-the-counter (OTC) drugs, recording dosage, frequency, and duration of treatment. Ask the patient what each tablet is for and when it is taken; this gives an indication of the patient's understanding of his or her problems and compliance.

Allergies

If the patient mentions an allergy, ask what exactly happened, and how long ago it happened.

Family history

When noting a family history (FH), it may be easier to draw a pedigree chart. Do any members of the family suffer from a respiratory disorder? Ask about atopy, asthma, eczema, and hayfever. Does anybody in the family smoke?

Social history

Social history (SH) is hugely important in the respiratory system. The patient's marital status and number of children should be recorded.

Home and social situation

Ask about accommodation:

- Type: house, flat (which floor), or bedsit.
- Heating: coal fire, gas fire, or central heating.
- Conditions: damp or dry.
- Number of people living in the accommodation.
- Area of town: gives an indication of socioeconomic class.
- Pets: dogs, cats, or birds.

Ask about the patient's financial situation: is he or she entitled to any state benefits (e.g. social support)? Enquire about diet and exercise.

Smoking and alcohol

Smoking? If yes, cigarettes, cigars, or pipe and for how long? Record the number or amount smoked daily. Has he or she ever stopped; if so, for how long?

Alcohol? If yes, convert the weekly intake into units if possible. One glass of wine or one-half pint of beer is equivalent to 1 unit.

Occupation

Present the patient's jobs in chronological order starting from the time the patient left school. Some respiratory conditions have a long latent period between time of exposure and presentation.

Enquire about occupational related disorders (e.g. asbestos exposure and mesothelioma). The length of each job and the job description need to be recorded.

Summarize the relevant points of the history to add clarity to the history and to ease presentation.

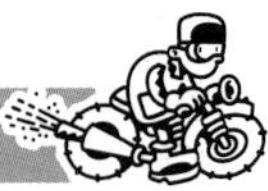

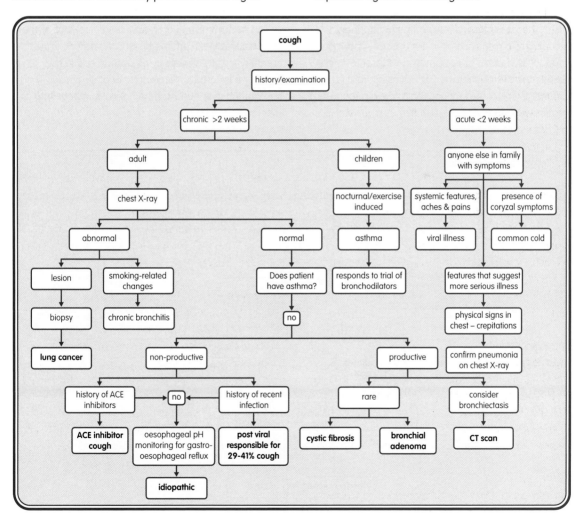

- **Describe how to take a respiratory history.**
- **Why is it important to take a detailed social history (in particular, an occupational history) of the patient?**

COMMON PRESENTING COMPLAINTS

The major problem with respiratory disorders is that the clinical findings often overlap considerably, thereby making a firm diagnosis difficult.

When a patient is seen, the whole clinical situation needs to be addressed before a diagnosis can be made. It is important to remember that extreme lung disease does not necessarily produce clinical signs.

Cough

A cough is the commonest manifestation of lower respiratory tract disease (Fig. 7.2). The cough reflex is a complex centrally mediated defence reflex, resulting from the appropriate chemical or mechanical stimulation of the larynx and the more proximal portion of the tracheobronchial tree. The basic pattern of a cough can be divided into four components:

- Rapid deep inspiration.
- Expiration against a closed glottis.

- **cough**
  - history/examination
    - chronic >2 weeks
      - adult
        - chest X-ray
          - abnormal
            - lesion → biopsy → **lung cancer**
            - smoking-related changes → chronic bronchitis
          - normal
            - Does patient have asthma? → no
              - non-productive
                - history of ACE inhibitors → **ACE inhibitor cough**
                - history of recent infection → **post viral responsible for 29-41% cough**
                - no (to both) → oesophageal pH monitoring for gastro-oesophageal reflux → **idiopathic**
              - productive
                - rare → **cystic fibrosis**; **bronchial adenoma**
                - consider bronchiectasis → **CT scan**
      - children → nocturnal/exercise induced → asthma → responds to trial of bronchodilators
    - acute <2 weeks
      - anyone else in family with symptoms
        - systemic features, aches & pains → viral illness
        - presence of coryzal symptoms → common cold
        - features that suggest more serious illness → physical signs in chest – crepitations → confirm pneumonia on chest X-ray

Fig. 7.2 Diagnostic algorithm of cough.

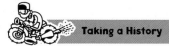

- Sudden glottal opening.
- Relaxation of expiratory muscles.

A cough may be a voluntary or involuntary response.

With the complaint of cough, it is important that the timing of the cough (morning or evening), its chronicity, and nature (i.e. productive or unproductive) are elicited.

Although severe coughing attacks rarely cause death, they may cause considerable distress for the patient.

The commonest cause of a chronic cough is cigarette smoking.

Wheeze

Wheezing is a common complaint, complicating many different disease processes (Fig. 7.3). It occurs in 20–30% of adults.

A wheeze is an audible expiratory noise with a definite pitch. Wheezes are classified as either monophonic, occurring as a result of bronchial stenosis, or polyphonic. Poylphonic wheezes are common in widespread airflow obstruction; it is the characteristic wheeze heard in asthmatics. A localized monophonic wheeze suggests a large airway obstruction (e.g. caused by a tumour).

The symptom of wheezing is not diagnostic of asthma, although asthma and chronic obstructive pulmonary disease are the commonest causes and they can be difficult to distinguish. However, the presence of wheeze is a poor indicator of disease severity.

An audible inspiratory noise is termed stridor and indicates narrowing of the larger airways, such as the larynx, trachea, and bronchus. It is very important that you differentiate between a wheeze and stridor because they imply disease in separate parts of the airway.

Breathlessness

Breathlessness is a very common reason for referral to a respiratory clinic (Figs 7.4–7.6).

Breathlessness (dyspnoea) is a subjective difficulty or distress in breathing. The patient may describe the symptom in a variety of ways. Common terms used are 'puffed', 'can't get enough air', and 'feeling suffocated'.

The symptom should be assessed in relation to the patient's lifestyle. From the history, the nature of the breathlessness can usually be ascertained (e.g. whether it is cardiac, respiratory, or other cause). The onset of the dyspnoea can be helpful in diagnosing a likely cause.

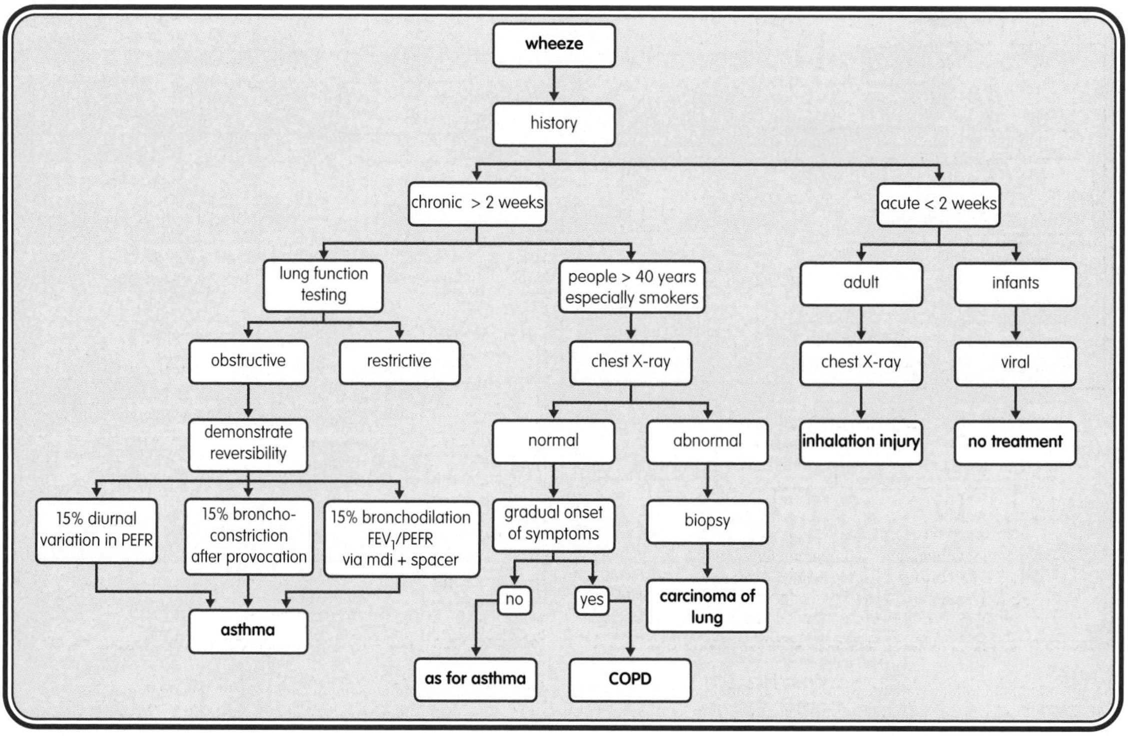

- **wheeze**
  - history
    - chronic > 2 weeks
      - lung function testing
        - obstructive
          - demonstrate reversibility
            - 15% diurnal variation in PEFR → **asthma**
            - 15% broncho-constriction after provocation → **asthma**
            - 15% bronchodilation FEV_1/PEFR via mdi + spacer → **asthma**
        - restrictive
      - people > 40 years especially smokers
        - chest X-ray
          - normal
            - gradual onset of symptoms
              - no → **as for asthma**
              - yes → **COPD**
          - abnormal
            - biopsy
              - **carcinoma of lung**
    - acute < 2 weeks
      - adult
        - chest X-ray
          - **inhalation injury**
      - infants
        - viral
          - **no treatment**

Fig. 7.3 Diagnostic algorithm of wheeze.

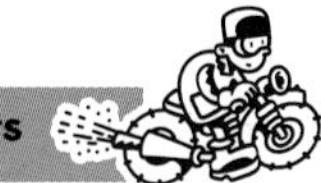

Conditions associated with dyspnoea, grouped according to onset		
Sudden onset	**Onset occurring over hours**	**Onset occurring over weeks**
Pulmonary embolism	Pneumonia	Chronic obstructive pulmonary disease (COPD)
Spontaneous pneumothorax	Exacerbation of asthma	Pleural effusion
Acute pulmonary oedema	Pulmonary oedema	Bronchial carcinoma
Inhalation of foreign body		Pulmonary fibrosis
Acute asthma		Anaemia

Fig. 7.4 Onset of dyspnoea.

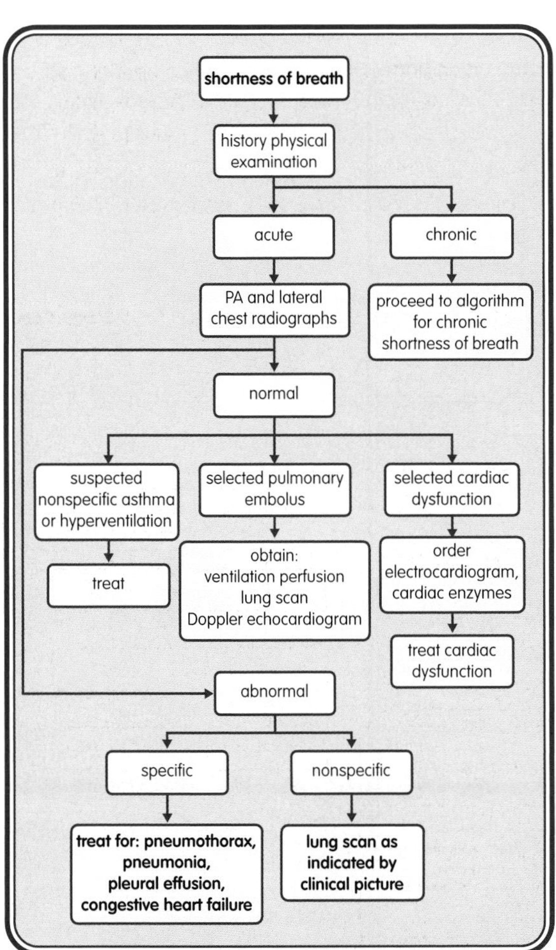

Fig. 7.5 Diagnostic algorithm of breathlessness. (Adapted with permission from *Clinical Medicine* 2e by H.L. Greene et al. Mosby Year Book 1996.)

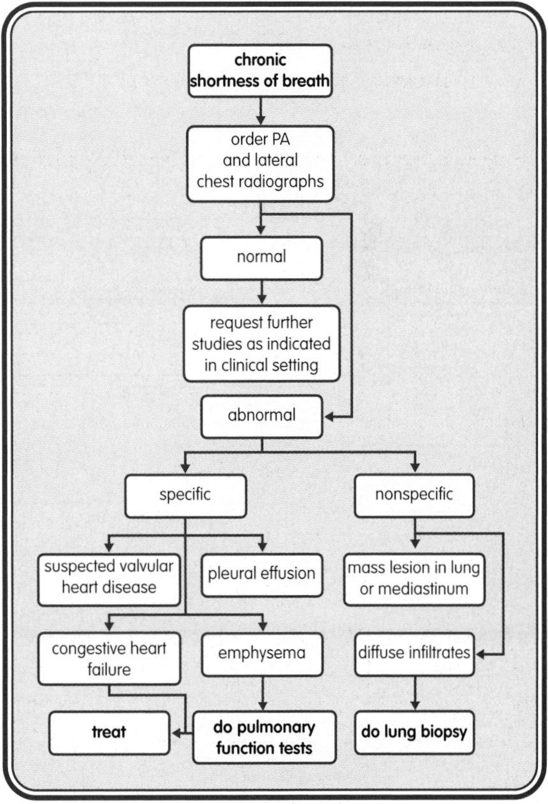

Fig. 7.6 Diagnostic algorithm of chronic breathlessness.(Adapted with permission from *Clinical Medicine* 2e by H.L. Greene et al. Mosby Year Book 1996.)

Haemoptysis

Haemoptysis is blood-stained sputum; this needs to be differentiated from other sources of bleeding within the oral cavity and haematemesis. This distinction is usually obvious from the history. Do not necessarily take the patient's word that they he or she has blood-stained sputum. Haemoptysis is not usually a solitary event and so the sputum sample should be inspected.

Haemoptysis is a serious and often alarming symptom that requires immediate investigation (Fig. 7.7). A chest radiograph is mandatory in a patient with haemoptysis, and the symptom should be treated as bronchogenic carcinoma until proved otherwise.

The common causes of haemoptysis are disease processes involving the respiratory mucosa (e.g. bronchitis, bronchiectasis, and bronchogenic carcinoma).

Sputum production

Everybody produces airway secretions. In a healthy nonsmoker, approximately 100–150 mL of mucus is produced every day. This mucus is transported up the airway's ciliary mucus escalator and swallowed by the patient. This process is not perceived by the patient. Only when there is excess mucus is it expectorated as sputum. Sputum is a nonspecific sign of disease (Fig. 7.8).

Sputum is normally clear and mucoid. Increased sputum volume may result from irritation of the respiratory tract (commonly caused by cigarette smoking or the common cold). Most bronchogenic carcinomas do not produce sputum. The exception is alveolar cell carcinoma, which produces copious amounts of mucoid sputum.

It is essential that the sputum is always inspected, and the volume, colour, consistency, and odour of the

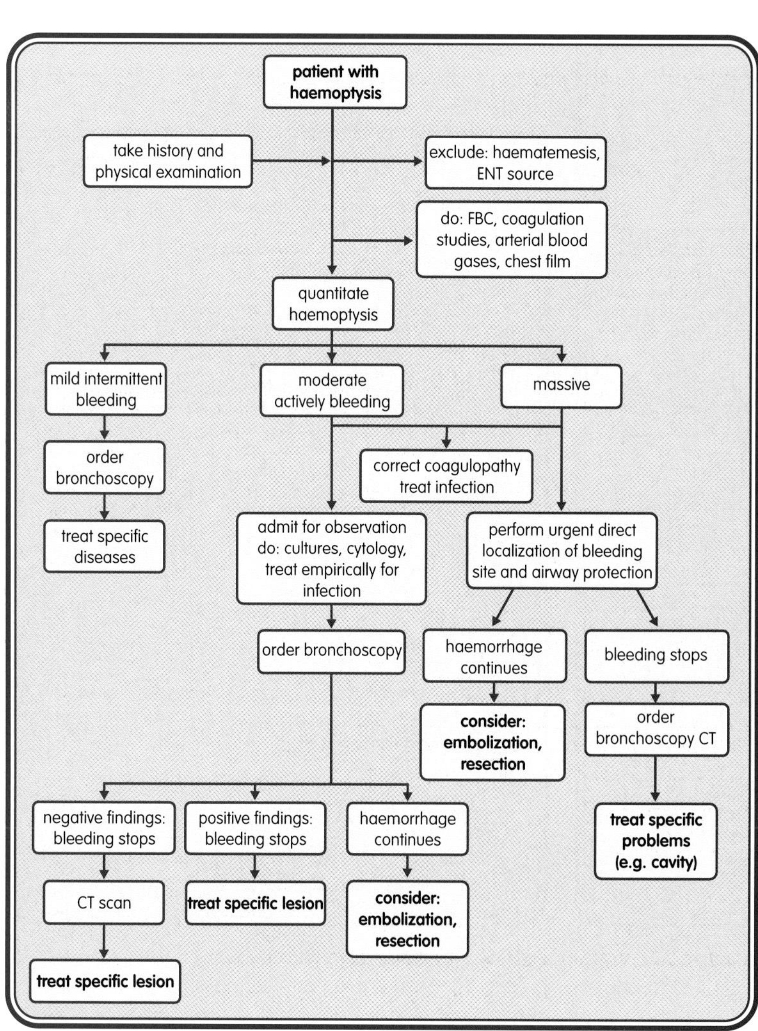

Fig. 7.7 Diagnostic algorithm of haemoptysis. (Adapted with permission from *Decision making in Medicine* by H.L. Greene, W.P. Johnson and M.J. Maricic. Mosby Year Book, 1993.)

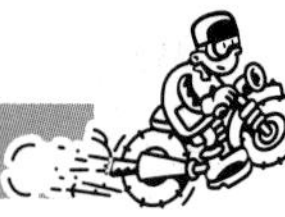

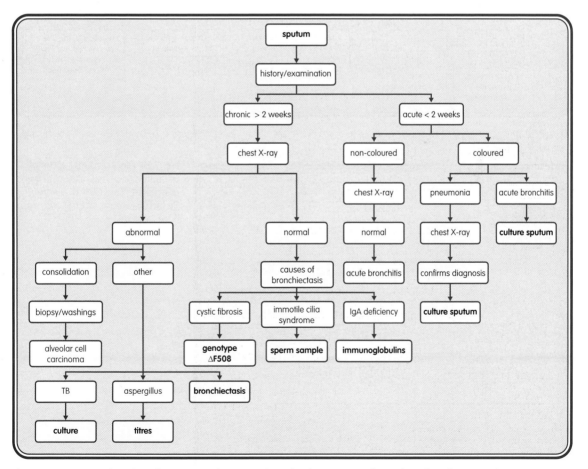

sputum noted. Yellow–green sputum implies infection and is caused by the presence of cellular material including bronchial epithelial cells and eosinophil or neutrophil granulocytes. A large production of yellow–green sputum is characteristic of bronchiectasis; anaerobic infection produces foul-smelling sputum.

Clubbing

Clubbing is a physical finding on examination which is characterized by painless, bulbous enlargement of the distal digit of the fingers, accompanied by softening of the nail-bed and loss of the nail-bed angle. The toes may also be affected. Clubbing takes time to develop and its presence can alert the doctor to the possibility of serious underlying pathology (Fig. 7.9). The early signs of clubbing are best seen in the thumb and index finger. Clubbing is usually symmetrical.

The causes of clubbing are:

- Pulmonary origin: 75%
- Cardiac origin: 10%
- Hepatic/gastrointestinal origin: 10%
- Miscellaneous: 5%

Before every clinical examination, the student should be able to list the common causes of clubbing relevant to the different systems.

Cyanosis

Cyanosis is indicated by a blue discoloration of the mucous membrane or the skin, typically at the peripheries.

Cyanosis develops when the level of deoxygenated haemoglobin rises above 5 g/dL. Bright sunlight is the best light source in which to examine the patient for signs of cyanosis.

Cyanosis can be difficult to determine in dark-skinned people.

- **sputum**
  - history/examination
    - chronic > 2 weeks
      - chest X-ray
        - abnormal
          - consolidation
            - biopsy/washings
              - alveolar cell carcinoma
          - other
          - → TB → **culture**
          - → aspergillus → **titres**
          - → **bronchiectasis**
        - normal
          - causes of bronchiectasis
            - cystic fibrosis → **genotype ΔF508**
            - immotile cilia syndrome → **sperm sample**
            - IgA deficiency → **immunoglobulins**
    - acute < 2 weeks
      - non-coloured
        - chest X-ray
          - normal
            - acute bronchitis
      - coloured
        - pneumonia
          - chest X-ray
            - confirms diagnosis
              - **culture sputum**
        - acute bronchitis
          - **culture sputum**

Fig. 7.8 Diagnostic algorithm of sputum production. (Adapted with permission from *Clinical Medicine* 2e by H.L. Greene et al. Mosby Year Book 1996.)

Peripheral cyanosis

Peripheral cyanosis is typically seen in fingernails and fingers. It results from vasoconstriction and stasis of blood in the extremities (Fig. 7.10).

The cause of peripheral cyanosis is poor blood flow through the capillaries; therefore, the skin temperature is cool. In central cyanosis, the skin temperature tends to be warm.

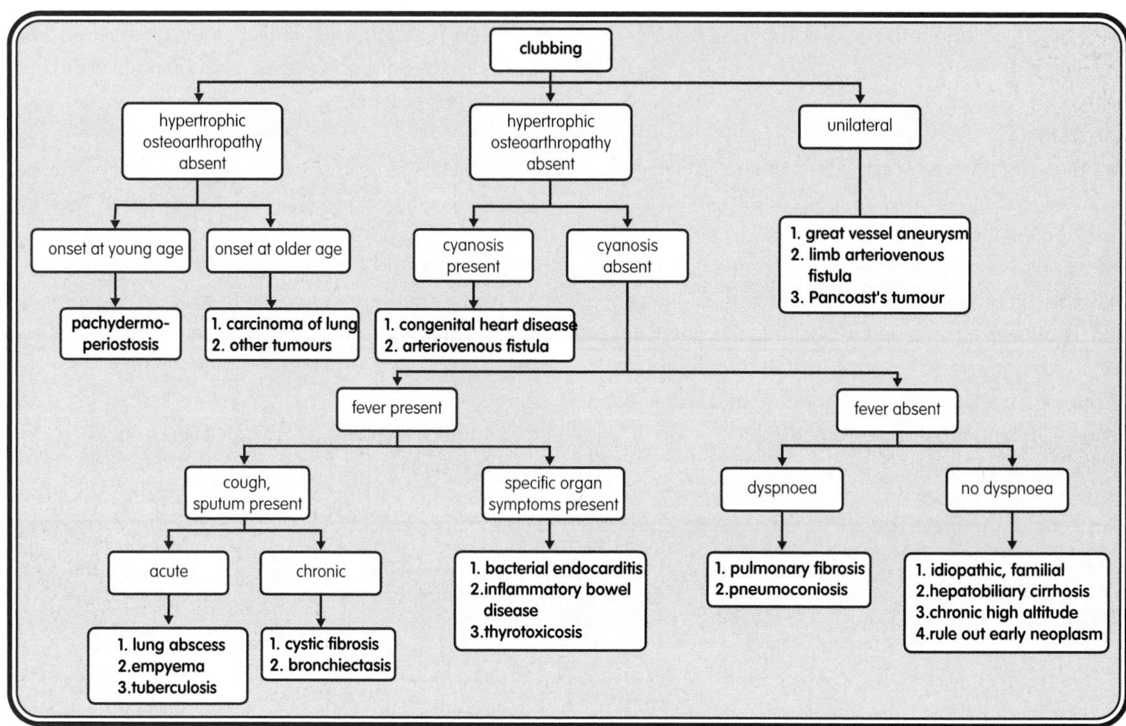

Fig. 7.9 Diagnostic algorithm of clubbing. (Adapted with permission from *Clinical Medicine* 2e by H.L. Greene et al. Mosby Year Book 1996.)

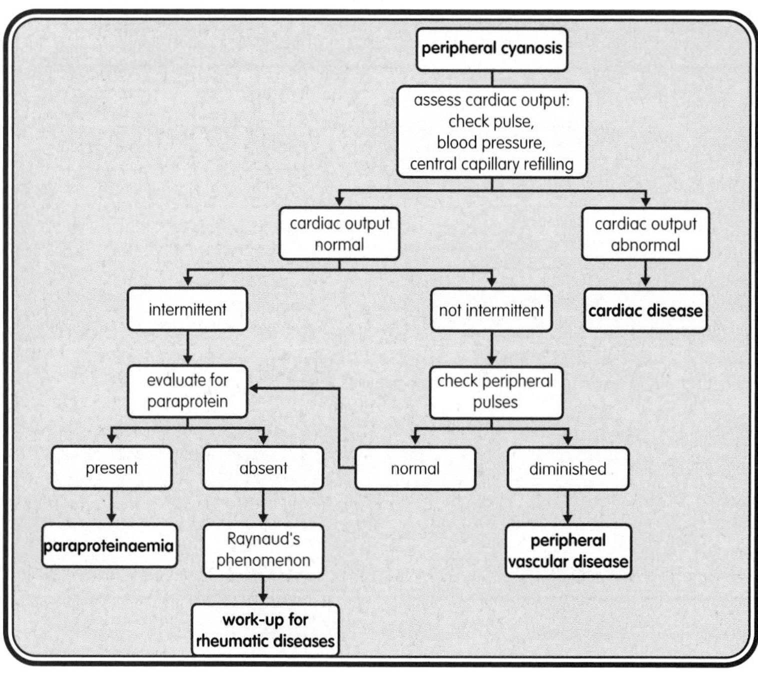

Fig. 7.10 Diagnostic algorithm of peripheral cyanosis. (Adapted with permission from *Clinical Medicine* 2e by H.L. Greene et al. Mosby Year Book 1996.)

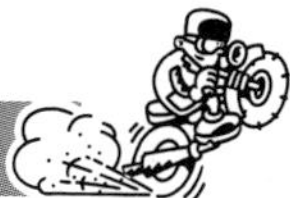

Central cyanosis

Central cyanosis is present when the tongue is cyanosed. It has either cardiac or respiratory causes (Fig. 7.11). If the problem is cardiac in origin, breathing oxygen will not relieve the cyanosis.

Central cyanosis is caused by a decrease in pulmonary venous saturation.

Respiratory failure

Respiratory failure is caused by failure to oxygenate the blood or failure to remove carbon dioxide by ventilation. A patient who has respiratory failure will usually have signs of underlying disease in addition to the symptoms caused by the respiratory failure (Fig. 7.12).

central cyanosis
→ confirm in proper lighting
→ check skin temperature
- not warm → **peripheral cyanosis**
- warm → central cyanosis → check pulse, blood pressure, capillary refilling confirm normal cardiac output → check arterial blood gases
  - PO_2<37mmHg SaO_2 < 70%
    - signs or symptoms of cirrhosis → **intrapulmonary shunts**
    - no signs or symptoms of cardiopulmonary disease → PFTs chest radiograph → PFTs and chest radiograph normal PCO_2 increased → **central hypoventilation**
    - signs or symptoms of COPD, interstitial lung disease, kyphoscoliosis → PFTs chest radiograph
      - PFTs and chest radiograph show COPD PCO_2 increased → **COPD**
      - PFTs show restriction chest radiograph shows interstitial disease kyphoscoliosis PCO_2 increased → **restrictive lung disease**
    - signs or symptoms of congenital heart disease history physical examination → chest radiograph electrocardiogram echocardiogram cardiac catheterization → **congenital heart disease**
  - PO_2>37mmHg SaO_2 > 70% → check haemoglobin concentration
    - increased → **work-up for polycythaemia**
    - not increased → **haemaglobin electrophoresis for methaemoglobin, sulphaemoglobin**
  - PO_2>37mmHg SaO_2 < 70% → **P_{50} (curve shifted right)**

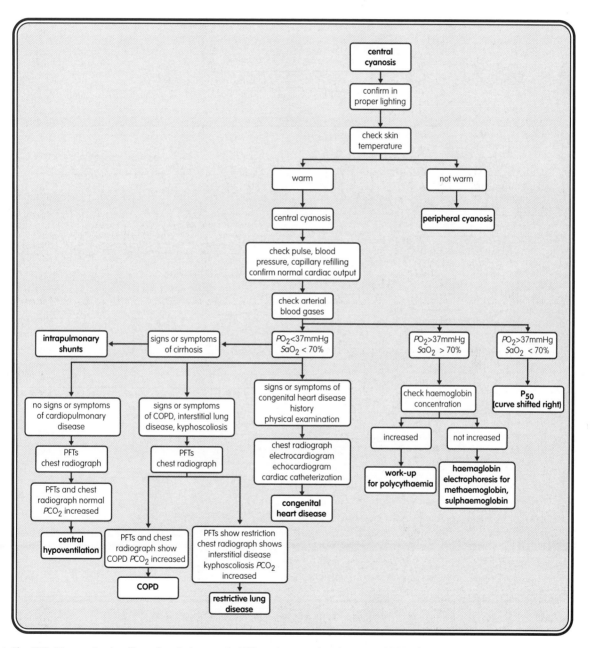

Fig. 7.11 Diagnostic algorithm of central cyanosis. PFTs, pulmonary function tests; COPD, chronic obstructive pulmonary disease. (Adapted with permission from *Clinical Medicine* 2e by H.L. Greene et al. Mosby Year Book 1996.)

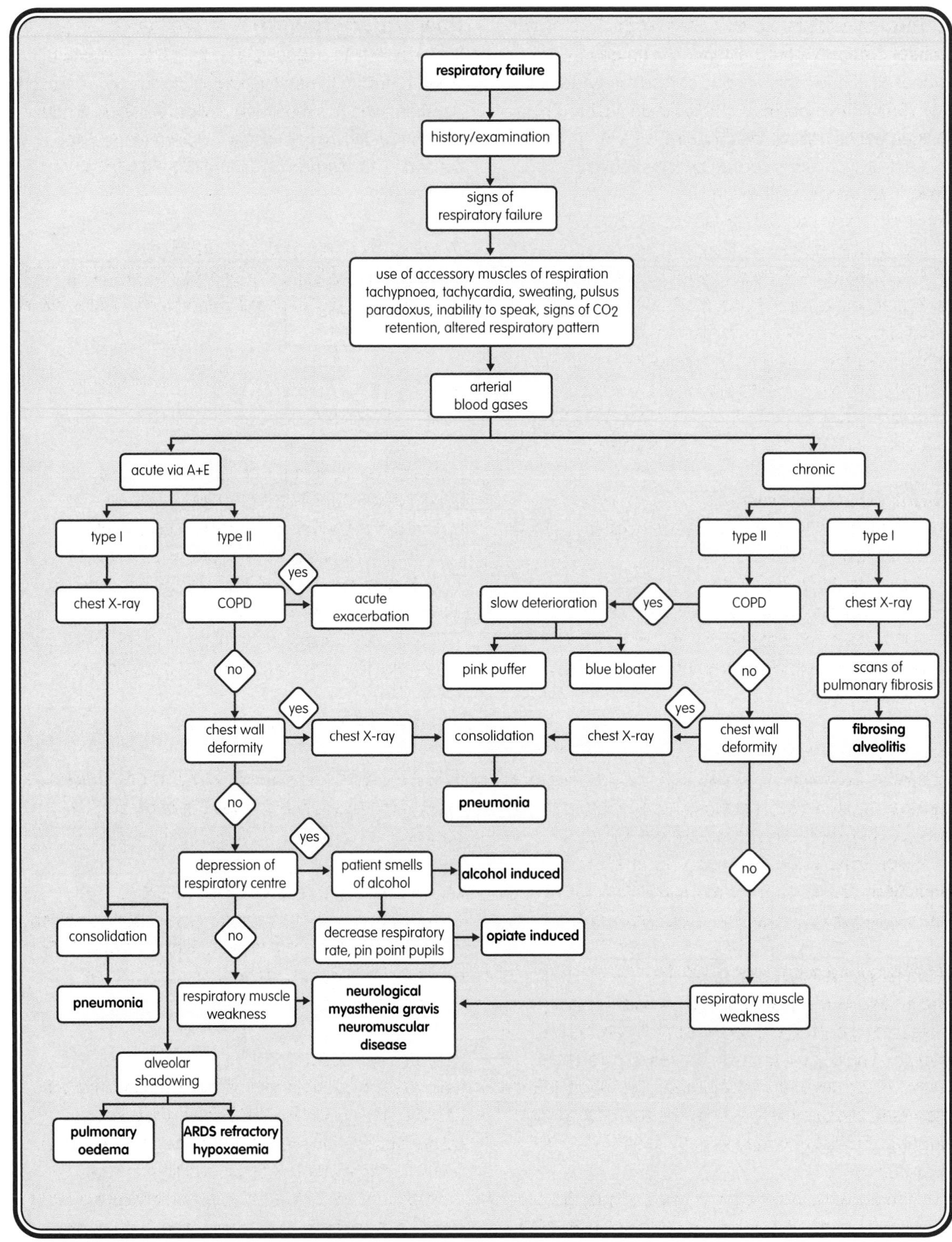

Fig. 7.12 Diagnostic algorithm of respiratory failure. ARDS, adult respiratory distress syndrome. (Adapted with permission from *Clinical Medicine* 2e by H.L. Greene et al. Mosby Year Book 1996.)

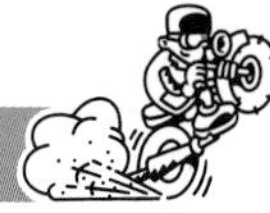

Respiratory failure can be diagnosed on the clinical picture of the patient and following blood gas analysis.

Classification of respiratory failure

Respiratory failure can be classified into two types.

Type I respiratory failure

The features of type I respiratory failure are:

- Acute hypoxaemia.
- P_aO_2 low (<8 kPa), P_aCO_2 normal or low.
- The patient is hypoxic. As the P_aO_2 falls, the patient will become cyanotic, confused, and restless.
- Causes of type I respiratory failure include diseases that damages the lung tissue, alveolar hypoventilation, ventilation:perfusion mismatch, right-to-left shunts, and abnormal diffusion.

Type II respiratory failure

The features of type II respiratory failure are:

- Ventilatory failure.
- P_aO_2 low, P_aCO_2 high (>7 kPa).
- The patient is hypoxic and hypercapnic. As the P_aCO_2 rises, the patient will have warm peripheries; a flapping tremor may develop when P_aCO_2 >8 kPa.

Causes of type II respiratory failure include alveolar ventilation insufficient to remove carbon dioxide caused by reduced ventilatory effort or by the inability to overcome increased resistance to ventilation.

Respiratory failure is treated by treating the underlying cause. Chronic obstructive pulmonary disease is a common cause of respiratory failure.

Solitary pulmonary nodule

The finding of a solitary pulmonary nodule on a plain chest radiograph is not an uncommon event. The nodule, which is commonly referred to as a coin lesion, is usually well circumscribed, less than 6 cm in diameter, lying within the lung. The rest of the lung appears normal and the patient is often asymptomatic.

If the patient is older than 35 years of age, then malignancy should be at the top of the list of possible differential diagnoses (Fig. 7.13). If the lesion is static for a long period of time, as determined by reviewing previous radiographs, then it is likely to be a benign lesion. However, a slow-growing nodule in an elderly patient is likely to be malignant.

The causes of a solitary pulmonary nodule are vast; however, the commonest causes are malignancy, hamartoma, tuberculoma, fungal granuloma, and artefact.

Arterial blood gas analysis

Blood gas analysis of an arterial blood sample is measured using a standard automated machine, which measures:

- P_aO_2.
- P_aCO_2.
- Oxygen saturation.

Furthermore, blood pH, standard bicarbonate, and base excess, can all be calculated.

Blood gas analysis is mandatory in all acute pulmonary conditions. Blood gas analysis should always be repeated soon after starting oxygen to assess response to treatment.

The assessment of blood gases occurs in two parts:

- Degree of arterial oxygenation—is the patient hypoxic?
- Acid–base balance disturbances.

Before accurate interpretation of the results, a detailed history of the patient including a detailed drug history is needed.

Disturbances of acid–base balance

Both acidosis and alkalosis can occur, both of which can be respiratory or metabolic (Figs 7.14 and 7.15). In addition, compensatory changes may also be present.

Respiratory acidosis

Respiratory acidosis is caused by retention of carbon dioxide; subsequently, P_aCO_2 and hydrogen ion concentration increase. If chronic, then compensation occurs, with renal retention of bicarbonate in an attempt to maintain the hydrogen ion concentration at normal values. In this case, the patient has primary respiratory acidosis with compensatory metabolic alkalosis.

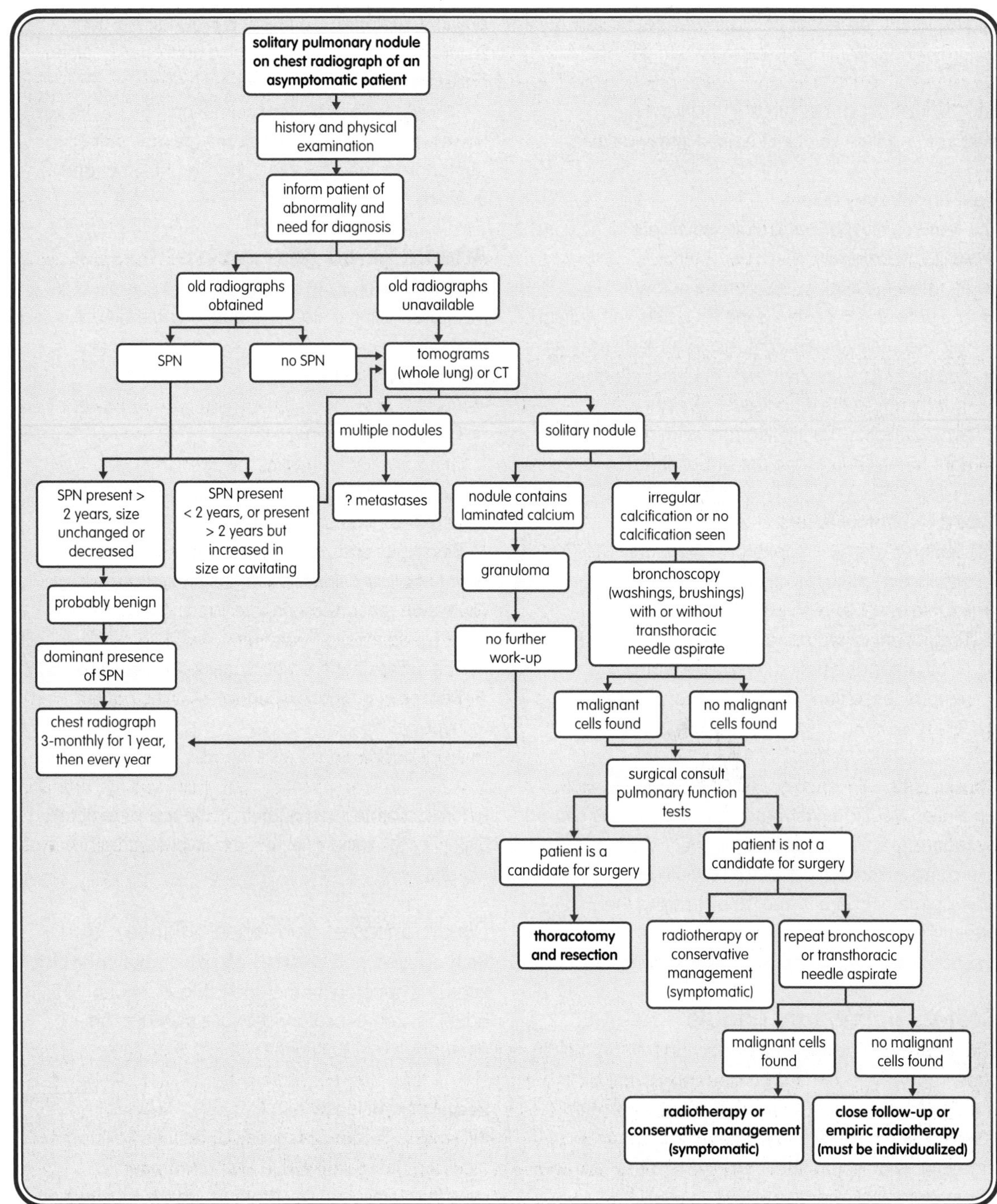

Fig. 7.13 Diagnostic algorithm of solitary pulmonary nodule. (Adapted with permission from *Clinical Medicine* 2e by H.L. Greene et al. Mosby Year Book 1996.)

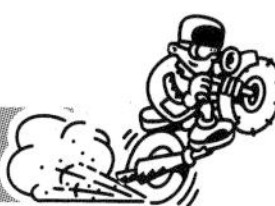

Diagnosis of acid–base balance disturbances					
Measurement	**Normal range**	**Respiratory acidosis**	**Respiratory alkalosis**	**Metabolic acidosis**	**Metabolic alkalosis**
pH	7.35–7.45	Decreased	Increased	Decreased	Increased
P_aCO_2	4.8–6.1 kPa	Increased	Decreased	Decreased	Increased
HCO_3^-	22–26 mmol/L	Increased	Decreased	Decreased	Increased

Fig. 7.14 Diagnosis of acid–base balance disturbances.

Common causes of acid-base disturbances	
Disturbance	**Causes**
Respiratory acidosis	Ventilatory failure Chronic bronchitis Emphysema
Respiratory alkalosis	Artificial ventilation Hypoxaemia Hyperventilation
Metabolic acidosis	Chronic renal failure Renal tubular acidosis Lactic acidosis
Metabolic alkalosis	Vomiting High intestinal obstruction Iatrogenic causes

Fig. 7.15 Table of common causes of acid–base disturbances.

Respiratory alkalosis

This is the opposite of acidosis; carbon dioxide and hydrogen ion concentrations are low. Renal compensation is rare in this condition.

Metabolic acidosis

Metabolic acidosis is caused by excessive acid production; it may also arise from chronic renal failure or after loss of a large amount of alkali.

Respiratory compensation occurs: the patient hyperventilates to blow off the excess carbon dioxide, thereby producing a compensatory respiratory alkalosis.

Metabolic alkalosis

Metabolic alkalosis is much rarer than metabolic acidosis. It is commonly caused by loss of acid (e.g. during vomiting). Respiratory compensation is often minimal.

- **What are the causes of common acid–base disturbances?**
- **What are the normal ranges of pH, P_aCO_2, and HCO_3^-?**
- **How does acid–base balance help classify respiratory failure?**
- **How does the body compensate for acid–base balance disturbances?**

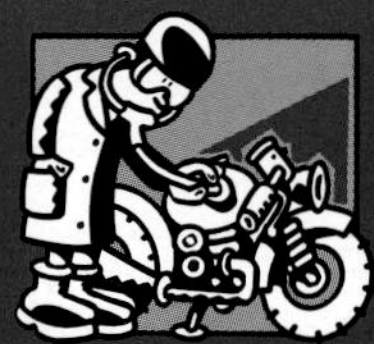

8. Examination of the Patient

GENERAL INSPECTION

Overview

As with any examination, it is important that you:

- Introduce yourself if you are only examining the patient.
- Wash your hands before you begin and when you finish the examination.
- Explain to the patient what you are going to do.

The structure of the examination is inspection, palpation, percussion, and auscultation. For a respiratory examination, patients should be fully exposed to the waist, comfortable, and sat at 45°, with their hands by their sides. The initial observation is vital: stand at the end of the bed and look at the locker for sputum pots, inhalers, and charts. Note any drip stands that are present, venous cannulae, or bandages.

General inspection and inspection of the thorax can practically be carried out together, but are discussed separately here.

The figures below will describe the main tests performed, signs observed, and diagnostic inference for:

- Cachexia (Fig. 8.1).
- Inspection of the skin (Fig. 8.2).
- Dyspnoea (Fig. 8.3).
- Breathing rate (Fig. 8.4).
- Pattern of breathing (Fig. 8.5).
- Hoarse voice (Fig. 8.6).

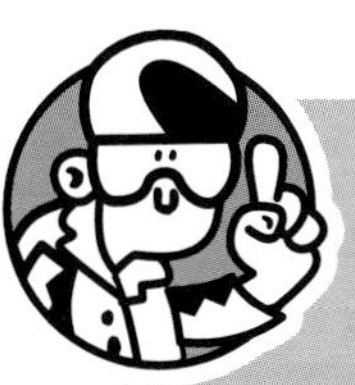

In clinical examinations, purposefully walk to the end of the bed to observe the patient; this emphasizes that you are observing the patient and also gives you thinking time. Give a running commentary of what you are doing, this needs practice as you will be nervous.

Cachexia		
Test performed	**Signs observed**	**Diagnostic inference**
observe muscle bulk and general condition of the skin	generalized muscle wasting and lack of nutrition; pallor; dry and wrinkled skin	malignant disease bronchial carcinoma chronic disease renal disease hepatic disease cardiac failure tuberculosis other anorexia nervosa malnutrition emotional disturbance

Fig. 8.1 Tests, signs, and diagnostic inferences found in cachexia.

Inspection of skin		
Test performed	**Signs observed**	**Diagnostic inference**
observe the general state of the skin	steroidal skin: shiny excessive bruising thin	prolonged use of corticosteroids: chronic obstructive pulmonary disease asthma fibrosing alveolitis systemic disease (e.g. Crohn's disease)
	generalized dryness and scaling of skin	ichthyosis vulgaris acquired ichthyosis hypothyroidism sarcoidosis
	thin skin	ageing Cushing's syndrome topical or systemic steroid use
observe the colour of the skin	pale skin	pallor anaemia leukaemia shock
	light brown coloured spots on skin	café-au-lait spots neurofibromatosis tuberous sclerosis

Fig. 8.2 Tests, signs, and diagnostic inferences found when inspecting the skin.

Dyspnoea		
Test performed	**Signs observed**	**Diagnostic inference**
assess if the patient is short of breath	patient sitting forward with elbows supported; accessory muscles of respiration in use; intercostal recession present on inspiration and patient exhibits nasal flaring	pulmonary causes of dyspnoea: asthma pneumothorax chronic obstructive pulmonary disease bronchiectasis laryngeal tumour other causes of dyspnoea: myocardial infarction cardiac failure mitral stenosis thyrotoxicosis

Fig. 8.3 Tests, signs, and diagnostic inferences found in dyspnoea.

Abnormal ventilation rate		
Test performed	**Signs observed**	**Diagnostic inference**
discretely count the respiratory rate while feeling the patient's pulse	14–20 breaths per minute	normal
	>20 breaths per minute (tachypnoea)	anxiety pain infection pneumothorax pulmonary embolism
	<14 breaths per minute (bradypnoea)	hypothyroidism increased intracranial pressure

Fig. 8.4 Tests, signs, and diagnostic inferences found when checking the breathing rate.

Abnormal patterns of breathing		
Test performed	**Signs observed**	**Diagnostic inference**
examine the pattern of breathing	hyperventilation with deep sighing respirations (Kussmaul's respiration)	diabetic ketoacidosis aspirin overdose acute massive pulmonary embolism
	increased rate and volume of respiration followed by periods of apnoea (Cheyne–Stokes respiration)	terminal disease increased intracranial pressure
	prolongation of expiration	airflow limitation

Fig. 8.5 Tests, signs, and diagnostic inferences found in the pattern of breathing.

Hoarseness		
Test performed	**Signs observed**	**Diagnostic inference**
when talking to the patient, assess the voice	rough, hoarse quality of voice	heavy smoker recurrent laryngeal nerve palsy laryngeal foreign body or tumour upper respiratory tract infection

Fig. 8.6 Tests, signs, and diagnostic inferences found in hoarse voice.

- **Why is the initial observation of the patient important?**
- **Describe the visible effects of long-term steroid use.**
- **List the causes of tachypnoea.**
- **List the different patterns of breathing and their significance.**

HANDS AND LIMBS

Examination of the hands

Clubbing is an important sign of respiratory disease (Figs 8.7 and 8.8). The figures below describe the main tests performed, signs observed, and diagnostic inference for:

- Nail staining (Fig. 8.9).
- Peripheral cyanosis (Fig. 8.10).
- Muscle wasting (Fig. 8.11).
- Rheumatoid hands (Fig. 8.12).
- Hypertrophic pulmonary osteoarthropathy (HPOA) (Fig. 8.13).
- Hand tremor (Fig. 8.14).
- Hand temperature (Fig. 8.15).

Examination of the limbs

The figures below describe the main tests performed, signs observed, and diagnostic inference for:

- Brachial pulse (Fig. 8.16).
- Pulsus paradoxus (Fig. 8.17).
- Axillary lymph nodes (Fig. 8.18).

Know the causes of clubbing before any clinical examination. Note that chronic bronchitis does not cause clubbing.

Clubbing		
Test performed	**Sign observed**	**Diagnostic inference**
view the nail from the side against a white background (e.g. a bed sheet); rock the nail from side to side on the nail-bed; look at the nail-bed and nail angle. place nails back to back; a diamond-shaped area is evident between them if clubbing does not exist.	increase in the soft tissues of the nail-bed and fingertip, with increased sponginess of the nail-bed loss of angle between nail and nail-bed transverse curvature of nail increases in final stages, whole tip of the finger becomes clubbed clubbing may also affect the toes bones are normal	pulmonary causes: tumour (bronchial carcinoma, mesothelioma) chronic pulmonary sepsis (empyema, lung abscess, bronchiectasis, cystic fibrosis) fibrosing alveolitis asbestosis hypertrophic pulmonary osteoarthropathy cardiac causes: congenital bacterial endocarditis other causes: idiopathic causes cirrhosis inflammatory bowel disease

Fig. 8.7 Tests, signs, and diagnostic inferences found in clubbing.

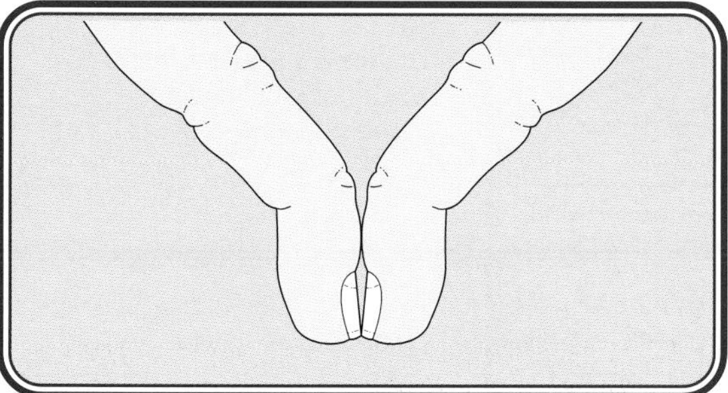

Fig. 8.8 How to inspect the fingers for clubbing. Normal fingers: note diamond-shaped area.

Staining of the nails		
Test performed	**Sign observed**	**Diagnostic inference**
look at the hands for any colour changes to the nails or subungual tissue	yellow or brown discoloration of the skin and nails	nicotine staining caused by: heavy smoking way in which the patient holds cigarette
	green discoloration	infection: pseudomonas aspergillus candida

Fig. 8.9 Tests, signs, and diagnostic inferences found in stained fingers.

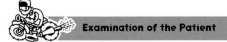

Peripheral cyanosis		
Test performed	**Sign observed**	**Diagnostic inference**
observe the fingertips for any discoloration	blue discoloration of the fingertips and cold peripheries	peripheral cyanosis in the absence of central cyanosis is caused by poor peripheral circulation others causes: Raynaud's disease Buerger's disease circulatory disturbance mitral stenosis pulmonary stenosis

Fig. 8.10 Tests, signs, and diagnostic inferences found in peripheral cyanosis.

Muscle wasting		
Test performed	**Sign observed**	**Diagnostic inference**
look at the dorsal aspect of the hand for any reduction in muscle bulk always compare both hands together	muscle wasting: note the distribution and if it is unilateral or bilateral	localized: unilateral – Pancoast's tumour bilateral – disuse atrophy; rheumatoid arthritis generalized: diabetes thyrotoxicosis anorexia nervosa

Fig. 8.11 Tests, signs, and diagnostic inferences found in muscle wasting.

Rheumatoid hands		
Test performed	**Sign observed**	**Diagnostic inference**
look at the hands for signs of rheumatoid disease	ulnar deviation of fingers swan-neck or boutonniere deformity Z-deformity of thumb subluxation of proximal phalanx wasting of small muscles	rheumatoid disease, which may affect the lung: pulmonary nodules pleural effusion

Fig. 8.12 Tests, signs, and diagnostic inferences found in rheumatoid hands.

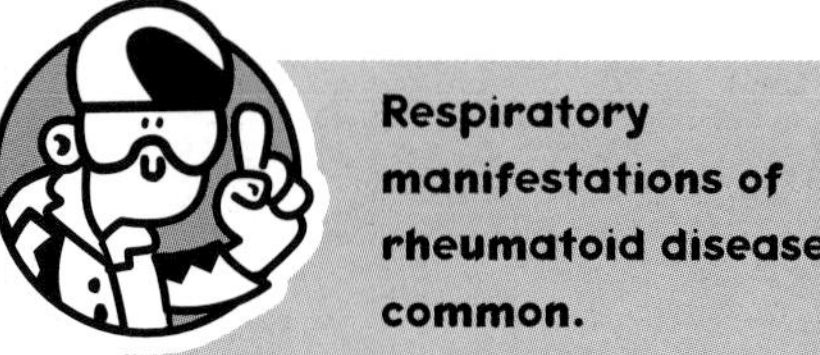

Respiratory manifestations of rheumatoid disease are common.

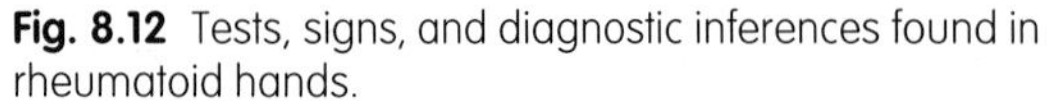

Hypertrophic pulmonary osteoarthropathy		
Test performed	**Sign observed**	**Diagnostic inference**
apply pressure to the wrist	tenderness on palpation of the wrist; the pain is over the shafts of the long bones adjacent to the joint arthralgia and joint swelling	hypertrophic pulmonary osteoarthropathy, a nonmetastatic complication of malignancy – subperiosteal new-bone formation in the long bones of the lower limbs and forearms; clubbing is also present – 90% of cases are associated with bronchogenic carcinoma, especially squamous cell carcinoma other causes: rheumatoid arthritis systemic sclerosis

Fig. 8.13 Tests, signs, and diagnostic inferences found in hypertrophic pulmonary osteoarthropathy.

Hand tremor		
Test performed	**Sign observed**	**Diagnostic inference**
ask patient to hold fingers outstretched and spread in front; place a piece of paper on the dorsal aspect of the hands; observe hands at eye level from the side	very fine finger tremor on outstretched fingers; finger tremor is made more obvious by placing a piece of paper on top of the hands	• stimulation of β-receptors by bronchodilator drugs especially nebulized drugs • thyrotoxicosis
ask patient to hold arm outstretched in front; fully extend the wrists; apply pressure to hands; leave patient like this for 30 seconds	flapping tremor (asterixis) against your hands, which is coarse and irregular in nature; maximum activity at wrist and metacarpophalangeal joints	CO_2 retention hepatic failure encephalopathy metabolic diseases subdural haematoma

Fig. 8.14 Tests, signs, and diagnostic inferences found in hand flap.

Abnormal hand temperature		
Test performed	**Sign observed**	**Diagnostic inference**
feel the temperature of the patient's hands	warm	CO_2 retention thyrotoxicosis
	cold	hypothyroidism poor peripheral circulation

Fig. 8.15 Tests, signs, and diagnostic inferences found when testing hand temperature.

Abnormal brachial pulse		
Test performed	**Sign observed**	**Diagnostic inference**
use the index finger with or without the middle finger to palpate the radial or brachial artery; note the pulse rate, rhythm, character, and volume	rate <90 beats per minute	normal
	rate >90 beats per minute (tachycardia)	pain shock infection thyrotoxicosis sarcoidosis pulmonary embolism drugs e.g. salbutamol iatrogenic causes
	full, exaggerated arterial pulsation (bounding pulse)	CO_2 retention thyrotoxicosis fever anaemia hyperkinetic states

Fig. 8.16 Tests, signs, and diagnostic inferences found when testing the brachial pulse.

Pulsus paradoxus		
Test performed	**Sign observed**	**Diagnostic inference**
measure blood pressure using a sphygmomanometer: cuff pressure is reduced and systolic sound is heard; this initially occurs only in expiration; with further reduction of cuff pressure you can hear systole in inspiration as well; the pressure difference between the initial systolic sound in expiration and when it is present throughout the breathing cycle is what is measured	pulse volume decreases with inspiration, the reverse of normal in normal individuals systolic blood pressure falls 3–5 mmHg with inspiration; a fall >10 mmHg is significant large fall in systolic blood pressure during inspiration	severe asthma: the measured pressure difference between inspiration and expiration is an indirect measurement of respiratory muscle contractile force other causes: cardiac tamponade massive pulmonary embolism fall is exaggerated when venous return to the right heart is impaired

Fig. 8.17 Tests, signs, and diagnostic inferences found in pulsus paradoxus.

Enlarged axillary lymph nodes		
Test performed	**Sign observed**	**Diagnostic inference**
Method 1: face the patient; place the patient's right arm on your right arm; patient's arm must be relaxed; palpate axilla with left hand; place the patient's left arm on your left arm; palpate left axilla	enlarged lymph node (axillary lymphadenopathy)	localized spread of viral or bacterial infection tuberculosis human immunodeficiency virus (HIV) infection actinomycosis cytomegalovirus (CMV) infection measles
Method 2: ask the patient to place hands behind head; palpate axilla by placing your fingers high up in axilla; press tips of fingers against chest wall; move fingers down over ribs		axial lymphadenopathy is often present in breast carcinoma

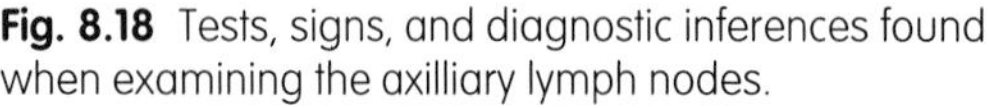

Fig. 8.18 Tests, signs, and diagnostic inferences found when examining the axilliary lymph nodes.

It is often easier and less obvious to count the respiratory rate while the pulse is being taken. Patients' respiration changes once they are aware of it being observed.

- **Describe the common causes of clubbing and how to look for clubbing.**
- **Describe the significance of unilateral muscle wasting of the hand.**
- **How would you palpate for axillary lymphadenopathy?**
- **How might you elicit a fine tremor of the hand?**

HEAD AND NECK

Examination of the face

The figures below describe the main tests performed, signs observed and the diagnostic inference for:

- Observation of the face (Fig. 8.19).
- Examination of the eyes (Fig. 8.20).
- Ptosis (Fig. 8.21).
- Anaemia (Fig. 8.22).
- Fundoscopy (Fig. 8.23).
- Central cyanosis (Fig. 8.24).
- *Candida* infection (Fig. 8.25).

Examination of the neck

The figures below describe the tests performed, signs observed, and diagnostic inference for:

- Tracheal position (Figs 8.26 and 8.27).
- Cervical lymphadenopathy (Fig. 8.28).
- Anatomy of the neck with its lymph node distribution (Fig. 8.29).
- Jugular venous pressure (Fig. 8.30).
- Height of the jugular venous pulse (Fig. 8.31).
- Tracheal tug (Fig. 8.32).

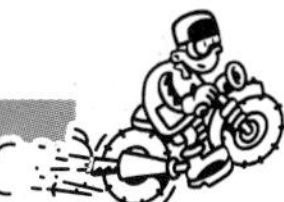

Observation of the face		
Test performed	**Sign observed**	**Diagnostic inference**
observe the patient's face	oedema cyanosis puffy eyes fixed, engorged neck veins	superior vena cava obstruction: bronchial carcinoma lymphoma mediastinal goitre fibrosis
	features associated with Cushing's syndrome: moon face plethora acne hirsute oral candidiasis	long-term administration of steroids: chronic obstructive pulmonary disease asthma ectopic secretion of adrenocorticotropic hormone by a small-cell bronchogenic carcinoma

Fig. 8.19 Tests, signs, and diagnostic inferences found when observing the face.

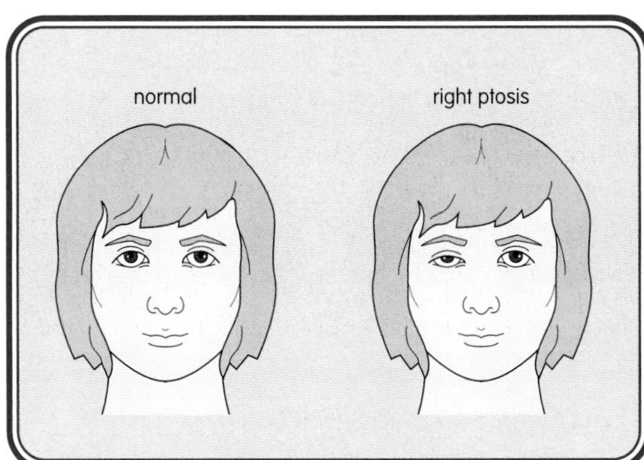

Fig. 8.21 Typical appearance of a patient with ptosis.

Examination of the eyes		
Test performed	**Sign observed**	**Diagnostic inference**
look at the eyes, noting the position of the eyelid and pupil size; always compare with the other side if an abnormality is present, check that the pupils are reactive to light	dropping of upper eyelid so that upper part of iris and pupil are covered (ptosis)	third nerve palsy (with dilated pupil) Horner's syndrome (with small reactive pupil): involvement of the sympathetic chain on the posterior chest wall by an apical bronchial carcinoma; T1 wasting and sensory loss also occur idiopathic (usually in young females) myasthenia gravis (with bilateral ptosis) dystrophia mitochondrial disease (rare)
	small pupil	old age Horner's syndrome Argyll Robertson pupil: miotic and responsive to accommodation effort, but not to light disease in pons cerebrovascular accident drugs (e.g. opiates)

Fig. 8.20 Tests, signs, and diagnostic inferences found when examining the eyes.

Opiate overdose produces bilateral pinpoint pupils. Treat with naloxone.

Anaemia		
Test performed	**Sign observed**	**Diagnostic inference**
ask patient to look up, then evert lower lid of eye note the colour of mucous membrane	pale mucous membrane	indication of anaemia; however, anaemia can only be conclusively diagnosed by measuring haemoglobin levels

Fig. 8.22 Tests, signs, and diagnostic inferences found in anaemia.

Fundoscopy		
Test performed	**Sign observed**	**Diagnostic inference**
look at the patient's eyes using an ophthalmoscope	flattened swollen optic disc with blurred edges (papilloedema)	carbon monoxide poisoning increase in intracranial pressure benign intracranial pressure cerebral metastases

Fig. 8.23 Tests, signs, and diagnostic inferences found when performing a fundoscopy.

Central cyanosis		
Test performed	**Sign observed**	**Diagnostic inference**
good natural light is needed ask the patient to stick tongue out look at the mucous membranes of the lips and tongue	blue discoloration to skin and mucous membrane central cyanosis cannot be accurately identified in black and Asian patients	diseases caused by marked ventilation–perfusion mismatch will cause central cyanosis: severe pulmonary fibrosis chronic bronchitis right–left heart shunts pneumonia respiratory failure bronchiectasis chronic obstructive pulmonary disease

Fig. 8.24 Tests, signs, and diagnostic inferences found in central cyanosis.

Candidiasis		
Test performed	**Sign observed**	**Diagnostic inference**
ask the patient to open their mouth; look for signs of infection	white coating of the mouth	*Candida albicans* infection: steroid use antibiotics idiopathic

Fig. 8.25 Tests, signs, and diagnostic inferences found in *Candida* infection.

Tracheal position		
Test performed	**Sign observed**	**Diagnostic inference**
stand at the front of the patient; pressing gently, place one finger on the trachea judge if the finger slides to one side (tracheal deviation gives an indication of the position of the upper mediastinum; however, the only conclusive method of judging the position is chest radiography)	central trachea	normal
	deviation of the trachea away from the midline	pulled to side of collapse pushed away from mass or fluid contralateral side to tension pneumothorax

Fig. 8.26 Tests, signs, and diagnostic inferences found when checking the tracheal position.

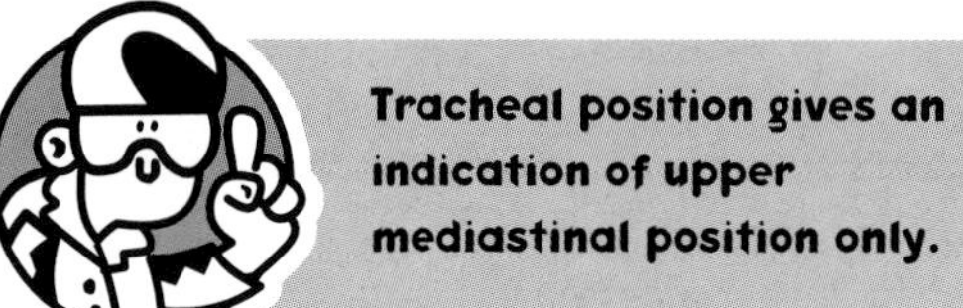

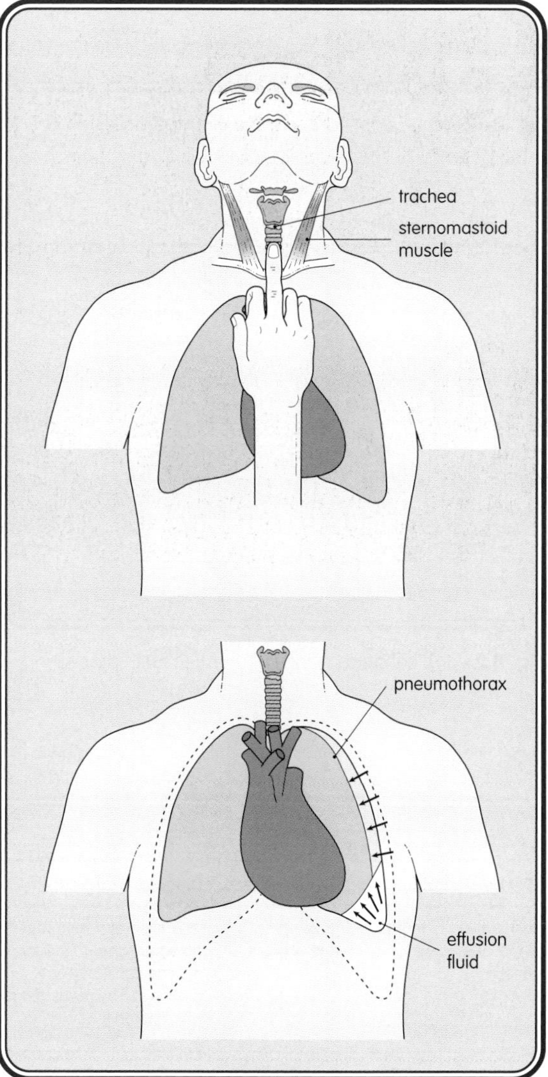

Fig. 8.27 Palpation to determine tracheal position.

Cervical lymphadenopathy		
Test performed	**Sign observed**	**Diagnostic inference**
examine the cervical chain of lymph nodes from behind the patient; it helps if the neck is slightly flexed; most patients extend neck to try and help you know the nodes which you are feeling using both hands, start at the mandibular ramus, palpate the submandibular nodes then anterior chain nodes, supraclavicular nodes, and posterior chain nodes in a Z-fashion	cervical lymphadenopathy note number of palpable nodes describe as for any lump	infection carcinoma tuberculosis sarcoidosis hard node: calcified soft, matted node: tuberculous

Fig. 8.28 Tests, signs, and diagnostic inferences found in cervical lymphadenopathy.

Develop a set system of palpating the lymph nodes of the neck (as mentioned above). Sit the patient up and examine from behind with both hands.

Before a clinical examination, learn the lymph nodes of the neck and into which set of nodes different structures drain.

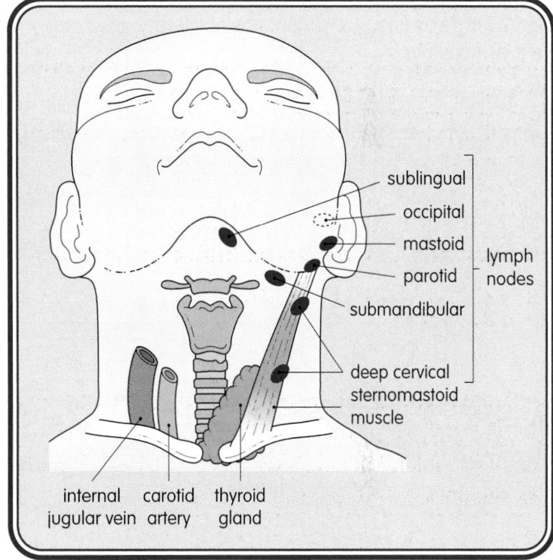

Fig. 8.29 Anatomy of the neck including lymph node distribution.

Jugular venous pressure		
Test performed	**Sign observed**	**Diagnostic inference**
patient must be at 45° looking straight ahead; good light is needed; ask patient to rest head comfortably against a pillow, neck slightly flexed; the patient's neck must be relaxed, as it is impossible to assess jugular venous pressure if the sternomastoid muscles are tensed	elevated jugular venous pressure	resting pressure in thorax is raised: • tension pneumothorax • severe hyperinflation in asthma
a normal jugular pulse becomes visible just above the clavicle between the two heads of sternocleidomastoid; jugular venous pressure is difficult to assess and needs much practice; if the jugular pulse is not seen, try the hepatojugular reflex: apply pressure to the liver, increasing venous return to the heart, and so increasing the jugular venous pressure	elevated nonpulsatile jugular venous pressure	superior vena cava obstruction, usually caused by malignant enlargement of the right bronchus
	elevated pulsatile jugular venous pressure	paratracheal lymph nodes cor pulmonale
time against the contralateral pulse and measure the height of the pulse above the heart (giving a measure of pressure); the normal height of the pulse above the atrium is <4 cm	depressed jugular venous pressure	shock dehydration severe infection

Fig. 8.30 Tests, signs, and diagnostic inferences found when checking the jugular venous pressure.

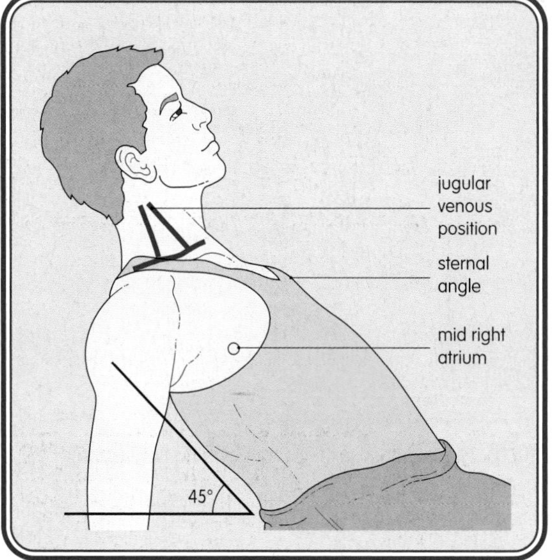

Fig. 8.31 Measurement of the height of the jugular venous pressure.

Tracheal tug		
Test performed	**Sign observed**	**Diagnostic inference**
measure the distance (in finger breadths) between the sternal notch and cricoid cartilage during a full inspiration	three or four finger breaths	normal
	reduced distance	air flow limitation

Fig. 8.32 Tests, signs, and diagnostic inferences found in tracheal tug.

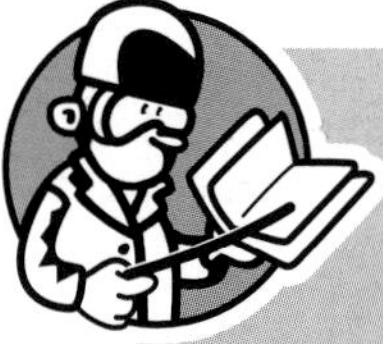

- **What are the differences between third nerve palsy and Horner's syndrome?**
- **Describe the principles of the hepatojugular reflex.**
- **Name the lymph nodes of the neck.**
- **Describe the relevance of tracheal position in tension pneumothorax.**

THE THORAX

Observation of the thorax

The figures below describe the tests performed, signs observed, and diagnostic inference for:

- Thoracic scars (Fig. 8.33).
- Chest wall deformities (Fig. 8.34).
- Chest wall movement (Fig. 8.35).
- Chest wall diameter (Fig. 8.36).
- Radiotherapy tattoos (Fig. 8.37).
- Spinal curvature (Fig. 8.38), and scoliosis and kyphosis (Fig. 8.39).

Palpation

The figures below describe the tests performed, signs observed, and diagnostic inference for:

- Chest expansion (Fig. 8.40).
- Apex beat (Fig. 8.41).
- Tactile vocal fremitus (Fig. 8.42).

Percussion

The correct method of percussion is shown in Fig. 8.43; the tests, signs, and diagnostic inferences encountered when performing percussion in the thorax are described in Fig. 8.44.

Thoracic scars		
Test performed	**Sign observed**	**Diagnostic inference**
look at the thorax for any obvious scars, remembering to look at the front and back of the chest, axilla, and under the breasts	scars present from previous operations	median sternotomy (most open-heart surgery; cardiopulmonary bypass) posteriolateral thoracotomy (ligation of posterior descending artery; lung and oesophageal resections) lateral thoracotomy (pneumothorax) left thoracotomy (closed mitral valvotomy)

Fig. 8.33 Tests, signs, and diagnostic inferences found in thoracic scars.

Chest wall deformities		
Test performed	**Sign observed**	**Diagnostic inference**
look at the sternum and its relationship to the ribs	depressed in pectus excavatum (funnel chest)	benign condition requiring no treatment. On chest radiograph, the heart may be displaced and appear enlarged
	prominent in pectus carinatum (pigeon chest)	may be secondary to severe childhood asthma

Fig. 8.34 Tests, signs, and diagnostic inferences found in chest wall deformities.

Chest wall movement		
Test performed	**Sign observed**	**Diagnostic inference**
observe chest wall movement during quiet tidal breathing and deep inspiration	overall movement of rib cage reduced	hyperinflation caused by: reduced pulmonary compliance (emphysema) reduced chest wall compliance (ankylosing spondylitis, M>F) weak inspiratory muscles (myaesthenia gravis)
	local chest wall movement reduced	pneumothorax pleural effusion pleural thickening pulmonary collapse

Fig. 8.35 Tests, signs, and diagnostic inferences found in chest wall movement.

Chest wall diameter		
Test performed	**Sign observed**	**Diagnostic inference**
observe the patient from the side; ask patient to fold arms and take a deep inspiration	anteroposterior diameter of chest < lateral diameter	normal
	anteroposterior diameter of chest > lateral diameter	hyperinflation asthma

Fig. 8.36 Tests, signs, and diagnostic inferences found in chest wall diameter.

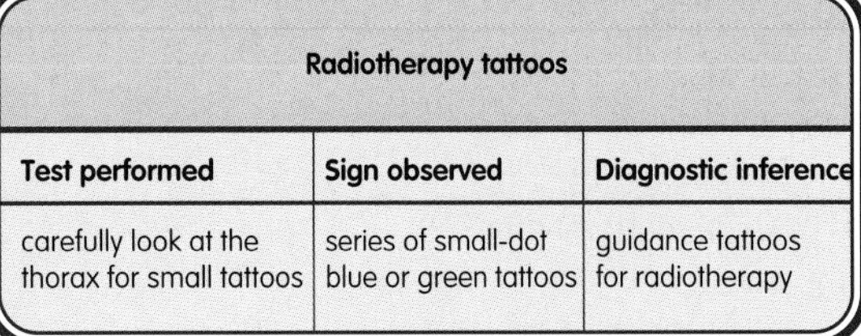

Radiotherapy tattoos		
Test performed	**Sign observed**	**Diagnostic inference**
carefully look at the thorax for small tattoos	series of small-dot blue or green tattoos	guidance tattoos for radiotherapy

Fig. 8.37 Tests, signs, and diagnostic inferences found in radiotherapy tattoos.

Scoliosis and kyphosis can lead to respiratory failure caused by compressional effects.

Spinal curvature		
Test performed	**Sign observed**	**Diagnostic inference**
ask the patient to stand; stand directly behind the patient and look at the curvature of the spine	increased lateral curvature of the spine (scoliosis)	structural abnormality developmental abnormality vertebral disc prolapse
next, stand at the side of the patient and again look at the curvature of the spine	increased forward curvature of the spine (kyphosis)	osteoporosis ankylosing spondylitis

Fig. 8.38 Tests, signs, and diagnostic inferences found in spinal curvature.

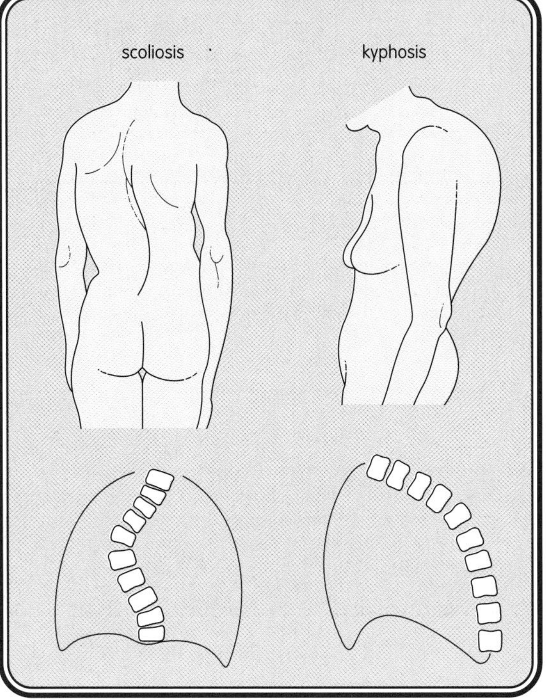

Fig. 8.39 Features of scoliosis and kyphosis.

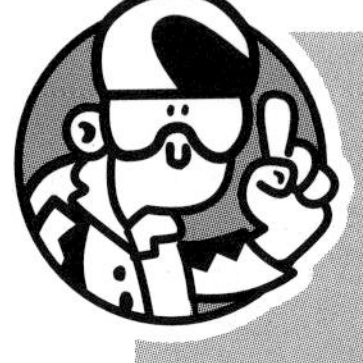

The apex beat position indicates lower mediastinal shift. In clinical examinations, beware of the patient with dextrocardia.

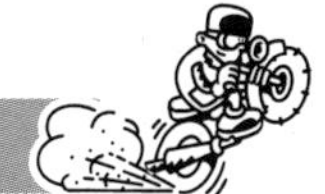

Chest expansion		
Test performed	**Sign observed**	**Diagnostic inference**
place the flat of both hands on the pectoral region of the chest; ask the patient to take a deep breath, and note any asymmetry	symmetrical rise of hands as chest expands	normal
	asymmetrical rise	unilateral pathology on the depressed side
put fingers of both hands as far around the chest as possible; bring thumbs together in the midline; keep thumbs off chest wall; ask patient to take a deep breath in; note distance between thumbs; examine both front and back	–	–
place a tape measure around the internipple line and measure the difference between inspiration and expiration	>4 cm expansion	normal
	<4 cm expansion	reduced expansion (see Fig. 8.35)

Fig. 8.40 Tests, signs, and diagnostic inferences found in chest expansion.

Apex beat		
Test performed	**Sign observed**	**Diagnostic inference**
slowly move your hand towards the midline from the lateral chest wall until you feel the apex beat palpate the chest wall with the flat of fingertips to detect the point of lowermost, outermost cardiac impulse	pulsation in fifth intercostal space midclavicular line	normal
	deviated pulsation; lower mediastinum displacement	left deviation: cardiomegaly pulmonary fibrosis scoliosis pectus excavatum bronchiectasis right deviation: pneumothorax pleural effusion dextracardia

Fig. 8.41 Tests, signs, and diagnostic inferences found in examination of the apex beat.

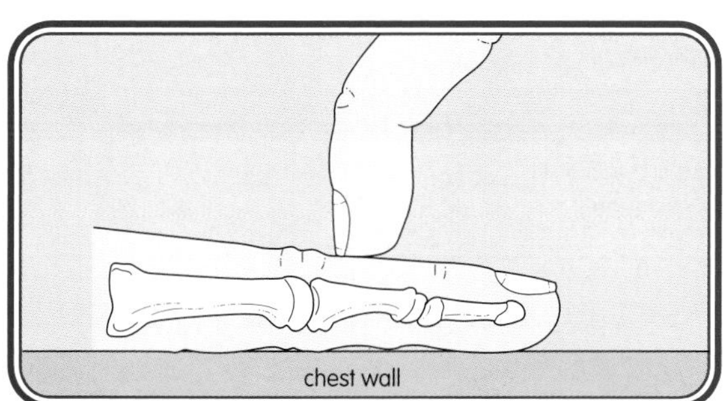

Fig. 8.43 Correct method of percussion (see text for explanation).

Tactile vocal fremitus		
Test performed	**Sign observed**	**Diagnostic inference**
place either the ulnar edge or the flat of your hand on the chest wall; ask the patient to repeatedly say '99' or '1, 2, 3'; repeat for front and back, comparing opposite zones the vibrations produced by the manoeuvre are transmitted through the lung substance and felt by the hand; alterations in disease are the same as for vocal resonance	increased resonance	solid areas of lung with open airways consolidation pneumonia tuberculosis extensive fibrosis
	decreased resonance	feeble voice pleural thickening blocked bronchus

Fig. 8.42 Tests, signs, and diagnostic inferences found in tactile vocal fremitus.

Percussion		
Test performed	**Sign observed**	**Diagnostic inference**
place your nondominant hand on the chest wall, palm downwards, with fingers slightly separated; the second phalanx of the middle finger should be in an intercostal space directly over the area to be percussed; strike this finger with the terminal phalanx of the middle finger of the other hand to achieve a good percussion note, the striking finger should be partially flexed and striked at right angles to the other finger; the striking movement must be a flick of the wrist on percussion you will hear a percussion note and feel vibrations percuss from top to bottom including axilla; to check for disease in the lung apices, percuss directly onto the clavicles; do not percuss more heavily than you need and always compare both sides, front and back dullness occurs as you percuss over the liver; note that the right diaphragm is higher than the left diaphragm	increased resonance (resonance depends on the thickness of the chest wall and the amount of air in the structures underlying it)	increased air in lung: • emphysema • large bullae • pneumothoracies • asthma
	dullness (solid lung tissue does not reflect sound as readily as aerated lung); if a dull area exists, map out its limits by percussing from the resonant to the dull area	consolidation: • fibrosis • collapse • pleural thickening • tuberculosis • extensive carcinoma
	stony dullness	fluid present: • pleural effusion

Fig. 8.44 Tests, signs, and diagnostic inferences found when doing percussion of the thorax.

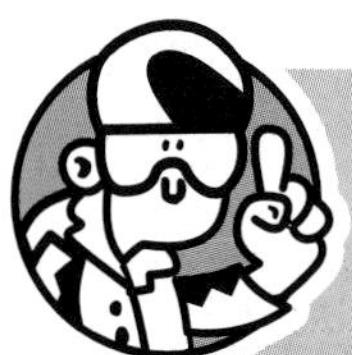

When percussing, remember that the upper lobe predominates anteriorly and the lower lobe predominates posteriorly.

Auscultation

The figures below describe the tests performed, signs observed, and diagnostic inference for:

- Auscultation of the thorax (Fig. 8.45).
- Stridor (Fig. 8.46).
- Wheeze (Fig. 8.47).
- Pleural rub (Fig. 8.48).
- Crackles (Fig. 8.49).

Auscultation of the thorax		
Test performed	**Sign observed**	**Diagnostic inference**
ask the patient to take breaths through an open mouth: a quick demonstration will remove any confusion using the diaphragm of the stethoscope, listen in sequence over the chest starting from top and working downwards; remember to auscultate the axilla; when you auscultate the back, ask the patient to put hands on their shins if possible: this rotates the patient's scapula out of the way	vesicular breath sounds (rustling quality heard in inspiration and the first part of expiration)	breath sounds are produced in the larger airways where flow is turbulent; sounds are transmitted through smaller airways to the chest wall; vesicular breath sounds are normal
		if vesicular breath sounds are reduced or absent: • airway obstruction • asthma • chronic obstructive pulmonary disease • tumour
you must appreciate the intensity and quality of breath sounds and added sounds	bronchial breath sounds (described in relation to timing; a gap exists between inspiration and expiration, which are of equal duration; harsh clear breath sounds)	normal, if heard at the tip of the scapula; otherwise caused by: • consolidation • pneumonia • lung abscess
		if inaudible: • severe emphysema • bullae • pneumothorax • pleural effusion

Fig. 8.45 Tests, signs, and diagnostic inferences found in auscultation of the thorax.

Stridor		
Test performed	**Sign observed**	**Diagnostic inference**
listen to the patient's breath sound; this may be heard best without the stethoscope	loud inspiratory sound	large airway narrowing (larynx, trachea, main bronchi): • laryngotracheobronchitis • epiglotitis • laryngitis

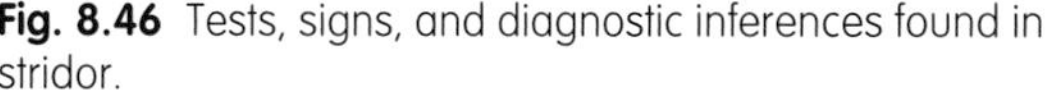

Fig. 8.46 Tests, signs, and diagnostic inferences found in stridor.

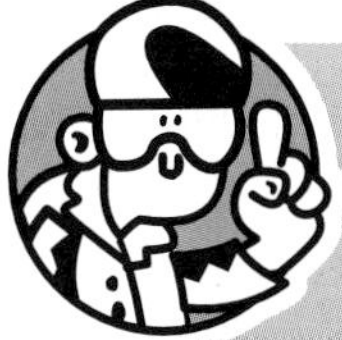

With auscultation always think BAR [B—Breath sounds; A—Added sounds; R—vocal Resonance]. Added sounds that disappear when the patient coughs are not significant.

Wheeze		
Test performed	**Sign observed**	**Diagnostic inference**
listen to the patient breathing	prolonged musical sound	none: the amount of wheeze is not a good indicator of the degree of airway obstruction
	polyphonic sound (many musical notes), mainly in expiration	small airway obstruction: narrowing caused by combination of smooth muscle contraction; inflammation within airways; increased bronchial secretions
	monophonic sound	large airway obstruction: a worrying finding, suggesting a single narrowing (e.g. tumour)

Fig. 8.47 Tests, signs, and diagnostic inferences found in wheeze.

Pleural rub		
Test performed	**Sign observed**	**Diagnostic inference**
listen to the patient breathing	leathery creaking sound associated with each breath inspiratory and expiratory sound that is not shifted by cough; reoccurs at the same time in each respiratory cycle	caused by inflamed surfaces of pleura rubbing together: • pneumonia • pulmonary embolism • emphysema • pleurisy

Fig. 8.48 Tests, signs, and diagnostic inferences found in pleural rub.

Crackles		
Test performed	**Sign observed**	**Diagnostic inference**
listen to the patient breathing crackles may be mimicked by rolling hair on your temple between two fingers; timing during the respiratory cycle is of huge significance	nonmusical, short, uninterrupted sounds heard during inspiration	crackles represent equalization of intraluminal pressure as collapsed small airways open during inspiration
	early inspiratory crackles	diffuse airflow limitation chronic obstructive pulmonary disease pulmonary oedema
	late inspiratory crackles	conditions that largely involve alveoli: • fibrosis • fibrosing alveolitis • bronchiectasis

Fig. 8.49 Tests, signs, and diagnostic inferences found in crackles.

Vocal resonance

The figures below describe the tests, signs, and diagnostic inference for vocal resonance (Fig. 8.50) and whispering pectoriloquy (Fig. 8.51); Fig. 8.52 summarizes the signs found on examination of the respiratory system.

Vocal resonance		
Test performed	**Sign observed**	**Diagnostic inference**
auscultatory equivalent to vocal fremitus; place the stethoscope on to the chest and ask the patient to repeatedly say '99' or '1, 2, 3'	normal lung attenuates high-frequency notes; normally, booming low-pitched sounds are heard	as for vocal fremitus

Fig. 8.50 Tests, signs, and diagnostic inferences found in vocal resonance.

Whispering pectoriloquy		
Test performed	**Sign observed**	**Diagnostic inference**
place the stethoscope on to the chest and ask the patient to repeatedly whisper '99' or '1, 2, 3'	words are clear and seem to be spoken right into the listener's ears (whispering pectoriloquy)	whispered speech cannot usually be heard over healthy lung; solid lung tissue conducts sound better than normally aerated lung, indicating consolidation, cavitation, tuberculosis, or pneumonia

Fig. 8.51 Tests, signs, and diagnostic inferences found in whispering pectoriloquy.

Signs found on examination of the respiratory system					
	Consolidation	**Pneumothorax**	**Pleural effusion**	**Lobar collapse**	**Pleural thickening**
Chest radiograph	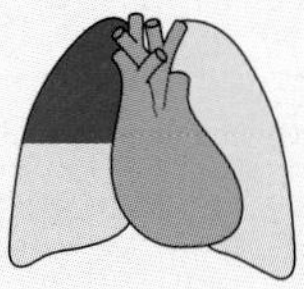	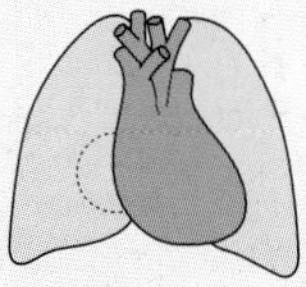	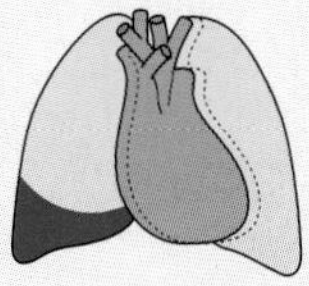	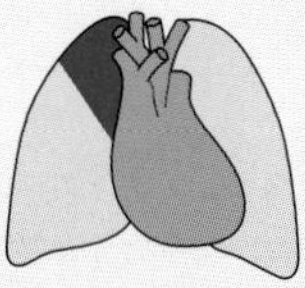	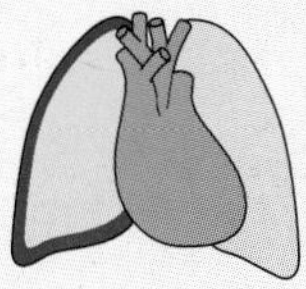
Mediastinal shift	none	none (simple), away (tension)	none or away	towards	none
Chest wall excursion	normal or decreased	normal or decreased	decreased	decreased	decreased
Percussion note	normal or decreased	increased	decreased (stony)	decreased	decreased
Breath sounds	increased (bronchial)	decreased	decreased	decreased	decreased
Added sounds	crackles	click (occasional)	rub (occasional)	none	none
Tactile vocal fremitus or vocal resonance	increased	decreased	decreased	decreased	decreased

Fig. 8.52 Summary table of signs found on examination of the respiratory system.

- **Name the common scars seen on the thorax and the possible operations that the patient may have undergone.**
- **List the surface markings of the lungs for percussion.**
- **Describe the relationship between added sounds and disease.**
- **How does lung disease alter examination findings?**

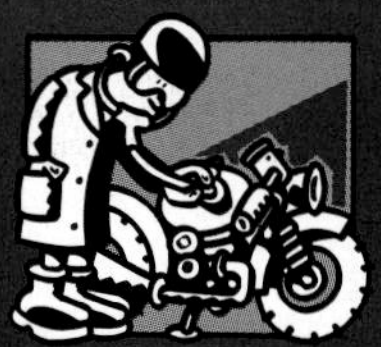

9. Further Investigations

INVESTIGATIONS OF RESPIRATORY FUNCTION

Tests of ventilation

Tests of pulmonary function identify restrictions in lung volume or obstructions in the airways; they are used to monitor patient response to treatment.

Forced expiration

Peak expiratory flow rate

Peak expiratory flow rate (PEFR) is a simple and cheap test that measures the maximum expiratory rate in the first 10 ms of expiration. Normal PEFR is 400–650 L/min in healthy adults.

Before measuring PEFR (Figs 9.1 and 9.2), the practitioner should instruct the patient:

- Take a full inspiration to maximum lung capacity.
- Seal the lips tightly around the mouthpiece.
- Blow out forcefully into the peak flow meter, which is held horizontally.

The best of three measurements is recorded and plotted on the appropriate graph. At least two recordings per day are required to obtain an accurate pattern.

PEFR is reduced in conditions that cause airway obstruction:

- Asthma, where there is wide diurnal variation in PEFR (Fig. 9.3).
- Chronic obstructive pulmonary disease.
- Upper airway tumours.

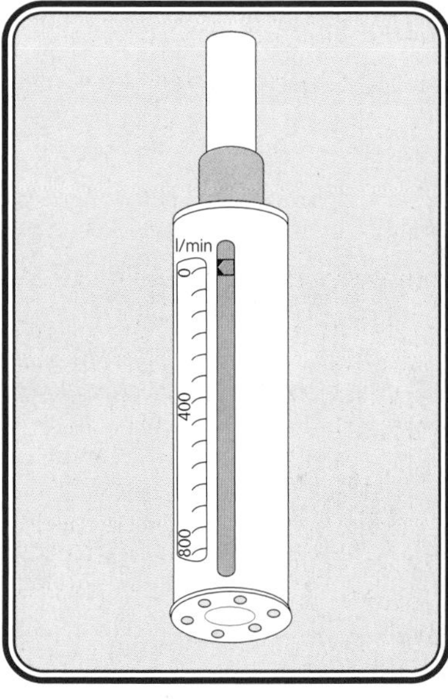

Fig. 9.2 Peak flow meter.

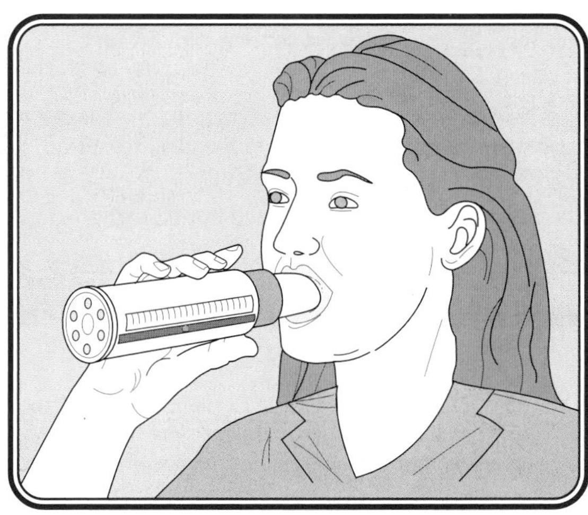

Fig. 9.1 Patient performing peak expiratory flow rate test.

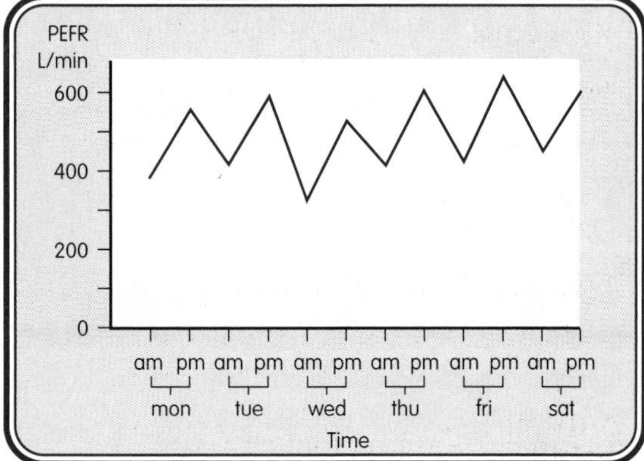

Fig. 9.3 Typical peak expiratory flow rate graph for an asthmatic patient.

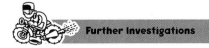

Other causes of reduced PEFR include expiratory muscle weakness, inadequate effort, and poor technique. PEFR is not a good measure of air flow limitation because it measures only initial expiration; it is best used to monitor progression of disease and response to treatment.

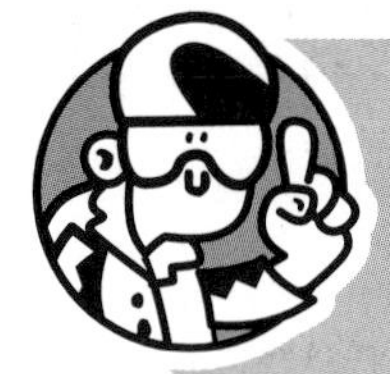

Visit an asthma nurse and ask her to explain how to perform PEFR tests properly.

Forced expiratory volume and forced vital capacity

Spirometry can measure the forced expiratory volume in one second (FEV_1) and the forced vital capacity (FVC). From these measurements, the FEV_1:FVC ratio can be calculated, which is a more useful measurement than FEV_1 or FVC alone. The FEV_1:FVC ratio is an excellent measure of airway limitation.

FEV_1 and FVC are related to height, age, and sex of the patient.

FEV_1 is the volume of air expelled in the first second of a forced expiration, starting from full inspiration. FEV_1 is greater than 70% of FVC in normal subjects. FVC is a measure of total lung volume exhaled; the patient is asked to exhale with maximal effort after a full inspiration.

Using the FEV_1:FVC ratio, we can differentiate obstructive from restrictive lung disease. In restrictive disease:

- No airway obstruction occurs.
- Both FEV_1 and FVC are reduced in proportion to each other.
- FEV_1:FVC ratio is normal.

Whereas, in obstructive diseases:

- High intrathoracic pressures generated by forced expiration cause premature closure of the airways with trapping of air in the chest.
- FEV_1 is reduced much more than FVC.
- FEV_1:FVC ratio is reduced.

Flow–volume loops

Flow–volume loops are constructed from maximal expiratory and inspiratory manoeuvres. The loop shape can identify the type and distribution of airway obstruction. After a small amount of gas has been exhaled, flow is limited by:

- Elastic recoil force of the lung.
- Resistance of airways upstream to collapse.

Flow–volume loops are useful in diagnosing upper airway obstruction (Fig. 9.4). In restrictive diseases:

- Maximum flow rate is reduced.
- Total volume exhaled is reduced.
- Flow rate is high during latter part of expiration because of increased lung recoil.

In obstructive diseases:

- Flow rate is low in relation to lung volume.
- Expiration ends prematurely because of early airway closure.
- Scooped out appearance is often seen after point of maximum flow.

Lung volumes

Neither functional residual capacity nor residual volume can be measured with simple spirometry. Alternative techniques have to be employed.

Helium dilution

The patient is connected to a spirometer containing a mixture of 10% helium in air. Helium is used because it is an insoluble, inert gas that does not cross the alveolar–capillary membrane. At the end of an expiration, the patient begins to breathe from the closed spirometer; after several breaths, the helium concentration in the spirometer and lung becomes equal.

The helium concentration is known at the start of the test and is measured when equilibrium has occurred. The dilution of helium is related to total lung capacity. Residual volume can be calculated by subtracting vital capacity from total lung capacity.

The helium dilution method measures only gas that is in communication with the airways.

Body plethysmography

The patient sits in a large air-tight box and breathes through a mouthpiece. At the end of a normal expiration, a shutter closes the mouthpiece and the patient is asked to make respiratory efforts. As the patient tries to inhale, box pressure increases. Using Boyle's law, lung volume can be calculated.

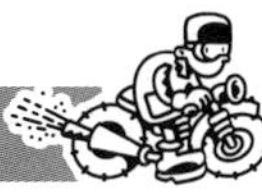

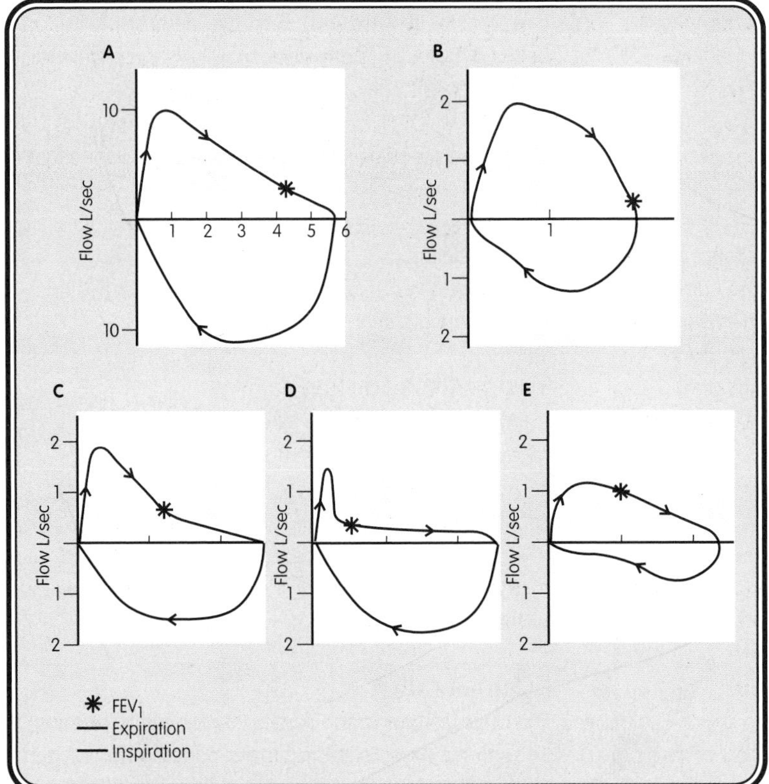

Fig. 9.4 Typical flow–volume loops. (A) Normal. (B) Restrictive defect (phrenic palsy). (C) Volume-dependent obstruction (e.g. asthma). (D) Pressure-dependent obstruction (e.g. severe emphysema). (E) Rigid obstruction (e.g. tracheal stenosis).

This method measures all intrathoracic gas including cyst, bullae, and pneumothoraces. In contrast to the helium dilution method, body plethysmography defines the extent of noncommunicating airspace within the lung; this is important in subjects with chronic obstructive pulmonary disease (e.g. emphysema).

Nitrogen washout

Nitrogen is completely displaced from the lungs during a period breathing 100% O_2.

Total volume of gas exhaled and its nitrogen concentration are measured. The concentration of nitrogen in the lung before washout is 80%. The concentration of nitrogen left in the lung can be measured by a nitrogen meter at the lips measuring end expiration gas. Assuming no net change in the amount of nitrogen, total lung volume can be calculated. Nitrogen washout measures only gas in communication with the airways.

Fowler's dead space

Fowler's dead space method measures the volume of the conducting airways, the anatomical dead space.

The patient inspires 100% O_2. On expiration, the nitrogen concentration rises as the deadspace gas (100% O_2) is washed out by alveolar gas (a mixture of nitrogen and oxygen). As pure alveolar gas is expired, nitrogen concentration reaches a plateau (the alveolar plateau). Nitrogen concentration is plotted against expired volume; deadspace is the volume at which the two areas under the plot are equal (see Chapter 3, Fig. 3.7).

In a healthy person, the physiological and anatomical deadspaces are nearly equal; however, in patients with alveoli disease and nonfunctioning alveoli (e.g. in emphysema), physiological deadspace may be up to 10 times that of the anatomical deadspace.

Tests of diffusion

Oxygen and carbon dioxide pass by diffusion between the alveoli and pulmonary capillary blood. The diffusing capacity of carbon monoxide (CO) measures the ability of gas to diffuse from inspired air to capillary blood, and also reflects the uptake of oxygen from the alveolus into the red blood cells. Carbon monoxide is used because:

- It is highly soluble.
- It combines rapidly with haemoglobin.

Two tests can be used to determine diffusion: the single-breath test and the steady-state method.

Single-breath test

The patient takes a single breath from residual volume to total lung capacity. The inhaled gas contains 0.28% carbon monoxide and 13.5% helium. The patient is instructed to hold his or her breath for 10 secs before expiring. The concentration of helium and carbon monoxide in the final part of the expired gas mixture is measured and the diffusing capacity of carbon monoxide is calculated. You need to know the haemoglobin level before the test.

Steady-state method

The patient breathes a low concentration of carbon monoxide for 30 secs until a steady state is reached. The rate of disappearance of carbon monoxide from alveolar gas is measured along with alveolar concentrations.

In practice, the transfer factor is used in preference to the diffusing capacity. In the normal lung, the transfer factor accurately measures the diffusing capacity of the lungs whereas, in diseased lung, diffusing capacity also depends on:

- Area and thickness of alveolar membrane.
- Ventilation:perfusion relationship.

Transfer factor

Transfer factor (T_LCO) is defined as the amount of carbon monoxide transferred per minute, corrected for the concentration gradient of carbon monoxide across the alveolar capillary membrane (Fig. 9.5).

The transfer factor is reduced in conditions where there are:

- Fewer alveolar capillaries.
- Ventilation:perfusion mismatching.
- Reduced accessible lung volumes.

Gas transfer is a relatively sensitive but nonspecific test, useful at detecting early disease in lung parenchyma; transfer coefficient is a better test. The transfer coefficient (*K*CO) is corrected for lung volumes and is useful in distinguishing causes of low T_LCO due to loss of lung volume:

- T_LCO and *K*CO are low in emphysema and fibrosing alveolitis.
- T_LCO is low, but *K*CO is normal in pleural effusions and consolidation.

Tests of blood flow

Contraction of the right ventricle pumps blood along the pulmonary arteries to the capillary bed, where gas exchange takes place. At any one time, pulmonary capillaries hold only about 10 mL of blood.

Pulmonary blood flow can be measured by two methods: the Fick method and the indicator dilution technique.

Fick method

The amount of oxygen taken up by the blood passing through the lungs is related to the difference in oxygen content between arterial and mixed venous blood. Oxygen consumption is measured by collecting expired gas in a large spirometer and measuring its oxygen concentration.

Indicator dilution technique

Dye is injected into the venous circulation; the concentration and time of appearance of the dye in the arterial blood are recorded.

With severe exercise, pulmonary blood flow is greatly increased, so time for oxygenation of red blood cells is less. In normal subjects breathing air, there is generally no fall in end capillary PO_2.

Conditions that affect the transfer factor

	Decreased transfer factor	Increased transfer factor
Pulmonary causes	emphysema; loss of lung tissue; diffuse infiltration	pulmonary haemorrhage
Cardiovascular causes	low cardiac output; pulmonary oedema	thyrotoxicosis
Other causes	anaemia	polycythaemia

Fig. 9.5 Conditions that affect the transfer factor.

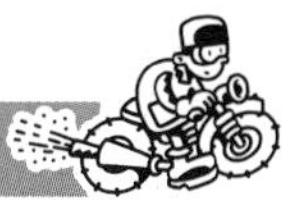

If the blood–gas barrier is thickened by disease, oxygen diffusion is impeded, so a measurable difference between the PO_2 in alveolar gas and end capillary blood may occur.

Testing ventilation:perfusion relationships

Regional differences of ventilation and blood flow can be measured using radioactive xenon.

Detection of pulmonary perfusion

Radioactive particles larger than the diameter of the pulmonary capillaries are injected intravenously, where they remain for several hours. Tc^{99m}-labelled macro-aggregated albumin (MAA) is used. A gamma camera is then used to detect the position of the MAAs. The pattern indicates the distribution of pulmonary blood flow.

Detection of ventilation

Ventilation is detected by inhalation of a gas or aerosol labelled with the radioisotope, Xe^{133}. The patient breathes and rebreathes the gas until it comes into equilibrium with other gases in the lung.

Finding of a nonperfused but ventilated zone is suggestive of pulmonary embolus. Poor perfusion with poor ventilation occurs in conditions such as asthma and emphysema; pulmonary embolus cannot be diagnosed if such a pattern is obtained—pulmonary angiography is then indicated.

Inequality of ventilation

Single-breath method

The single-breath method is similar to the method for measuring anatomic dead space. In patients with lung disease, it is noted that alveolar nitrogen concentration continues to rise during expiration because of uneven dilution of the alveolar nitrogen by inspired oxygen. This is caused by the poorly ventilated alveoli emptying last.

The change in nitrogen percentage concentration occurring between 750 mL and 1250 mL of expired volume is used as an index of uneven ventilation.

Testing mechanisms of breathing

Lung compliance

Compliance is a measure of distensibility (Fig. 9.6). It is defined as the volume change per unit of pressure across the lung.

Lung compliance is measured by introducing a balloon into the oesophagus to estimate intrapleural pressure. A lung of high compliance expands to a greater extent than one of low compliance when both are exposed to the same transpulmonary pressure.

To measure compliance:

- The patient breathes out from total lung capacity into a spirometer in steps.
- Oesophageal pressure is measured simultaneously.
- The lung is given time to stabilize for a few seconds after each step, so that equalization of pressure is achieved at a number of lung volumes throughout inspiration and expiration.
- A pressure–volume curve is obtained, which displays the elastic behaviour of the lung.

Airway resistance

A large proportion of the resistance to air flow is offered by the upper respiratory tract. Airways resistance is defined as the pressure difference required between the alveolus and mouth required to produce airflow of 1 L/s. Several methods have been used to measure airway resistance, but plethysmography is the best way because:

- It is accurate.
- It is easy.
- It also measures thoracic gas volume.

The patient is seated in a constant pressure within the body plethysmograph and instructed to pant. The pressure within the plethysmograph changes: during inspiration the volume increases whereas during expiration it decreases. The greater the airway resistance, the greater are the pressure swings in the chest and plethysmograph. Alveolar pressure can be obtained from the box pressure by suitable calibration.

Causes of altered lung compliance

Reduced compliance	Increased compliance
pulmonary venous pressure increased	old age
alveolar oedema	emphysema
fibrosis	bronchoalveolar drugs
airway closure	

Fig. 9.6 Causes of altered lung compliance.

Airway resistance should be related to lung volume or the transpulmonary pressure at time of measurement. Increase in airway resistance can be due to extrathoracic or intrathoracic causes. Intrathoracic causes may be extrapulmonary or intrapulmonary.

Obstruction may be caused by:

- Accumulation of material within lumen (e.g. a foreign body).
- Thickening of epithelial or subepithelial tissue (e.g. in oedema).
- External compression (e.g. by a tumour).
- Increased bronchomotor tone (e.g. in asthma).

Dynamic compliance

Lung compliance can be measured during tidal breathing. Intrapleural pressures are measured at the end of inspiration and expiration, when there is no airflow. This method is an unsatisfactory method for measuring airway compliance in patients with airway disease, as the abnormal region may continue inhaling while the rest of the lung has begun to exhale. This dynamic compliance decreases as breathing frequency increases because ventilation is distributed to airways that offer the least resistance.

Dynamic compliance is a test to measure airway resistance, not compliance. Resistance of the normal bronchial tree is mainly caused by large airways, so considerable small-airway disease can be present before alterations in total airway resistance are detected. Changes in resistance in the peripheral small airways cause uneven time constants and hence a change of dynamic compliance with breathing frequency; thus, it is possible to detect the presence of small-airway disease. In the presence of obstruction, the dynamic compliance falls as the frequency of breathing increases. This frequency dependence of compliance can provide evidence for narrowing of small lung airways.

Closing volume

Closing volume allows detection of early disease in the small airways (Fig. 9.7). Using the single-breath nitrogen washout method, four phases are recognized according to the composition of exhaled breath:

1. Pure deadspace.
2. Mixture of deadspace and alveolar gas.
3. Pure alveolar gas.
4. Towards the end of expiration, an abrupt increase in nitrogen concentration is seen.

The lung volume above residual volume at which closure of lung airways first occurs is indicated by the start of phase 4. Phase 4 is caused by preferential emptying of the apex of the lung after the lower zone airways have closed. Closing volume is usually expressed as a percentage of vital capacity. In young subjects, closing volume is approximately 10% of vital capacity and increases with age, being approximately 40% of vital capacity at 65 years of age. Small amounts of diseases in the small airways increase the closing volume (e.g. in chronic obstructive pulmonary disease).

Closing volume arises from regional differences in expansion ratios and is strongly associated with cigarette smoking.

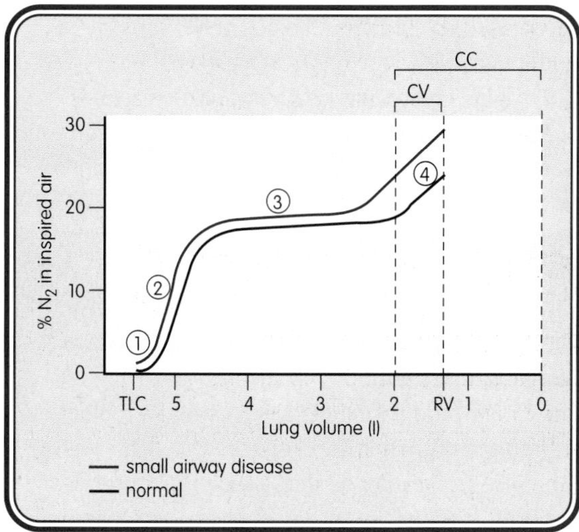

Fig. 9.7 Closing volume. Airways in lower lung zones close at low lung volumes and only those alveoli at top of lungs continue to empty. Because concentration of nitrogen in alveoli of upper zones is higher, the slope of the curve abruptly increases (phase 4). Phase 4 begins at larger lung volumes in individuals with even minor degrees of airway obstruction, increasing closing volume. CV = closing volume; CC = closing capacity; TLC = total lung capacity. (Courtesy of The Ciba Collection of Medical Illustrations, illustrated by Frank H. Netter, 1979.)

- What is the importance of spirometry in differentiating obstructive from restrictive disorders?
- Describe the differences between obstructive and restrictive lung disease.
- Describe how to accurately perform a PEFR test.
- List the uses and limitations of the PEFR test.
- Interpret and draw abnormal flow volume loops.
- Discuss the implications of an abnormal transfer factor test result.
- How can airway compliance and resistance be calculated?

ROUTINE INVESTIGATIONS

Haematology

In the associated figures, you will find some of the commonly performed haematological tests:

- Full blood count (Fig. 9.8).
- Differential white blood cell count (Fig. 9.9).
- Other haematological tests (Fig. 9.10).

Clinical chemistry

In the asscoiated figures, you will find some of the commonly performed biochemical tests:

- Blood tests (Fig. 9.11).
- Arterial blood gases (Fig. 9.12).

If malignancy is suspected, you should also perform liver function tests and test alkaline phosphatase as an indicator of metastases. In addition, endocrine tests should be performed for paraneoplastic manifestations.

Microbiology

Microbiological examination is possible with samples of sputum, bronchial aspirate, pleural aspirate, throat swabs, and blood. The aim of examination is to identify bacteria, viruses, or fungi.

Tests to request are microscopy, culture, and drug sensitivity. The microbiological findings should be interpreted in view of the whole clinical picture.

Differential white blood cell count			
		Diagnostic inference	
Cell type	**Normal values**	**Increased values**	**Decreased values**
white blood cell	$4–11 \times 10^9$/L	bacterial infections malignancy pregnancy	viral infections drugs systemic lupus erythematosus overwhelming bacterial infection
neutrophil	$2.5–7.5 \times 10^9$/L 60–70%	bacterial infections malignancy pregnancy	viral infections drugs systemic lupus erythematosus overwhelming bacterial infection
eosinophil	$0.04–0.44 \times 10^9$/L 1–4%	allergic reactions asthma sarcoidosis pneumonia	steroid therapy

Fig. 9.8 Tests performed and diagnostic inference for full blood count.

Bacterial samples

Blood culture

A blood culture should always be performed in patients with fever and lower respiratory tract infection. Collect a large volume of blood and divide it equally into two bottles of nutrient media, 20 mL of blood per culture bottle. Collect two or three cultures over 24 hours.

Blood cultures identify systemic bacterial and fungal infections. Results may be positive while sputum culture is negative.

Upper respiratory specimens

Microscopy is generally unhelpful because of the abundant commensals of the upper respiratory tract, which contaminate samples.

Differential white blood cell count			
		Diagnostic inference	
Cell type	**Normal values**	**Increased values**	**Decreased values**
white blood cell	4–11 × 10^9/L	bacterial infections malignancy pregnancy	viral infections drugs systemic lupus erythematosus overwhelming bacterial infection
neutrophil	2.5–7.5 × 10^9/L 60–70%	bacterial infections malignancy pregnancy	viral infections drugs systemic lupus erythematosus overwhelming bacterial infection
eosinophil	0.04–0.44 × 10^9/L 1–4%	allergic reactions asthma sarcoidosis pneumonia eosinophilic granulomatosus	steroid therapy
monocyte	0.2–0.8 × 10^9/L 5–10%	tuberculosis	chronic infection
lymphocyte	1.5–4.0 × 10^9/L 25–30%	infection cytomegalovirus infection toxoplasmosis tuberculosis	tuberculosis

Fig. 9.9 Tests performed and diagnostic inference for differential white blood cell count.

Other haematological tests			
		Diagnostic inference	
Test performed	**Normal values**	**Increased values**	**Decreased values**
C-reactive protein (CRP)	Normal < 4 mg/L Changes more rapidly than erythrocyte sedimentation rate	Acute infection; inflammation; same as erythrocyte sedimentation rate	Levels often normal in malignancy
Anti-streptolysin O (ASO) titre	Normal < 200 IU/mL	Confirms recent streptococcal infection	

Fig. 9.10 Other haematological tests and their diagnostic inference.

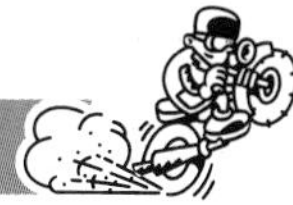

Throat specimens can be collected using Dacron or calcium alginate swab. The tonsils, posterior pharynx, and any ulcerated areas are sampled. Avoid contact with tongue and saliva, as this can inhibit identification of group A streptococci.

A sinus specimen is collected with a needle and syringe. The specimen is cultured for aerobic and anaerobic bacteria. Common pathogens of sinuses are *Streptococcus pneumoniae, Haemophilus influenzae, Mycoplasma catarrhalis, Staphylococcus aureus,* and anaerobes.

Lower respiratory specimens
Techniques used to collect samples include expectoration, cough induction with saline, bronchoscopy, bronchial alveolar lavage, transtracheal aspiration, and direct aspiration through the chest wall.

Biochemical blood tests			
		Diagnostic inference	
Test performed	**Normal values**	**Increased values**	**Decreased values**
urea	2.5–6.7 mmol/L	>7 mmol/L indicates a poor prognosis in pneumonia	
potassium	3.5–5.0 mmol/L		adrenocorticotropic hormone (ACTH) secreting tumour β-agonists
angiotensin converting enzyme (ACE)	10–70 U/L	sarcoidosis	
calcium	2.12–2.65 mmol/L	malignancy sarcoidosis squamous cell carcinoma of the lung	
glucose	3.5–5.5 mmol/L	adrenocorticotropic hormone (ACTH) secreting tumour long-term steroid use pancreatic dysfunction	

Fig. 9.11 Biochemical blood tests and their diagnostic inference.

Arterial blood gases			
		Diagnostic inference	
Test performed	**Normal values**	**Increased values**	**Decreased values**
pH	7.35–7.45	alkalosis hyperventilation	acidosis CO_2 retention
P_aO_2	>10.6 kPa		hypoxic
P_aCO_2	4.7–6.0 kPa	respiratory acidosis (if pH decreased)	respiratory alkalosis (if pH increased)
base excess	±2 mmol/L	metabolic alkalosis	metabolic acidosis
standardized bicarbonate	22–25 mmol/L	metabolic alkalosis	metabolic acidosis

Fig. 9.12 Tests performed and diagnostic inference for arterial blood gases

Sputum

Obtain the sample before antibiotic treatment is started. Collect into a sterile container, and inspect the sample macroscopically then microscopically to rule out contamination with upper airway bacteria.

Request Gram stain, Ziehl–Neelson stain, and anaerobic cultures. Culture on Lowenstein–Jensen medium to detect tuberculosis. A sputum sample is valuable in diagnosing suspected pneumonia, tuberculosis, and aspergillosis, or if the patient presents with an unusual clinical picture. Normal sputum is of limited usefulness; induced sputum is better.

Failure to isolate an organism from the sputum is not uncommon.

Resistance to commonly used antibiotics is often found in bacteria responsible for respiratory tract infections; therefore, antibiotic sensitivity testing is vital.

Viral samples

Because of the small size of viral particles, light microscopy provides little information: it is able to visualize viral inclusions and cytopathic effects of viral infection.

Viral serology

Viral serology is the most important group of tests in virology. Serological diagnoses are obtained when viruses are difficult to isolate and grow in cell culture.

Specimens should be collected early in the acute phase because viral shedding for respiratory viruses lasts 3–7 days; however, symptoms commonly persist for longer. A repeated sample should be collected 10 days later.

Specimens should be tested serologically only after the second sample has been received. The laboratory measures antibody type and titre in response to the viral infection: a four-fold increase in titre (rising titre) taken over 10 days is significant.

Viral serology also identifies the virus and its strain or serotype, and is able to evaluate the course of infection.

Coxiella bunetti, Mycoplasma pneumoniae, and *Legionella* are difficult to culture; therefore, results of serology must be used.

Cell culture

Specimens for cell cultures are obtained from nasal washings, throat swabs, nasal swabs, and sputum. Viruses cannot be cultured without living cells.

Fungal samples

Fungal infections may be serious, especially in the immunocompromised patient, where they can cause systemic infection; invasive fungal infections require blood culture. Repeated specimens from the site need to be taken to rule out contaminants in cultures.

Common fungal infections are *Candida* and *Aspergillus*. Microscopic identification may be difficult for *Aspergillus* because it is common in the environment. Culture is rarely helpful in identifying *Aspergillus;* the *Aspergillus precipitans* test is of more use.

Histopathology

Histopathology is the investigation and diagnosis of disease from the examination of tissues.

Histopathological examination of biopsy material

The histopathological examination is a vital test in cases of suspected malignancy, allowing a definitive diagnosis to be made. Biopsy material is obtained from:

- Bronchoscopy.
- Pleural biopsy.
- Lymph node biopsy.

Histological features of malignant neoplasms are:

- Loss of cellular differentiation.
- Abundant cells undergoing mitosis, many of which are abnormal.
- High nuclear:cytoplasm ratio.
- Cells or nuclei varying in shape and size.

Other uses of histopathology include identification of cellular responses to injury, acute inflammation and sequelae, chronic inflammation, disorders of growth, and thromboembolic disorders.

Cytological examination of sputum

Cytological examination is useful in diagnosing bronchial carcinoma and has the advantage of being a noninvasive, quick test; however, it is dependent upon adequate sputum production. Sputum is obtained by:

- Induction–inhalation of nebulized hypertonic saline.
- Transtracheal aspiration.
- Bronchoscopy.
- Bronchial washings.

Examine exfoliated cells (in the sputum, pleural fluid, bronchial brushings/washings, or fine-needle aspirate of lymph nodes and lesions) primarily for signs of malignancy.

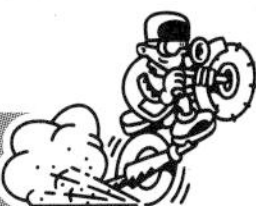

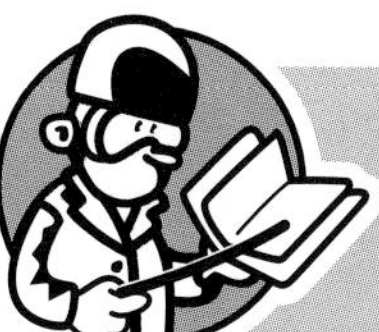

- Summarize the basic haematological tests performed.
- Describe the role of the microbiology laboratory in diagnosing infection.
- What is the main use of the histopathology laboratory in diagnosing respiratory disease?

IMAGING OF THE RESPIRATORY SYSTEM

Plain radiography

The plain film radiograph is of paramount importance in the evaluation of pulmonary disease. The standard radiographic examinations of the chest are described below.

Posteroanterior erect radiograph (PA chest)

In the posteroanterior erect radiograph, X-rays travel from the posterior of the patient to the film, which is held against the front of the patient (Fig. 9.13). The scapula can be rotated out of the way, and accurate assessment of cardiac size is possible. The radiograph is performed in the erect position because:

- Gas passes upwards, making the detection of pneumothorax easier.
- Fluid passes downwards, making pleural effusions easier to diagnose.
- Blood vessels in mediastinum and lung are represented accurately.

Lateral radiograph

Lateral views help to localize lesions seen in posteroanterior views; they also give good views of the mediastinum and thoracic vertebrae (Fig. 9.14). Valuable information can be obtained by comparison with older films, if available.

In women of reproductive age, radiography should be performed within 28 days of last menstruation.

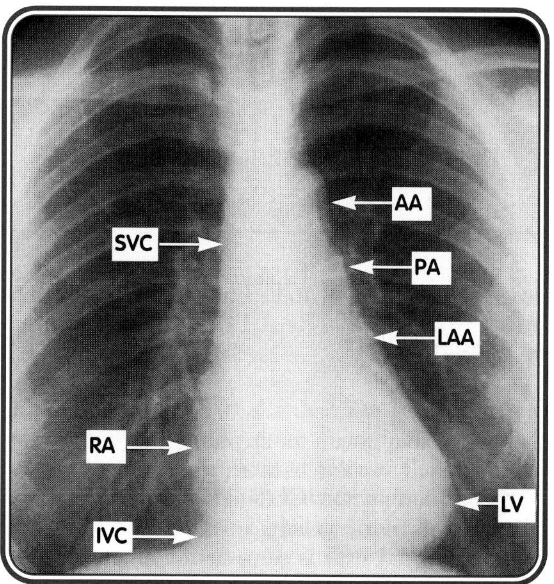

Fig. 9.13 Normal posteroanterior chest radiograph. The lungs are equally transradiant, the pulmonary vascular pattern is symmetrical. AA = aortic arch; SVC = superior vena cava; PA = pulmonary artery; LAA = left artrial appendage; RA = right atrium; LV = left ventricle; IVC = inferior vena cava. (Courtesy of Dr D. Sutton and Dr J. W. R. Young.)

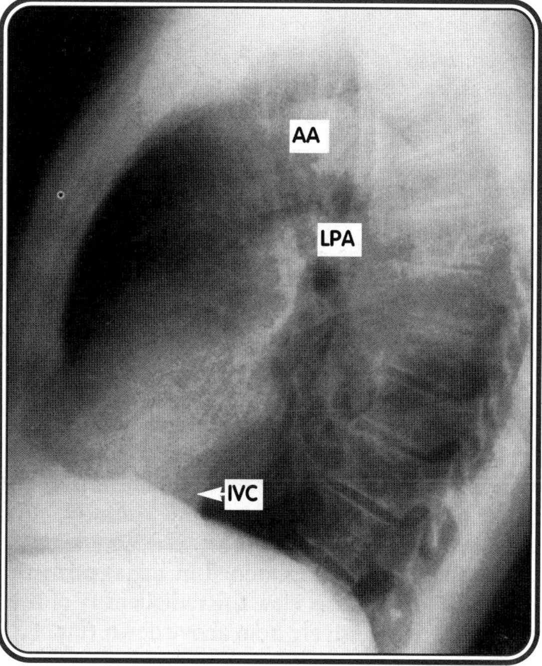

Fig. 9.14 Normal lateral chest radiograph. AA = aortic arch; LPA = left pulmonary artery; IVC = inferior vena cava. (Courtesy of Dr D. Sutton and Dr J. W. R. Young.)

Routine check

Always view chest radiographs on a viewing box and follow a set routine for reporting plain films.

Clinical data

Take down the following details:

- Patient's name.
- Age and sex.
- Clinical problem.
- Date of radiography.

Technical qualities

Note that radiographs contain right- or left-side markers.

With good penetration of X-rays, you should just be able to see the vertebral bodies through the cardiac shadow. In overpenetration, the lung fields appear too black. Conversely, in underpenetration, the lung fields appear too white.

Note the projection (AP, PA, or lateral; erect or supine). To deduce whether the patient was straight or rotated, compare the sternal ends of both clavicles.

With adequate inspiration, you should be able to count six ribs anterior to the diaphragm. Make sure that the whole lung field is included.

Heart and mediastinum

When examining the cardiac shadow, observe the position, size, and shape of the heart. Are the cardiac borders clearly visible?

Note whether the trachea is central or deviated to either side. Identify blood vessels and each hilum.

Other

Note the following points:

- Diaphragm—visible behind the heart. Costophrenic angles acute and sharp.
- Lungs—divide the lungs in to zones (upper, middle, and lower); compare like with like.
- Bones—ribs, clavicles, sternum, thoracic vertebra.
- Finally, recheck the apices, behind the heart, and hilar and retrodiaphragmatic regions.

Lateral radiograph

On a lateral radiograph, note the following:

- Diaphragms—right hemidiaphragm seen passing through heart border.
- Lungs—divide lungs into area in front, behind, and above the heart.
- Retrosternal space—an anterior mass will cause this space to be white.
- Fissures—horizontal fissure (faint white line that passes from midpoint of hilum to anterior chest wall); oblique fissure (passes from T4/5 through hilum to the anterior third of the diaphragm).
- Hilum.
- Bones—check vertebral bodies for shape size and density; check sternum.

Patterns of collapse

Atelectasis (collapse) is loss of volume of a lung, lobe, or segment for any cause. The most important mechanism is obstruction of a major bronchus by tumour, foreign body, or bronchial plug.

The silhouette sign can help localize the lesion (Fig. 9.15).

The silhouette sign	
Nonaerated area of lung	**Border that is obscured**
Right upper lobe	Right border of ascending aorta
Right middle lobe	Right heart border
Right lower lobe	Right diaphragm
Left upper lobe	Aortic knuckle and upper left cardiac border
Lingula of left lung	Left heart border
Left lower lobe	Left diaphragm

Fig. 9.15 The silhouette sign.

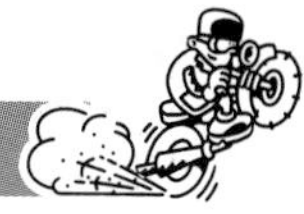

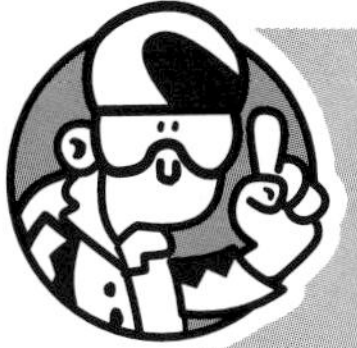

Follow a set pattern for reading radiographs; in that way, you will not miss anything.

Signs of lobar collapse

Signs of lobar collapse are:

- Decreased lung volume.
- Displacement of pulmonary fissures.
- Compensatory hyperinflation of remaining part of the ipsilateral lung.
- Elevation of hemidiaphragm on ipsilateral side.
- Mediastinal and hilar displacement. Trachea pulled to side of collapse.
- Radiopacity (white lung).
- Absence of air bronchogram.
- Posteroanterior and lateral radiographs are required. Compare with old films where available.

Specific signs related to lobe involvement

Upper lobe collapse

In the right lung, a posteroanterior film is most valuable in making the diagnoses; the collapsed lobe lies adjacent to mediastinum (Fig. 9.16A).

In the left lung, a lateral film is most valuable in making diagnoses; the lobe collapses superiomedially and anteriorly (Fig. 9.16B)

Lower lobe

Similar for both sides, collapse causes rotation and visualization of the oblique fissure on posteroanterior film.

Middle lobe collapse

Lateral film is most valuable in making diagnosis. Thin, wedge-shaped opacity between horizontal and oblique fissures is seen.

Alveolar processes

Alveolar processes are shown as fluffy ill-defined areas of opacity, appearing rapidly after the onset of symptoms (Figs 9.17 and 9.18). There are two patterns of distribution:

- Segmental or lobar distribution.
- Bat's-wing distribution.

Peripheral lung fields may be spared (e.g. in pulmonary oedema). Air bronchograms may be seen, because they are delineated by surrounding consolidated lung.

Interstitial patterns

Three types of interstitial pattern exist (linear, nodular, and honeycomb), and overlap may occur.

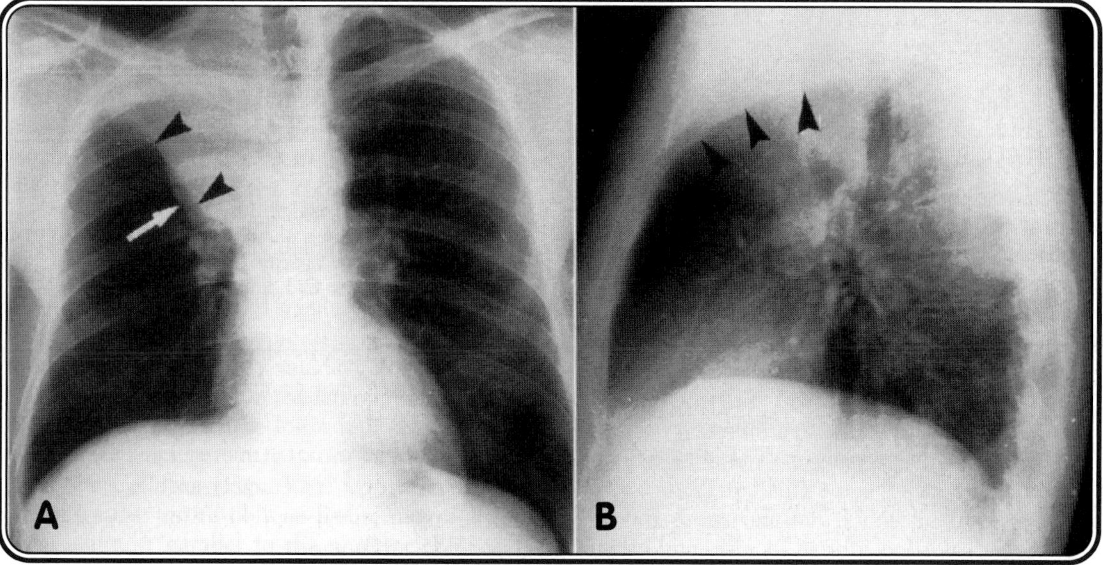

Fig. 9.16 (A and B) Right upper lobe collapse. The horizontal and oblique fissures (black arrowheads) are displaced. There is a mass (white arrow) at the right hilum. Courtesy of Dr D Sutton and Dr J W R Young.

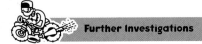

Radiological distribution of alveolar processes		
	Bat-wing pattern	
Segmental pattern	**Acute**	**Chronic**
pneumonia	pulmonary oedema	atypical pneumonia
pulmonary infarct	pneumonia	lymphoma
segmental collapse	pulmonary haemorrhage	sarcoidosis
alveolar cell carcinoma		pulmonary alveolar proteinosis
		alveolar cell carcinoma

Fig. 9.17 Radiological distribution of alveolar processes.

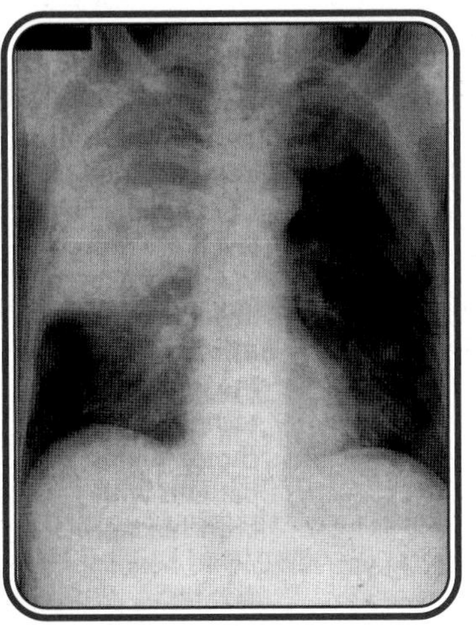

Fig. 9.18 Consolidation of the right upper lobe. (Courtesy of Professor C.D. Forbes and Dr W.F. Jackson.)

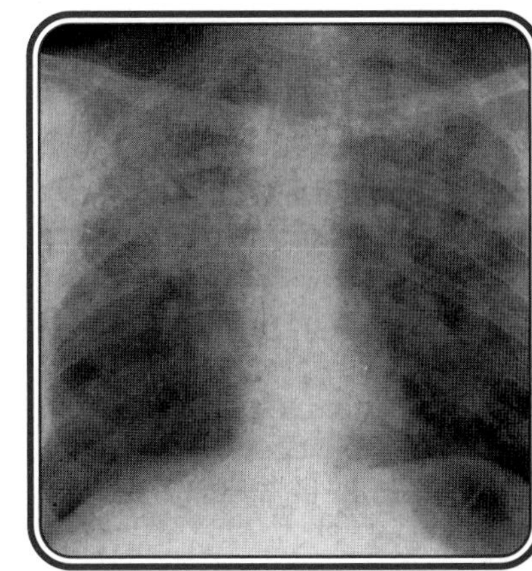

Fig. 9.19 Tuberculosis in a Greek immigrant to the UK. This film shows multiple areas of shadowing, especially in the upper lobes, and several lesions have started to cavitate. (Courtesy of Professor C.D. Forbes and Dr W.F. Jackson.)

Linear pattern

A linear pattern is seen as a network of fine lines running throughout the lungs. These lines represent thickened connective tissue and are termed Kerley A and B lines:

A Upper lobes—long, thin lines.

B Lower lobes—short, thin horizontal lines 1–2 cm in length.

Nodular pattern

This pattern is seen as numerous well-defined small nodules (1–5 mm) evenly distributed throughout the lung.

Honeycomb pattern

A honeycomb pattern indicates extensive destruction of lung tissue, with lung parenchyma replaced by thin-walled cysts. Pneumothorax may be present. Normal pulmonary vasculature is absent.

Pulmonary nodules

Solitary nodules

Solitary nodules can be caused by:

- Malignant tumour—bronchial carcinoma or secondary deposits.
- Infection—tuberculosis (Fig. 9.19) or pneumonia.
- Benign tumour—hamartoma.

It is important to take into account clinical history and compare with a past chest radiograph if available. You should be able to distinguish carcinoma from other causes:

- Size of lesion—if lesions is >4 cm diameter, be suspicious of malignancy.

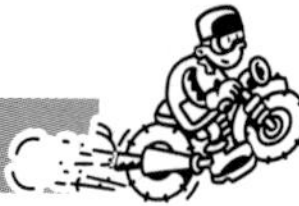

- Margin—an ill-defined margin suggests malignancy.
- Cavitation indicates infection or malignancy.
- Calcification—unlikely to be malignancy.
- Presence of air bronchogram—sign of consolidation, not malignancy.

Multiple pulmonary nodules

Metastases are usually seen as well-defined nodules varying in size, which are more common at the periphery of lower lobes (Fig. 9.20); cavitation may be present. Abscesses are cavitated with thick and irregular wall. Cysts are often large.

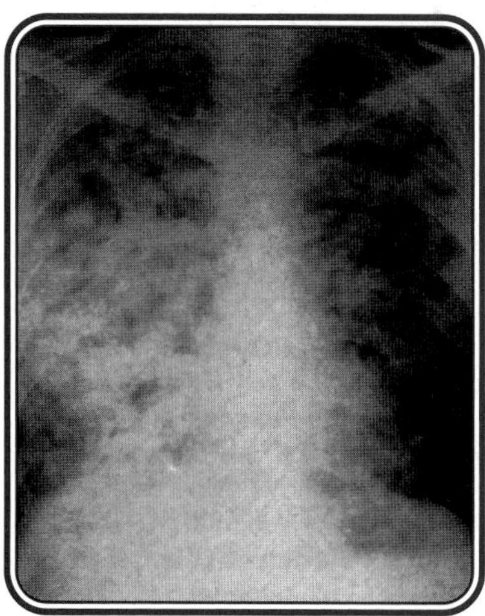

Fig. 9.20 Snowstorm mottling in both lung fields. In this case, the underlying diagnosis was testicular seminoma, with disseminated haematogenous metastases. (Courtesy of Professor C.D. Forbes and Dr W.F. Jackson.)

Other nodules:

- Rheumatoid nodules.
- Wegener's granulomatous.
- Multiple arteriovenous malformations.

Hilar masses

Normal hilar complex includes:

- Proximal pulmonary arteries and bifurcations.
- Bronchus.
- Pulmonary veins.
- Lymph nodes, not seen unless enlarged.

Hilar size varies from person to person, so enlargement is difficult to diagnose (Fig. 9.21). Radiological features of the hilum are:

- Concave lateral margin.
- Equal radiopacity.
- Left hilum lies higher than right.

Posteroanterior film is most valuable in assessing hilar shadow, but you must always consult the lateral film. Technical qualities of the film need to be adequately assessed before conclusions can be made because

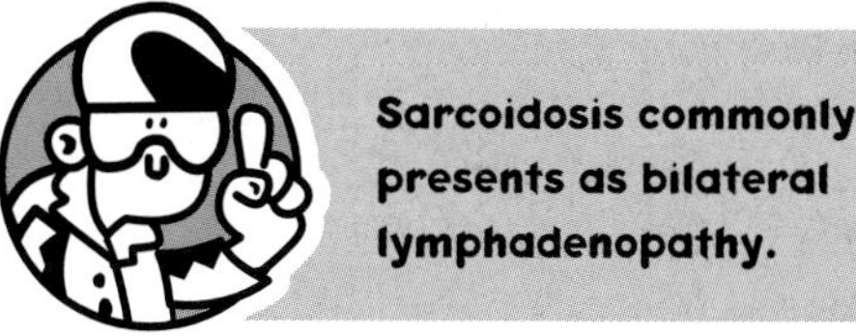

Sarcoidosis commonly presents as bilateral lymphadenopathy.

Causes of hilar enlargement

	Bilateral enlargement	
Unilateral enlargement	**Enlarged lymph nodes**	**Enlarged vessels**
bronchial carcinoma	lymphomas	left-to-right cardiac shunts
metastatic malignancy	sarcoidosis	pulmonary arterial hypertension
lymphomas	cystic fibrosis	chronic obstructive pulmonary disease
primary tuberculosis	infectious mononucleosis	left heart failure
sarcoidosis	leukaemia	pulmonary embolism
pulmonary embolus		
pulmonary valve stenosis		

Fig. 9.21 Unilateral and bilateral causes of hilar enlargement.

patient rotation commonly mimics hilar enlargement.

Mediastinal masses

Characteristics of mediastinal masses include:

- Sharp concave margin.
- No air bronchogram.

Silhouette sign and lateral films are of most use in assessing mediastinal masses. Localization is important in predicting the nature of the mass. Mediastinal masses are frequently asymptomatic. Consider lesions according to their anatomical position (Fig. 9.22). It is advisable to perform computerized tomography (CT) where there is a doubt as to the nature of the lesion.

Anterior mediastinal masses

Characteristics of anterior mediastinal masses are:

- Hilar structures still visible.
- Mass merges with the cardiac border.
- A mass passing into the neck is not seen above the clavicles.
- Small anterior mediastinal masses are difficult to see on posteroanterior films.

Middle mediastinal masses

Characteristics of middle mediastinal masses are:

- Mass merges with hila and cardiac border.
- The majority of masses are caused by enlarged lymph nodes.

Posterior mediastinal masses

Characteristics of posterior mediastinal masses are:

- Cardiac border and hila are seen.
- Posterior aorta obscured.
- Vertebral changes may be present.

Pleural lesions

Pneumothorax

Pneumothorax is usually obvious on normal inspiratory posteroanterior films. Look carefully at upper zones, because air accumulates first here; you will see an area devoid of lung markings (black lung), with the lung edge outlined by air in the pleural space. Small pneumothoracies can be identified on the expiratory film and may be missed in the supine film.

Tension pneumothorax

Tension pneumothorax is seen as a displacement of the mediastinum and trachea to the contralateral side, depressed ipsilateral diaphragm, and increased space between the ribs.

Pleural effusions

Posteroanterior erect radiography is performed. The observed appearance is not related to the nature of the fluid. The absence of an air bronchogram points to a pleural effusion and away from malignancy.

Classically, there is a radiopaque mass at the base of the lung and blunting of the costophrenic angle, with the pleural meniscus higher laterally than medially. Large effusions can displace the mediastinum contralaterally. A horizontal upper border implies that a pneumothorax is also present.

Mesothelioma

Mesothelioma is a malignant tumour of the pleura, which may present as discrete pleural deposits or as a

Mediastinal masses		
Anterior masses	**Middle masses**	**Posterior masses**
retrosternal thyroid	bronchial carcinoma	neurogenic tumour
thymic mass	lymphoma	paravertebral abscess
dermoid cyst	sarcoidosis	oesophageal lesions
lymphomas	primary tuberculosis	aortic aneurysm
aortic aneurysm	bronchogenic cyst	

Fig. 9.22 Mediastinal masses.

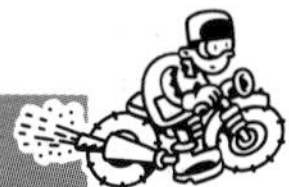

localized lesion.

Thickened pleura is observed with irregular medial margin on radiography; in 50% of cases, pleural plaques are elsewhere. Pleural effusions are common, usually containing blood (Fig. 9.23). Rib destruction is uncommon.

Vascular patterns

Normal vascular pattern

Lung markings are vascular in nature. Arteries branch vertically to upper and lower lobes. On erect films, upper lobe vessels are smaller than the lower lobe vessels. It is difficult to see vessels in the peripheral one-third of lung fields.

Pulmonary venous hypertension

On erect films, upper lobe vessels are larger than the lower lobe vessels. Pulmonary venous hypertension is associated with oedema and pleural effusions.

Pulmonary arterial hypertension

Pulmonary arterial hypertension is seen as bilateral hilar enlargement associated with long-standing pulmonary disease.

Pulmonary plethora

Pulmonary plethora is an increase in size and number of pulmonary vessels with vessels seen in peripheral one-third of lung fields. It is associated with left-to-right cardiac shunts.

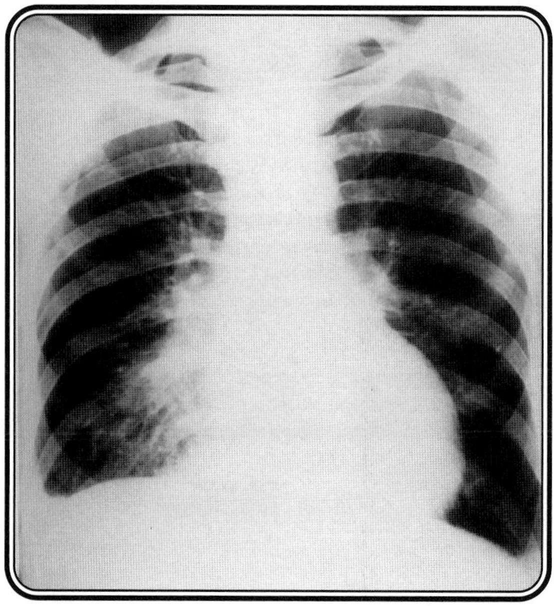

Fig. 9.23 Small pleural effusions. Both costophrenic angles are blunted. (Courtesy of Dr D. Sutton and Dr J.W.R. Young.)

Pulmonary oligaemia

Pulmonary oligaemia shows as a decrease in the size and number of pulmonary vessels, resulting in blackness to the lung fields. It is associated with right-to-left shunts.

Ventilation:perfusion scans and angiography

Radioisotope scans are used to depict pulmonary perfusion and ventilation. Ventilation:perfusion scans are the screening test of choice for the detection of pulmonary embolism. The finding of a nonperfused but ventilated zone is suggestive of pulmonary embolus.

Poor perfusion with poor ventilation occurs in conditions such as asthma and emphysema; pulmonary embolus cannot be diagnosed if such a pattern is obtained. Pulmonary angiography is then indicated.

Pulmonary angiography

Indications:

- When a ventilation:perfusion scan is inconclusive for pulmonary embolus.
- Before surgery or thrombolysis for pulmonary embolism.

Pulmonary angiography is more accurate than a ventilation:perfusion scan. The test is performed by injection of contrast media through a catheter introduced in the main pulmonary artery using the Seldinger technique. Obstructed vessels or filling defects can be seen clearly and emboli show as filling defects.

Computerized tomography

Computerized tomography (CT) is the imaging modality of choice for mediastinal and many pulmonary conditions. CT scans provide detailed cross-sectional images of the thorax. The images can be electronically modified to display different tissues (e.g. by using a bone setting compared with a soft-tissue setting).

The patient passes through a rotating gantry which has X-ray tubes on one side and a set of detectors on the other. Information from the detectors is analysed and displayed as a two-dimensional image displayed on visual display units, then recorded.

CT gives a dose of radiation approximately 100 times that of a standard plain film chest radiograph.

Applications of computerized tomography

Detection of pulmonary nodules

CT can evaluate the presence of metastases in a patient with known malignancy; however, it cannot distinguish between benign and malignant masses.

Mediastinal masses

CT is a useful technique in searching for lymphadenopathy in a person with primary lung carcinoma.

Carcinoma of the lung

CT can evaluate the size of a lung carcinoma, and detect mediastinal extension and staging.

Pleural lesions

CT is effective at detecting small pleural effusions and identifying pleural plaques (Fig. 9.24).

Vascular lesions

Contrast studies allow imaging of vascular lesions (e.g. aortic aneurysms).

High-resolution computerized tomography

High-resolution CT is useful in imaging diffuse lung disease: thinner sections show greater lung detail (Fig. 9.25). Contrast medium is not used.

Applications of high-resolution computerized tomography

Bronchiectasis

High-resolution CT has replaced bronchography. In dilated bronchi, the technique can show:

- Collapse.
- Scarring.
- Consolidation.

Interstitial lung disease

High-resolution CT is more specific than plain film radiography. Disorders that have specific appearances on high-resolution CT include sarcoidosis, occupational lung disease, and interstitial pneumonia.

High-resolution CT can be used for biopsy guidance.

Atypical infections

High-resolution CT provides diagnosis earlier than using plain chest radiography and is useful in monitoring disease and response to treatment. It also provides good delineation of disease activity and destruction.

High-resolution CT is used in imaging of patients with AIDS (e.g. PCP).

Diagnosis of lymphangitis carcinomatosa

High-resolution CT can be used in the diagnosis of lymphangitis carcinomatosa.

Magnetic resonance imaging

Magnetic resonance (MR) imaging uses the magnetic properties of the hydrogen atom to produce images.

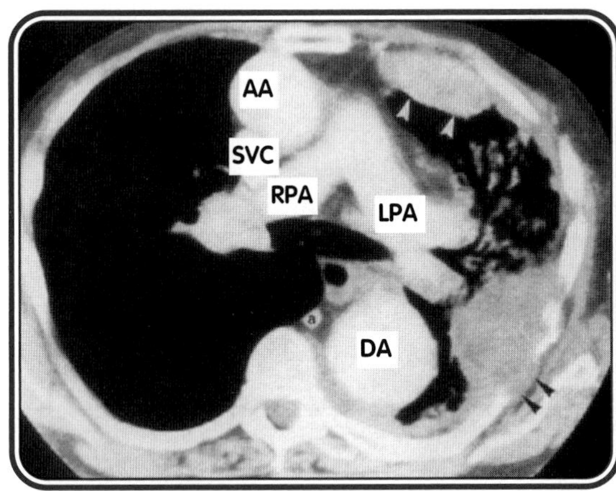

Fig. 9.24 CT scan of a pleural mass. Enhanced CT scan at level of bifurcation of main pulmonary artery. The left lung is surrounded by pleural masses (arrowheads), and the posterior mass is invading the chest wall. The vascular anatomy of the mediastinum is well shown. a = azygos vein; RPA = right pulmonary artery; LPA = left pulmonary artery; AA = ascending aorta; SVC = superior vena cava; DA = descending aorta. (Courtesy of Dr D. Sutton and Dr J.W.R. Young.)

Technical differences between CT and HRCT		
slice	**CT**	**HRCT**
thickness	5–10 mm	1 mm
spacing	10 mm	10–15 mm

Fig. 9.25 Technical differences between CT and high-resolution CT (HRCT).

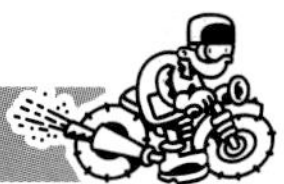

MR gives excellent imaging of soft tissues and the heart, but has limited use in the respiratory system. Flowing blood does not provide a signal for MR imaging, and vascular structures appear as hollow tubes. MR imaging can be used to differentiate masses around the aorta or in the hilar regions. It has the advantage of not using ionizing radiation and that the body may be viewed in transverse, sagittal, or coronal planes; however, the equipment, running costs, and maintenance costs are high.

- **Describe how to read a posteroanterior plain film chest radiograph.**
- **What are the differences between interstitial and alveoli appearances?**
- **What is the silhouette sign? What are its uses?**
- **Describe the differences between collapse and consolidation on chest radiographs.**
- **What are the uses and limitations of CT and MR imaging in respiratory imaging?**

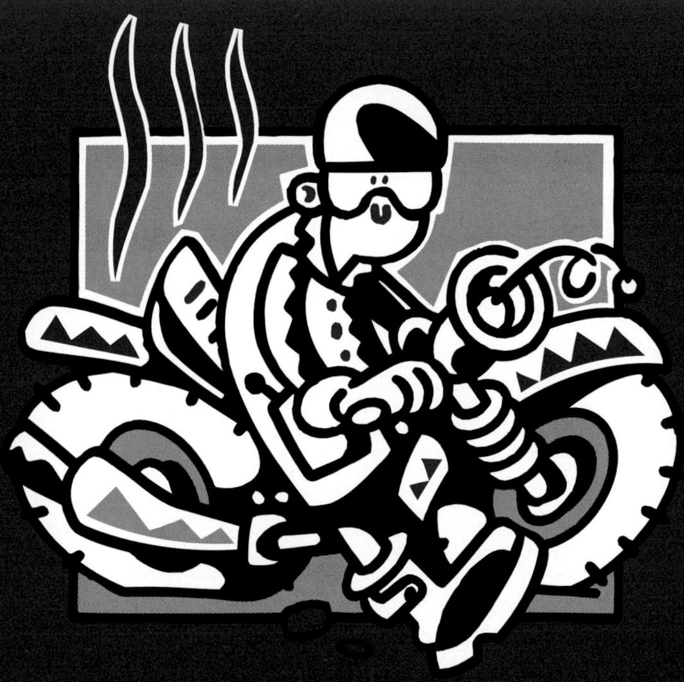

BASIC PATHOLOGY

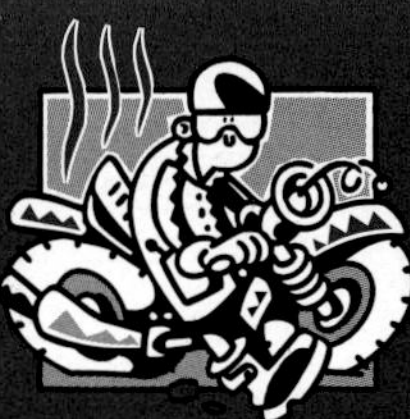

10. Pathology of the Upper Respiratory Tract

THE NOSE AND NASOPHARYNX

Inflammatory conditions

Infectious rhinitis (common cold)

The common cold is a highly contagious self-limiting condition, with the highest incidence in children. It is caused by a number of viral infections:

- Rhinovirus.
- Adenovirus.
- Parainfluenza virus.
- Respiratory syncitial virus.
- Influenza virus.

Symptoms of the common cold are nasal obstruction, rhinorrhoea, and sneezing.

Pathology

Acute inflammation with oedema, glandular hypersecretion, and loss of surface epithelium.

Treatment

Treat symptomatically with decongestants and analgesics. Antibiotics are useless because of viral aetiology.

Chronic rhinitis

Chronic rhinitis may follow an acute inflammatory episode. Predisposing factors include inadequate drainage of sinuses, nasal obstruction caused by polyps, and enlargement of the adenoids.

Allergic rhinitis

Allergic rhinitis is a common condition, affecting up to 30% of the Western population (Fig. 10.1). It is classified as either seasonal rhinitis (hayfever) or perennial rhinitis.

Seasonal rhinitis

Has a maximum prevalence in patients aged 10–20 years. It occurs during summer months. Approximately 20% of patients with allergic rhinitis also suffer from asthma.

Perennial rhinitis

The incidence of perennial rhinitis decreases with age. It is most common in patients aged 10–30 years. Four types of perennial rhinitis exist:

- Perennial rhinitis—mainly caused by Der p1 allergen in faecal particles of the house dust mite. Proteins from the urine and saliva of domestic pets also cause problems.
- Perennial nonallergic rhinitis with eosinophilia—no allergic extrinsic cause has been identified.
- Vasomotor rhinitis—patient may be suffering from nonspecific nasal hyperreactivity.
- Nasal polyps—causing nasal obstruction.

Aetiology

Rhinitis is caused by hypersensitivity to allergens; commonest allergens are highly soluble proteins or glycoproteins (e.g. from pollens, moulds, and dust mite).

Pathology

Symptoms are caused by a type I IgE mediated hypersensitivity reaction. IgE fixes onto mast cells in nasal mucous membranes. Upon re-exposure to allergen, an antigen–antibody reaction takes place on the surface of the mast cells. Mast cells degranulate and release histamine and leukotrienes.

Clinical features of rhinitis	
Seasonal rhinitis	**Perennial rhinitis**
Sneezing	Sneezing
Watery nasal discharge	Watery nasal discharge
Nasal irritation	Nasal blockage
Watery eyes	

Fig. 10.1 Clinical features of rhinitis.

Investigation

Diagnosis of rhinitis is clinical. Skin prick tests, nasal smears, and provocation tests can be used. Blood tests are:

- PRIST (plasma radioimmunosorbent test)—measures total plasma IgE levels.
- RAST (radioallergosorbent test)—measures specific serum IgE antibody.

Treatment

Treatment is by allergen avoidance and drug treatment with antihistamines, decongestants, anti-inflammatory drugs (e.g. corticosteroids), and sodium cromoglycate.

Acute sinusitis

Sinusitis is an inflammatory process involving the lining of paranasal sinuses. The maxillary sinus is most commonly clinically infected. The majority of infections are rhinogenic in origin and are classified as either acute or chronic.

Aetiology

The causes of acute sinusitis are:

- Secondary bacterial infection (by *Streptococcus pneumonia* or *Haemophilus influenzae*), often after upper respiratory tract viral infection.
- Dental extraction or infection.
- Swimming and diving.
- Fractures involving sinuses.

Clinical features

Symptoms occur over several days with yellow–green nasal discharge, malaise, sinus tenderness, pain that is worse on bending, and disturbed sense of smell. Acute sinusitis does not cause simple cheek swelling; if present, further investigation is needed.

Pathology

Hyperaemia and oedema of the mucosa occurs. Blockage of sinus otia and mucus production increases. Cilia stop beating; therefore, stasis of secretions leads to secondary infection.

Investigations

The investigations are:

- Blood—increased white cell count and erythrocyte sedimentation rate.
- Culture pus from nose.
- Radiology of paranasal sinuses—CT scan.

Treatment

Medical treatment is by analgesia, broad-acting antibiotic for 7 days, and a decongestant. Discourage smoking and alcohol consumption. If no response to two regimens of antibiotics, refer to ear, nose, and throat (ENT) specialist.

Chronic sinusitis

Chronic sinusitis is a chronic inflammation of the sinuses, usually occurring after recurrent acute sinusitis. Many patients are heavy smokers and work in dusty environments (Fig. 10.2).

Predisposing factors of sinusitis			
Acute factors		Chronic factors (same as for acute, in addition to the following)	
Local	**General**	**Local**	**General**
Pre-existing rhinitis	Debilitation	Pre-existing rhinitis	Debilitation
Nasal polyps	Immunocompromised	Anatomical variants	Atmospheric irritants
Nasal foreign bodies	Mucociliary disorders	Dental disease	
URTI		Recurrent sinus infection	
Nasal tumours			

Fig. 10.2 Predisposing factors of sinusitis.

Clinical features

Clinical features include a yellow–brown postnasal discharge, a foul taste in the mouth, blocked nose, pain over the bridge of the nose, and a frontal headache.

Pathology

The pathology of chronic sinusitis includes:

- An increase in vascular permeability.
- Oedema and hypertrophy of the mucosa.
- Goblet-cell hyperplasia.
- Chronic cellular infiltrate.
- Ulceration of the epithelium, resulting in granulation tissue formation.
- Irreversible disease of the sinus mucosa.

Investigations

The investigations are through sinus radiographs, high definition coronal section CT, and diagnostic endoscopy.

Treatment

This condition is difficult to treat. Treatments are:

- Medical—broad-acting antibiotics and decongestant.
- Surgical—antral lavage, inferior meatal intranasal antrostomy, and functional endoscopic sinus surgery.

Kartagener's syndrome

Kartagener's syndrome is a congenital mucociliary disorder caused by the absence of the ciliary protein dynein and characterized by sinusitis, dextrocardia, and bronchitis. Complications include recurrent sinusitis, otitis media, bronchitis, and infertility.

Necrotizing lesions

Mucomycosis

Mucomycosis is an opportunistic infection caused by *Rhizopus oryzae.* Spread of infection is by the inhalation of spores. The primary sites of infection are nasal turbinates; patients present with sinusitis, inflammation of the orbit with proptosis, and meningoencephalitis.

Pathology

An acute inflammatory reaction occurs, with invasion of blood vessels producing thrombi and ischaemic necrosis. Death occurs within several days of diagnosis.

Predisposing factors

Predisposing factors include diabetes mellitus (especially if acidotic), extensive burns, leukaemia, and lymphoma.

Treatment

Treatment is by systemic amphotericin B. Prognosis is poor.

Wegener's granulomatosis

Wegener's granulomatosis is a rare, necrotizing vasculitis of unknown aetiology affecting small arteries and veins. It classically involves the upper and lower respiratory tract and the kidneys (glomerulonephritis). Mucosal thickening and ulceration occur, producing the clinical features of rhinorrhoea, cough, haemoptysis, and dyspnoea.

If untreated, mortality after 2 years is 93%, but the disease responds well to cyclophosphamide 150–200 mg daily.

Malignant midline granuloma of the nose

Malignant midline granuloma of the nose is a T cell lymphoma that presents as an ulcerated lesion and which progressively destroys midfacial structures. The lesion consists of proliferating lymphocytes and macrophages. Treatment is by radiotherapy combined with surgical excision.

Neoplasms

Nasopharyngeal angiofibroma

Nasopharyngeal angiofibroma is a benign neoplasm occurring in childhood affecting boys more than girls. It arises unilaterally and frequently coincides with a pubertal growth spurt. The disease presents with epistaxis and nasal obstruction.

Pathology

An enlarging vascular tumour is present, which contains a fibrous component. The disease can cause

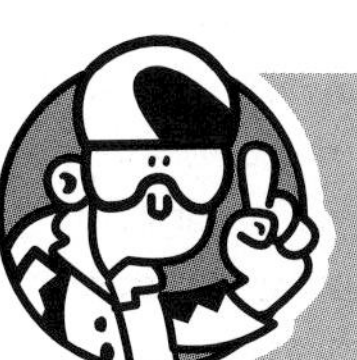

True benign tumours of the nose are uncommon.

bone erosion and destruction by pressure atrophy. The sphenopalatine foramen is always involved.

Investigations and treatment

Investigate by MR imaging or CT scanning. Surgical treatment is possible, but vascularity may be a problem. Radiotherapy is used only in unresectable cases.

Inverted papilloma

Inverted papilloma is a benign epithelial tumour affecting men and women in the ratio of 5:1. The disease accounts for 5% of all nasal tumours. Aetiology is unclear.

Pathology

A papilliferous exophytic mass arises from the lateral walls of nose. The epithelium invaginates into underlying tissue, and microcyst formation occurs resembling nasal polyps. Less than 2% of tumours undergo malignant change.

Plasmacytoma

Plasmacytoma is a malignant extramedullary lymphoma composed of plasma cells. It arises in the nasal septum or lateral wall and can occur as part of multiple myeloma. Patients present with an obstructing mass and localized mucosal thickening. Ten-year survival rates are greater than 50%.

Olfactory neuroblastoma

Olfactory neuroblastoma is a malignant epithelial tumour. It affects all ages, and there is an equal incidence in men and women; the median age of onset is 50 years. Olfactory neuroblastoma arises from neural crest stem cells. It presents with nasal obstruction and epistaxis. Neoplasm is unique to the nose, occurring only in the upper nasal cavity and always involving the cribriform plate.

Nasopharyngeal carcinoma

Nasopharyngeal carcinoma is commonly a poorly differentiated squamous cell carcinoma. Men are more likely to suffer from the disease, which usually presents in patients aged 50–70 years. The disease is common in South East Asia, and is associated with the Epstein–Barr virus and salted preserved fish.

Nasopharyngeal carcinoma presents with epistaxis, nasal obstruction, or a neck lump. Seventy per cent of patients have metastatic lymph node involvement at presentation. Overall 5-year survival rate is 35%. Treatment is by radiotherapy.

- **Describe the pathology and management of allergic rhinitis.**
- **List the clinical features of rhinitis.**
- **List the differences between acute and chronic sinusitis.**
- **Describe the presentation and management of nasal neoplasms.**

THE LARYNX

Inflammatory conditions

Acute laryngitis

Acute laryngitis is a common condition, usually caused by viral infection, although secondary infection with streptococci or staphylococci can occur. Patients typically present with a hoarse voice and feel unwell. Rarely, dysphagia and pain on phonation occur.

Acute laryngitis is usually a self-limiting condition. If symptoms persist, refer to an ENT specialist.

Chronic laryngitis

Chronic laryngitis is inflammation of the larynx and trachea associated with excessive smoking, continued vocal abuse, and excessive alcohol.

The mucous glands are swollen and the epithelium hypertrophied. Heavy smoking leads to squamous metaplasia of the larynx. Biopsy is mandatory to rule out malignancy. Management is directed at avoidance of aetiological factors.

Laryngotracheobronchitis (croup) and acute epiglottitis

The features of laryngotracheobronchitis (croup) and acute epiglottitis are described in Fig. 10.3.

Laryngotracheobronchitis (croup) and acute epiglottitis		
	Croup	**Epiglottitis**
Aetiology	Viral	Bacterial
Organism	Parainfleunza, respiratory syncitial virus	Group B haemophilus influenza
Age range	6 months to 3 years	3–7 years
Onset	Gradual over days	Sudden over hours
Cough	Severe barking	Minimal
Temperature	Pyrexia <38.5°C	Pyrexia >38.5°C
Stridor	Harsh	Soft
Drooling	No	Yes
Voice	Hoarse	Reluctant to speak
Able to drink	Yes	No
Active	Yes	No, completely still
Mortality	Low	High

Fig. 10.3 Features of laryngotracheobronchitis (croup) and acute epiglottitis.

Pathology

In laryngotracheobronchitis, there is necrosis of epithelium and formation of an extensive fibrous membrane on the trachea and main bronchi. Oedema of the subglottic area occurs, with subsequent danger of laryngeal obstruction.

In acute epiglottitis, there is an acute inflammatory oedema and infiltration by neutrophil polymorphs. No mucosal ulceration occurs.

Treatment

To treat laryngotracheobronchitis, keep the patient calm and hydrated. Nurse in a warm room in an upright position. Drug treatment, if required, includes steroids, oxygen, and nebulized adrenaline.

Acute epiglottitis is a medical emergency. Call for paediatric team, anaesthetist, and ENT surgeon. Never attempt to visualize the epiglottis. Keep calm and reassure the patient. Never leave the patient alone.

Reactive nodules

Reactive nodules are common, small, inflammatory polyps usually measuring less than 10 mm in diameter. They are also known as singer's nodules. They present in patients aged 40–50 years and are more common in men. Reactive nodules are caused by excessive untrained use of vocal cords. Patients present with hoarseness of the voice.

Pathology

Keratosis develops at the junction of the anterior and middle thirds of the vocal cord on each side. Oedematous myxoid connective tissue is covered by squamous epithelium. The reactive nodules may become painful because of ulceration.

Hyperplasia and keratosis

Hyperplasia

Benign hyperplasia

Benign hyperplasia is usually a response to injury; it is a thickening of the epithelium.

Atypical hyperplasia

Atypical hyperplasia is where individual cells have nuclear abnormalities. Atypical cells do not replace the full thickness of the epithelium.

Benign keratosis

Keratosis is caused by formation of keratohyaline granules in the cytoplasm of superficial epithelial cells.

Cytoplasm is replaced, the nucleus disappears, and only keratin is left. If the nucleus is retained, the condition is known as parakeratosis. Patients present with raised whitish plaques on vocal cord surfaces. Synonyms for this condition include hyperkeratosis, leukoplakia, chronic hypertrophic laryngitis, and pachyderma laryngitis.

Squamous cell carcinoma

Squamous cell carcinoma is the commonest malignant tumour of the larynx affecting men and women in the ratio of 5:1. The disease accounts for 1% of all male malignancies. Incidence increases with age, with peak incidence occurring in those aged 60–70 years. Patients presents with hoarseness, although dyspnoea and stridor are late signs.

Predisposing factors

Predisposing factors include alcohol and tobacco smoke (the condition is very rare in nonsmokers).

Pathology

Carcinoma of vocal cord appears first, which subsequently ulcerates. Carcinoma of larynx infiltrates and destroys surrounding tissue. Infection may follow ulceration.

Investigations

Investigations include chest radiography, full blood count, serum analysis (liver function tests for metastatic disease), direct laryngoscopy under general anaesthesia, and full paraendoscopy and bronchoscopy.

Treatment

Treatment is by radiotherapy and surgery.

Prognosis

Prognosis is poor if the tumour involves the upper part of the larynx or subglottic region.

Squamous papilloma

Squamous papilloma is the commonest benign tumour of larynx; it usually occurs in children aged 0–5 years, but can also affect adults.

Aetiology

The disease is caused by infection of the epithelial cells with human papillomavirus (HPV) types 6 and 11, and can be acquired at birth from maternal genital warts.

Clinical features

Clinical features include hoarseness of the voice and an abnormal cry (Fig. 10.4).

Pathology

Tumours may be sessile or pedunculated. They can occur anywhere on the vocal cords. Lesions are commoner at points of airway constriction (Figs 10.5A and B).

Investigation

Investigation include endoscopy, followed by histological confirmation.

Treatment

Surgical treatment is by removal with a carbon dioxide laser. Medical treatment is with alpha interferon.

Assume a hoarse voice is caused by laryngeal carcinoma until proved otherwise.

Features of squamous papilloma		
	Adult	**Child**
Incidence	Rare	Common
Number of lesions	Single mass	Multiple masses
Outcome	Surgical removal	Regress spontaneously at puberty

Fig. 10.4 Features of squamous papilloma.

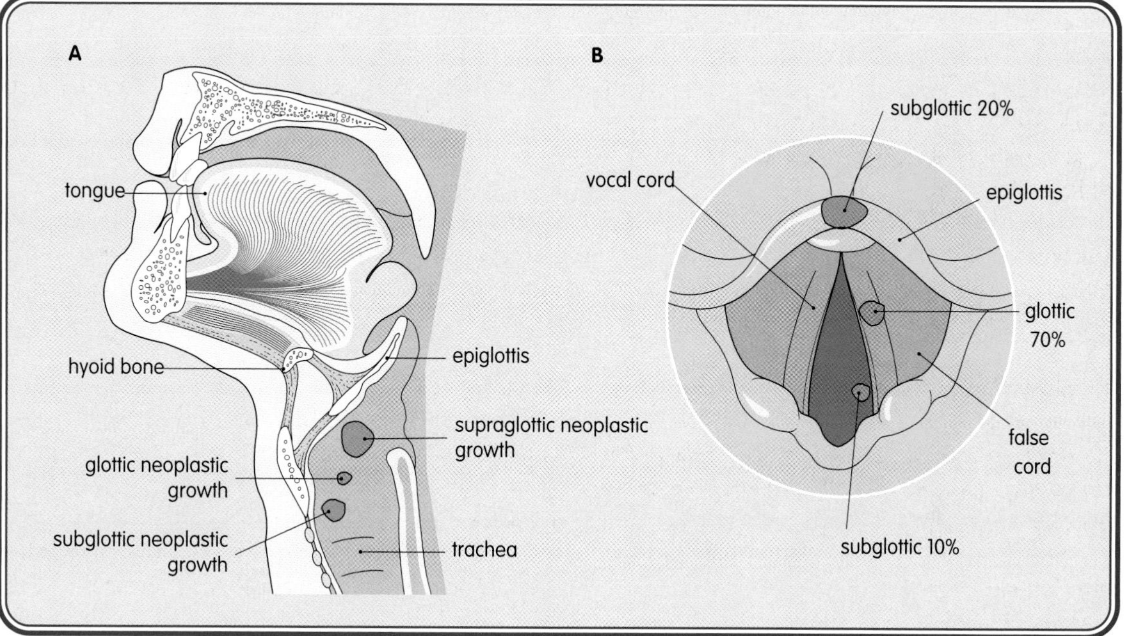

Fig. 10.5 Position of laryngeal carcinoma (A) and as seen on mirror examination (B).

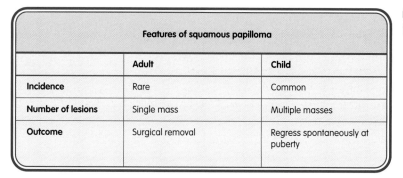

- **Describe the differences between croup and acute epiglottitis.**
- **Name the common tumours of the larynx.**
- **List the causes of hoarseness of the voice.**

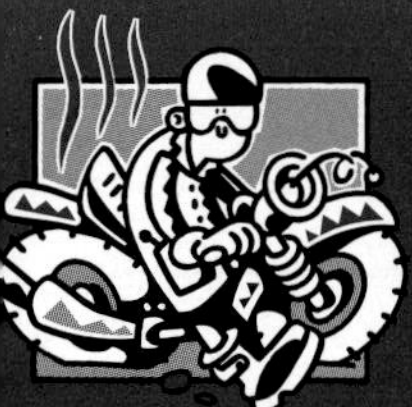

11. Pathology of the Lungs

CONGENITAL ABNORMALITIES

Congenital cysts

The respiratory system is an outgrowth of the ventral wall of the foregut. Bronchogenic cysts may result from abnormal budding of the tracheobronchial tree. They are lined by bronchial elements: cartilage, smooth muscle, and ciliated respiratory epithelium. Cysts are classified according to position:

- Central (mediastinal)—85%.
- Peripheral (intrapulmonary)—15%.

Cysts are usually single, spherical or oval, unilocular masses. They are mainly asymptomatic and can present at any age, although they are more common in men. Surgical excision is recommended. Radiologically, it is impossible to differentiate between a bronchogenic cyst and malignancy (Fig. 11.1).

Lobar sequestrations

Lobar sequestrations are masses of pulmonary tissue that do not communicate anatomically with the tracheobronchial tree (Fig. 11.2).

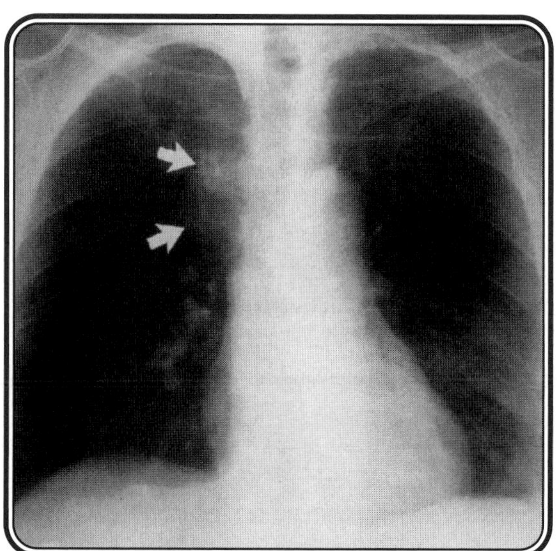

Fig. 11.1 Radiograph of a bronchogenic cyst. There is a right paratracheal mass (arrows). Courtesy of Dr D Sutton and Dr J W R Young.

Vascular abnormalities

Vascular abnormalities include absent pulmonary artery trunk, absent unilateral pulmonary artery, pulmonary artery stenosis, pulmonary arteriovenous malformations, anomalous origin of the left pulmonary artery, and anomalous pulmonary venous drainage.

Congenital lobar emphysema

Lobar emphysema is an overdistension of a lobe (usually an upper lobe) caused by intermittent bronchial obstruction. Symptoms in early life are caused by

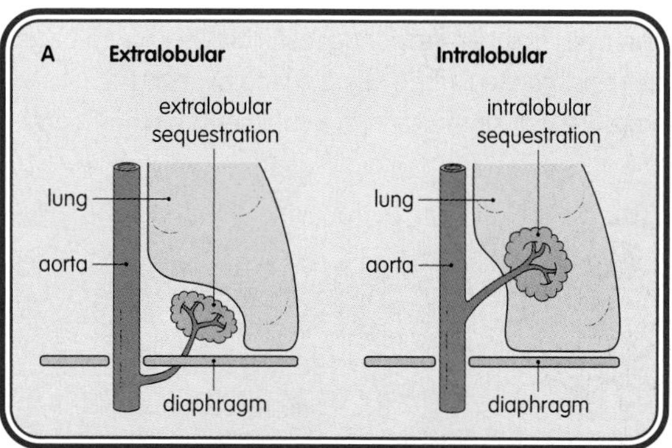

B **Comparison between intralobular and extralobular sequestrations**

	Intralobular	Extralobular
incidence	more common	less common
male-to-female ratio	1 : 1	4 : 1
side of thorax	60% left	90% left
arterial supply	70% thoracic aorta	40% thoracic aorta
venous drainage	pulmonary veins	systemic
position	within normal lung and its pleural covering	separate from normal lung in its own pleural cover
other congenital defects	uncommon	frequent

Fig. 11.2 (A and B) Differences between extralobular and intralobular sequestrations.

pressure effects. Pathogenesis includes defects in the bronchial cartilage, mechanical causes of bronchial obstruction, and idiopathic causes. Prognosis is good.

Agenesis and hypoplasia

Agenesis

Agenesis is a complete absence of one or both lungs with no trace of bronchial or vascular supply.

Hypoplasia

In hypoplasia, the bronchus is fully formed, but reduced in size; there is failure of alveolar development. Hypoplasia is associated with other congenital abnormalities such as Potter's syndrome and diaphragmatic hernia.

Abnormalities of trachea or bronchi

Abnormalities of trachea or bronchi include tracheal agenesis, tracheo-oesophageal fistula, tracheal stenosis, tracheal narrowing caused by extrinsic pressure, tracheomalacia, and tracheobronchomegaly.

- **How are congenital cysts formed?**
- **List the differences between intralobular and extralobular sequestrations.**
- **What is congenital lobar emphysema?**

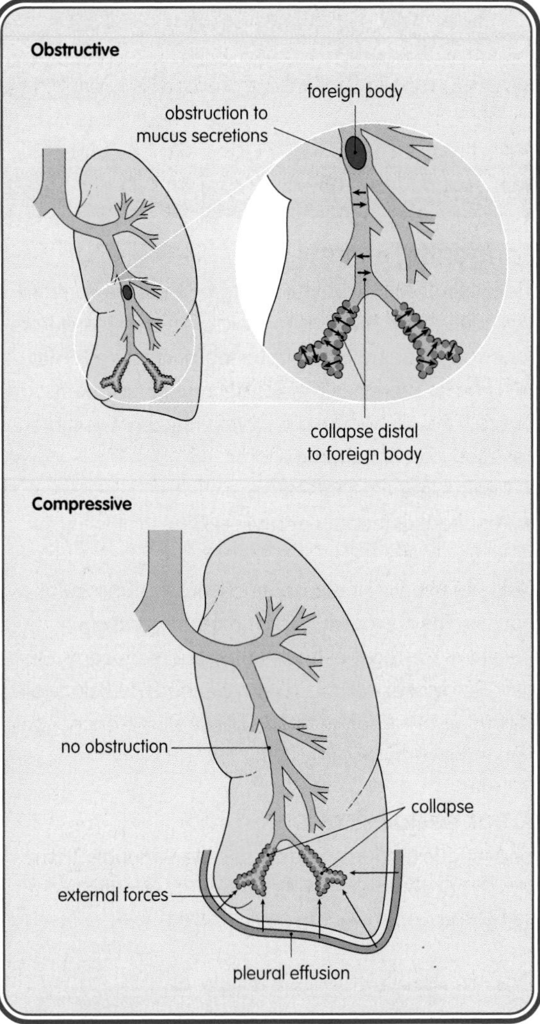

Fig. 11.3 Obstructive and compressive atelectasis.

ATELECTASIS

Atelectasis (from the Greek *ateles* imperfect + *ektasis* expansion) is classified as primary or secondary:

- Primary—lung fails to expand at birth.
- Secondary—caused by obstruction or compression (Fig. 11.3).

Obstructive atelectasis

Obstruction is the commonest cause of atelectasis; this is also known as resorptive atelectasis (Fig. 11.4).

Comparison of acute and chronic obstruction	
Acute	**Chronic**
inhalation and impaction of foreign bodies	tumours
mucus plugging of bronchi (e.g. after anaesthesia)	lymphadenopathy
after tracheostomy	aneurysm
lung infections	

Fig. 11.4 Causes of acute and chronic obstruction.

Obstructive atelectasis follows an acute and complete obstruction of a large bronchus. Air in the collapsed area of the lung is absorbed and secretions distal to the obstruction accumulate; subsequently, these bronchial secretions become infected and suppurate. Distal to the blockage, the bronchi mechanically distend.

If the collapse has been present for some time, irreversible pulmonary fibrosis occurs. Pulmonary artery branches may have narrowed lumens.

Compressive atelectasis

In compressive atelectasis, bronchial obstruction does not occur; therefore, bronchial secretions are free to drain up the bronchial tree. As such, the collapsed lung does not become seriously infected.

Compressive atelectasis results from external compression of the lung.

Causes of compression

Causes of compression include pleural effusion, haemothorax, empyema, pneumothorax, space-occupying intrathoracic lesion, and abdominal distension.

Haemodynamic and vascular changes occur. High inflation pressures on inspiration are required to overcome retractive forces. Re-expansion of the lung usually occurs after compression is resolved.

Patchy atelectasis

Depending on the cause, atelectasis may occur in a patchy or diffuse distribution.

- **Describe the two main ways in which atelectasis can occur.**
- **Classify and give examples of the causes of atelectasis.**
- **What are the long-term consequences of atelectasis?**

VASCULAR DISEASE

Pulmonary congestion and oedema

Pulmonary oedema is defined as an abnormal increase in the amount of interstitial fluid in the lung. It can be caused by:

- Increased venous hydrostatic pressures.
- Injury to alveolar capillary wall.
- Blockage of lymphatic drainage.
- Lowered plasma oncotic pressure (a rare cause).

Haemodynamic pulmonary oedema

Fluid movement between intravascular and extravascular compartments is governed by Starling forces (see Fig. 4.11). Net fluid flow through a capillary wall (out of the blood) is governed by:

- Hydrostatic pressure (arterial blood pressure) at the arteriole end of capillary bed.
- Capillary permeability.
- Opposing oncotic pressure exerted by serum proteins (mainly albumin); interstitial oncotic pressure may also contribute to the outflow.

Reabsorption of interstitial fluid is governed by:

- Plasma oncotic pressure (pulling pressure).
- Hydrostatic pressure in the interstitial space (tissue pressure).
- Fall in hydrostatic pressure at venous end of capillary.

Imbalances in Starling forces and a reduced plasma oncotic pressure will cause expansion of the interstitial spaces.

No pathological conditions cause a local reduction of plasma protein concentration within the lung capillaries. However, many conditions (e.g. left ventricular failure) cause an elevation of hydrostatic pressure. If left arterial pressure rises, so do pulmonary venous and capillary pressures, thereby raising hydrostatic pressure and causing oedema formation. Pulmonary oedema occurs only after the lymphatic drainage capacity has been exceeded. Lymphatic drainage can increase 10-fold without oedema formation. However, if lymphatic drainage is blocked (e.g. in cancer), oedema occurs more readily.

Oedema due to haemodynamic causes has a low protein content.

Oedema caused by microvascular injury

Capillary blood is separated from alveolar air by three anatomical layers:

- Capillary endothelium.
- Narrow interstitial layer.
- Alveolar epithelium.

Damage to capillary endothelium

Normal alveolar capillary endothelial cells are joined by tight junctions containing narrow constrictions. Many conditions can damage the pulmonary capillary endothelium, resulting in movement of fluid and a transcapillary leak of proteins. Interstitial oncotic pressure rises; thus, a natural defence against oedema formation is disabled.

After damage, fibrinogen enters and coagulates within the interstitium. Interstitial fibrosis subsequently occurs, leading to impaired lymphatic drainage. Oedema caused by microvascular damage characteristically has a high protein content.

Progression of pulmonary oedema

Fluid first accumulates in loose connective tissue around the bronchi and large vessels. Fluid then distends the thick, collagen-containing portions of the alveolar wall. The final stage of pulmonary oedema is accumulation of fluid within the alveolar spaces. If pulmonary oedema is chronic, recurrent alveolar haemorrhages lead to the accumulation of haemosiderin-laden macrophages along with interstitial fibrosis.

Clinical features

Clinical features of oedema are as follows:

- Acute breathlessness.
- Wheezing.
- Anxiety.
- Tachypnoea.
- Profuse perspiration.
- Productive of pink sputum while coughing.
- Peripheral circulatory shutdown.
- Tachycardia.
- Basal crackles and wheezes heard on auscultation.
- Respiratory impairment with hypoxaemia.
- Overloaded lungs predispose to secondary infection.

Treatment

The patient should be placed in sitting position and 60% O_2 administered. Intravenous diuretics give an immediate and delayed response. Morphine sedates the patient and causes systemic vasodilatation: if systemic arterial pressure falls below 90 mmHg do not use morphine. Aminophylline can be infused over 10 minutes, but should be used only when bronchospasm is present.

Adult respiratory distress syndrome (ARDS)

Adult respiratory distress syndrome (ARDS) is noncardiogenic pulmonary oedema defined as diffuse pulmonary infiltrates, refractory hypoxaemia, stiff lungs, and respiratory distress (Fig. 11.5). ARDS forms part of a systemic inflammatory reaction.

Aetiology

Causes are as follows:

- Gram-negative septicaemia.
- Trauma or shock.
- Infection (e.g. pneumonia).
- Pancreatitis.
- Gastric aspiration.
- Perforated viscus.
- Narcotic abuse.
- Disseminated intravascular coagulation.
- Oxygen toxicity.
- Gas inhalation.
- Ionizing radiation.

The underlying insult is damage to the alveolar capillary wall, leading to diffuse alveolar damage.

Precipitating mechanisms of ARDS

Mechanisms include pulmonary capillary hypoxaemia, microembolism, and loss of surfactant caused by pulmonary epithelium damage.

Pathology

The key feature of ARDS is noncardiogenic pulmonary oedema. Pulmonary venous and capillary engorgement occurs, leading to interstitial oedema. Pulmonary epithelium damage also occurs.

Pulmonary hypertension is common; hypoxic vasoconstriction redirects blood to better areas of oxygenation.

A protein-rich intra-alveolar haemorrhagic exudate promotes formation of hyaline membranes that line alveolar ducts and alveoli.

In long-standing cases, pulmonary fibrosis ensues and the alveolar walls become lined by metaplastic cuboidal epithelium.

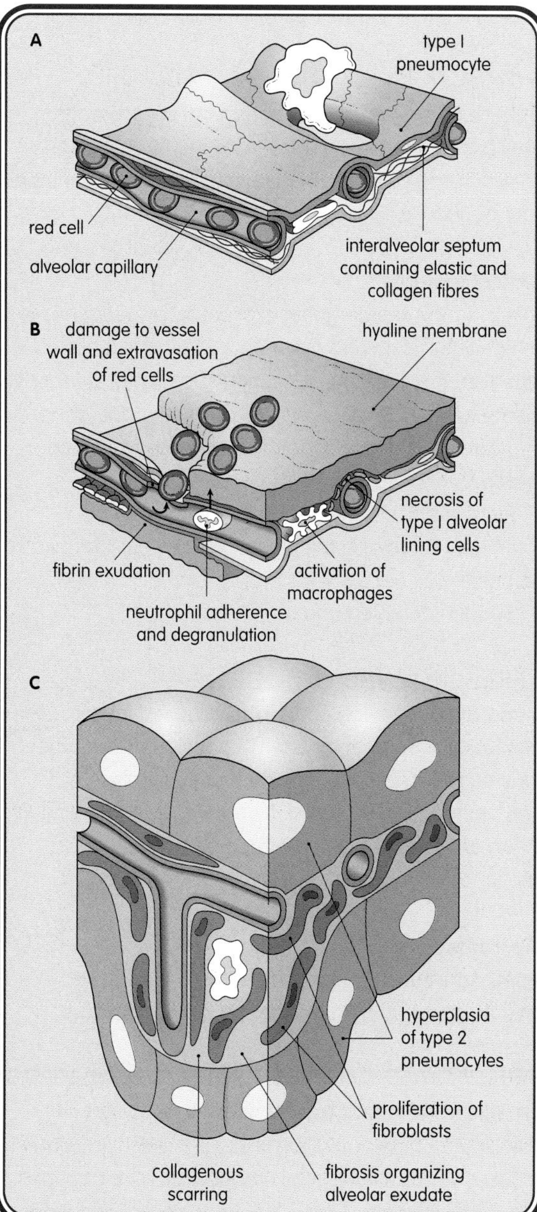

Fig. 11.5 Cell types in adult respiratory distress syndrome. (A) Normal alveolar wall; (B) acute phase of ARDS; (C) organisation phase of ARDS.

Resolution

Resolution occurs as follows:

- Resorption of oedema.
- Ingestion of red cells and hyaline membranes by alveolar macrophages.
- Regeneration of type II pneumocytes.

Clinical features

Features change during the progression of ARDS. Patients with ARDS present with:

- Tachypnoea, often unexplained.
- Dyspnoea.
- Pulmonary oedema—fine crackles throughout both lung fields.
- Arterial hypoxaemia, refractory to oxygen therapy.

Chest radiography shows bilateral diffuse shadowing.

Management

Treat underlying condition and provide supportive measures.

Treat as for pulmonary oedema: the aim is to achieve a negative fluid balance.

Provide cardiovascular support and mechanical ventilation (e.g. positive end expiratory pressure).

Prognosis

Prognosis is dependent upon cause, but mortality is generally greater than 50%.

Prognosis is poor in the elderly. With septic shock, mortality is 90%. With fat embolism, mortality is 10%.

Death is caused by cardiac arrhythmias with sepsis, usually from Gram-negative organisms.

Embolism, haemorrhage, and infarction

Vascular disease of the lungs can be caused by:

- Vessel obstruction.
- Vessel wall damage.
- Intravascular pressure variations.

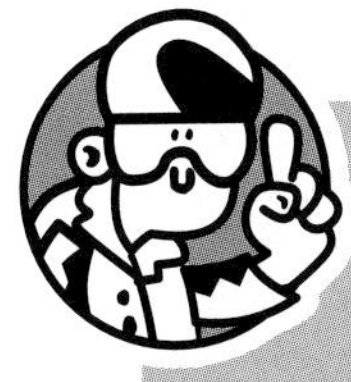

Adult respiratory distress syndrome is noncardiogenic pulmonary oedema.

Obstruction: pulmonary embolism

An embolus is an abnormal mass of material that is transported in the bloodstream from one part of the circulation to another and which impacts finally in the lumen of a vessel which has a calibre too small to allow passage. The end result of an embolus derived from venous thrombus is impaction in the pulmonary arterial tree. Most thrombi originate in the deep veins of the calf or pelvis.

This is a common condition: incidence of pulmonary emboli at autopsy has been reported to be 12%.

Pulmonary emboli rarely have a cardiac cause and are very rare in children.

Predisposing factors

Predisposing factors are:

- Immobilization (e.g. prolonged bed rest).
- In women, the oral contraceptive pill—risk is increased by cigarette smoking.
- Malignancy, especially pancreatic.
- Cardiac failure.
- Chronic pulmonary disease.
- Postoperative recovery.
- Fractures of the pelvis or lower limb.
- Hypercoaguable states (e.g. pregnancy).

Symptoms are related to the size of the embolus and the corresponding volume of lung tissue deprived of blood in addition to the presence or absence of congestion in the pulmonary circulation at the time of impaction.

Pulmonary embolism can be classified as massive, moderate, or small.

Massive pulmonary embolism

A massive pulmonary embolism is a clinical emergency. The embolus is typically derived from a thrombus that occludes a long venous segment in the lower limb. The calibre of the main pulmonary arteries is greater than the iliac and femoral veins; therefore, thrombi must loosely bundle together to block the pulmonary arteries (as seen in a saddle embolus, which occurs at the bifurcation of the left and right pulmonary arteries).

Within normal human lung, occlusion of more than 50% of the pulmonary vascular bed is necessary for a massive pulmonary embolism to prove fatal. Animal studies have shown that other factors in addition to obstruction are involved:

- Vagal reflex—induces spasm of coronary and pulmonary arteries.
- Reflex, causing cardiac arrest.
- Reflex, causing marked peripheral vasodilatation.
- Massive release of platelet-derived thromboxane, which can provoke bronchospasm in the pulmonary vasculature.

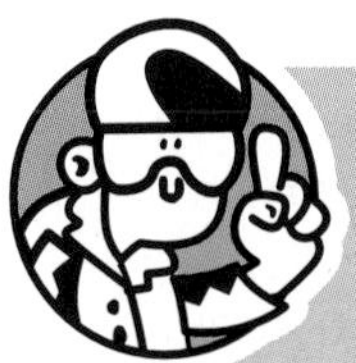

When a patient presents postoperatively with sudden-onset chest pain, pulmonary embolism should be at the top of the list of differential diagnoses.

Clinical features

This is a clinical emergency presenting as sudden-onset severe chest pain and dyspnoea. Often onset occurs when straining during defecation. Classically, a massive pulmonary embolism occurs 10 days after operation.

There are signs of shock: tachycardia, low blood pressure.

Right ventricular heave, gallop rhythm, and a prominent a-wave in the jugular venous pulse may also be noted.

Sudden death can occur.

Moderate pulmonary embolism

Moderate pulmonary embolism is caused by occlusion of a lobar or segmental artery. Perfusion of a segment may be reduced producing an area of localized necrosis.

An area of necrosis secondary to ischaemia is known as an infarct.

Clinical features

Pulmonary infarction presents with sudden-onset pleuritic chest pain. Cough with haemoptysis and dyspnoea are other symptoms.

Small pulmonary embolism

Small pulmonary embolism is usually clinically silent. It is caused by multiple small emboli occluding arterioles. Gradual occlusion of the pulmonary arterial bed leads to pulmonary hypertension.

Outcome

Thrombotic material is retracted within the wall of

vessels. A combination of retraction and organization leaves small fibrous cords.

If there is extensive retraction:

- Thrombotic mass becomes packed down onto a vessel wall (similar to a mural thrombus).
- Emboli become incorporated into the vessel wall.
- Increased intimal thickness occurs, causing decreased pulmonary vascular compliance and pulmonary hypertension.

Clinical features

Clinical features include effort dyspnoea, tiredness, and syncope. Basal crackles are heard on auscultation.

Other forms of emboli

Fat embolism

Fat embolism results from massive injury to subcutaneous fat or fracture of bones containing fatty marrow. Globules of lipid enter the torn vessels.

Air embolism

Air embolism arises during childbirth or abortion. These microemboli can cause tiny infarcts in several organs.

Tumour embolism

Tumour cells, like other particulate matter, become trapped in the pulmonary capillary bed. This is an important mechanism in the development of metastases.

Amniotic fluid embolism

Amniotic fluid embolism can occur during childbirth or abortion, and may be fatal. Small fragments of trophoblast are commonly found in lungs of pregnant women at autopsy, but do not cause any symptoms.

Investigations

Chest radiography and electrocardiography are usually normal. Electrocardiography may show signs of right ventricular strain (deep S waves in lead I, Q waves in lead III, and inverted T waves in lead III).

Arterial blood gases show arterial hypoxaemia and hypocapnia.

Radioisotope ventilation–perfusion scans demonstrate underperfused areas.

Treatment

Treatment is by avoidance of deep vein thromboses:

- Early mobilization of patients after operation.
- Use of tight elastic stockings.
- Leg exercises.
- Prophylactic anticoagulation.

Further emboli should be prevented (patients with a pulmonary embolism have a 30% chance of developing further emboli). Intravenous heparin is administered:

- Bolus: 10 000 IU.
- Continuous infusion: 1000–2000 IU/hour.

Oral anticoagulants are given after 48 hours, and heparin is reduced. Oral anticoagulants are continued for between 6 weeks and 6 months.

It is possible to break down thrombi:

- Fibrinolytic therapy.
- Intravenous streptokinase 250 000 IU infusion over 30 minutes.
- Intravenous streptokinase 100 000 IU hourly.

Surgery is performed only on massive pulmonary emboli.

Prognosis

Of clinical pulmonary emboli, 10% are fatal.

Vessel wall damage

Diseases of the lung caused by vessel damage are rare; the majority of such diseases are immunologically mediated (e.g. Goodpasture's syndrome). Pulmonary haemorrhage results from circulating antiglomerular basement membrane antibodies binding to cross-reacting antigens of the pulmonary basement membrane.

Pulmonary infarction

Less than 10% of pulmonary emboli cause infarction within the lung. Pulmonary infarction is usually a consequence of a moderate pulmonary embolism. Pulmonary infarction is rare in young people.

Predisposing factors

Predisposing factors for infarction include:

- Rise in pulmonary venous pressure.
- Mitral stenosis or left ventricular failure.
- Bronchial occlusion.
- Pleural effusion.
- Infection.

Pathology

A wedge-shaped section of the lung downstream from the blockage becomes necrotic. The base of the wedge is situated toward the pleural aspect of the lung. Pleural inflammation over the infarcted area is common. Organization of pulmonary infarcts precedes rapidly.

Lung infarcts are more common in the lower lobes; infarction is less common in the lungs than in other organs because of the lungs' dual blood supply.

Clinical features

Clinical features include sudden-onset pleuritic chest pain and dyspnoea.

Investigation

Blood tests show increases in erythrocyte sedimentation rate and lactate dehydrogenase (LDH) levels. Polymorphonuclear leucocytosis is present.

Arterial blood gas measurement reveals hypoxaemia, but normal PCO_2.

Ventilation–perfusion scans show other defects.

Pulmonary hypertension and vascular sclerosis

Pulmonary hypertension occurs when blood pressure in the pulmonary circulation exceeds 30 mmHg (Fig. 11.6). The condition is classified according to:

- Aetiology.
- Site of vascular lesion.

Pulmonary hypertension	
Aetiology	**Vascular lesion**
Cardiac disease	Precapillary (e.g. left-to-right shunt)
Hypoxia	Capillary (e.g. hypoxia)
Fibrosis	Postcapillary (e.g. left ventricular failure)
Miscellaneous	
Idiopathic (primary)	

Fig. 11.6 Classification of pulmonary hypertension. Note that pulmonary arterial changes depend on aetiology of the pulmonary hypertension.

Changes can occur with hypertension in the pulmonary artery tree:

- Muscular hypertrophy.
- Intimal proliferation.
- Capillary dilatation.

Effects of pulmonary hypertension

Effects of pulmonary hypertension include:

- Enlarged proximal pulmonary arteries.
- Right ventricular hypertrophy.
- Right arterial dilatation.
- Necrotizing arteritis.

Clinical features

Clinical features are as follows:

- Symptoms of the underlying cause.
- Chest pain and exertional dyspnoea.
- Syncope and fatigue.
- Prominent a-wave in jugular venous pulse.
- Right ventricular heave.
- Loud pulmonary component to second heart sound.
- Midsystolic ejection murmur.

Investigation

When investigating pulmonary hypertension, a possible cause should be sought.

A full blood count may show secondary polycythaemia. Chest radiography may reaveal right ventricular enlargement, pulmonary artery dilatation, or oligaemic peripheral lung fields.

Electrocardiography may indicate right ventricular hypertrophy, right-axis deviation, a prominent R wave in V1, or inverted T waves in the right precordial leads.

Radioisotope lung scans and echocardiography may also be useful.

Treatment

Treatment is dependent upon cause. Primary pulmonary hypertension is treated with anticoagulation therapy.

If the underlying cause of hypertension is untreatable, the patient will progress to cor pulmonale and death. Continuous oxygen therapy is beneficial in patients with cor pulmonale. Diuretics are used to treat fluid overload.

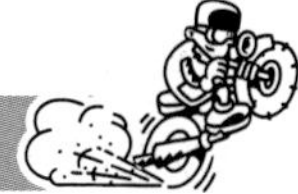

Heart–lung transplantation is recommended in young patients.

Prognosis is poor: 5-year survival rate is 40%.

Cardiac condition

Cardiac conditions that cause pulmonary hypertension include congenital cardiac shunts, such as left-to-right shunts (e.g. ventricular septal defects).

Direct transmission of systemic arterial pressure into pulmonary circulation occurs, initially causing:

- Hypertrophy of the medial coat of the small pulmonary arteries.
- Pulmonary arterioles develop a distinct muscular media, usually absent in pulmonary arterioles.

Cellular intimal proliferation of myofibroblasts in pulmonary arteries and arterioles then occurs. Organic occlusion of pulmonary arteries occurs, followed by dilatation of the pulmonary vasculature. Localized dilatation lesions are clusters of thin-walled branches of small pulmonary arteries arising proximal to the sites of occlusion. These form a collateral circulation to maintain blood flow to the capillary bed, and are known as angiomatoid lesions.

A proliferation of myofibroblasts and mesenchymal cells may arise in a plexiform pattern within angiomatoid lesions to form plexiform lesions.

Elevation of pulmonary arterial pressure

When pulmonary arterial pressure is elevated (e.g. in left ventricular failure), medial hypertrophy and intimal fibrosis of pulmonary arteries and muscularization of pulmonary arterioles occurs, resulting in pulmonary oedema. Plexiform lesions are not present. Persistent pulmonary congestion and oedema are associated with:

- Hyperplasia of granular pneumocytes.
- Development of interstitial fibrosis of the lung.

Hypoxia or chronic lung disease

An example of hypoxia is seen in Pickwickian syndrome.

Pulmonary hypertension is caused by poor respiration associated with gross obesity. Smooth muscle hypertrophy occurs in the media of the terminal portions of the pulmonary arterial tree, and pulmonary vascular resistance increases. Because insignificant intimal fibrosis occurs, the condition is largely reversible.

Pulmonary fibrosis

Early changes of pulmonary vasculature are initially muscular in type and reversible. Obliterative fibrosis of pulmonary arteries and arterioles occurs later, with irreversible increases in pulmonary vascular resistance.

Idiopathic

Idiopathic pulmonary hypertension is a rare condition of unknown aetiology, predominantly seen in women aged 20–30 years, but which may also occur in children aged less than 10 years. The condition may be familial.

Miscellaneous

In crotalaria spectabilis, overactivity of the sympathetic nervous system causes vasoconstriction.

- **List the causes of pulmonary oedema.**
- **Describe the management of pulmonary oedema.**
- **List the multifactoral aetiology of adult respiratory distress syndrome.**
- **Summarize the pathogenesis of pulmonary embolism.**
- **List the investigations required to diagnose pulmonary embolism.**
- **Describe the consequences of pulmonary hypertension.**

PULMONARY DISEASE

Obstructive and restrictive defects

Obstructive defects

Airway obstruction and resultant airflow limitation may be caused by local or diffuse lesions; examples include asthma, chronic bronchitis, and emphysema. Airways are widened distal to the diseased airway. Patients breathe deeply and slowly. Symptoms include coughing, wheezing, and dyspnoea.

Pulmonary function tests show the following results:

- Increased residual volume and total lung capacity.
- Reduced vital capacity, FEV_1, peak expiratory flow rate, and FEV_1:FVC ratio.

Restrictive defects

Examples of defects that restrict normal lung movement during respiration include pulmonary fibrosis, pleural disease, and consolidation. Patients' breathing is shallow and rapid.

Characteristically, all lung volumes are reduced. FEV_1:FVC ratio is normal, but vital capacity is decreased.

Chronic obstructive pulmonary disease

Chronic obstructive pulmonary disease (COPD) is a common progressive disease of the lungs involving many airways; it affects 17% of men and 8% of women aged 40–60 years. The disease is strongly associated with cigarette smoking.

'Pink puffers' and 'blue bloaters'		
	Pink puffer	**Blue bloater**
body size	thin	obese
chest hyperinflation	marked	present
predominant disease	emphysema	chronic bronchitis
postmortem finding	panacinar emphysema	centrilobular emphysema
cor pulmonale	absent	present
secondary polycythaemia	absent	present
cyanosis	absent	centrally
blood gases	low P_aCO_2	raised P_aCO_2

Fig. 11.7 'Pink puffers' and 'blue bloaters'.

Clinical presentation varies widely; two clinical groups of patient can be identified, although these represent the two ends of a spectrum of illness collectively known as COPD (Fig. 11.7).

Aetiology

Cigarette smoking is the major aetiological factor; all others are minor in comparison. Cigarette smoking has three major effects:

- Impairs ciliary movement.
- Causes mucus gland hypertrophy.
- Alters the structure and function of alveolar macrophages.

Atmospheric pollution, occupational exposure, and recurrent bronchial infections are also implicated. Recurrent bronchial infections are frequent causes of acute exacerbations; their role in development rather than progression of the condition is less clear.

Clinical features

Clinical features are as follows (Fig. 11.7):

- Productive cough.
- Breathlessness, becoming severe as the disease progresses.
- Wheezing with mild disease.
- Recurrent low-grade infective exacerbations.

Emphysema

Emphysema is a permanent enlargement of the air spaces distal to the terminal bronchiole accompanied by destruction of their walls. Classification is based on anatomical distribution (Fig. 11.8).

Centriacinar (centrilobular) emphysema

Septal destruction and dilatation occurs, limited to central portion of acinus, with free communication between all orders of respiratory bronchioles. The upper lung lobes are affected more commonly than the lower lobes. Histologically, there are dilated air spaces and chronic inflammation centred around the bronchi and bronchioles. Respiratory bronchiolitis is frequently present. This form of emphysema occurs predominantly in male smokers and is associated with chronic bronchitis ('blue bloater') (Fig. 11.8B).

Panacinar (panlobular) emphysema

Panacinar (panlobular) emphysema is a characteristic lesion of α_1 antitrypsin deficiency. Loss of lung

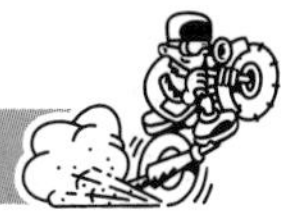

parenchyma, including pulmonary capillaries, occurs. The whole of the acinus is involved distal to the terminal bronchioles, usually affecting lower lobes.

Enlarged air spaces may become cystic and form bullae. This form of emphysema is not usually associated with chronic bronchitis (Fig. 11.8C).

Irregular emphysema

Irregular emphysema is associated with scarring and damage affecting lung parenchyma, commonly found around old healed tuberculosis scars in the lung apices. Air trapping caused by fibrosis is thought to be the pathogenesis.

Irregular emphysema overlaps clinically with paraseptal emphysema (Fig. 11.8D).

Paraseptal (distal acinar) emphysema

In paraseptal (distal acinar) emphysema, alveolar wall destruction is restricted to the periphery of the acinus, with the upper lobes more frequently affected. If dilated airspace measures more than 10 mm in diameter, the condition is termed bullous (Fig. 11.8E).

α_1 antitrypsin deficiency

α_1 antitrypsin is an acute-phase serum protein produced in the liver, which functions as an antiprotease and inhibits the action of:

- Neutrophil elastase—an enzyme released during an inflammatory response, which is capable of destroying alveolar cell wall tissue.
- Trypsin.
- Collagenase.

In α_1 antitrypsin deficiency, serum levels of the enzyme are reduced. This is an autosomal dominant condition, where homozygous individuals develop severe panacinar emphysema.

α_1 antitrypsin deficiency develops at an early age (before 40 years of age) with equal distribution between sexes. The homozygous state has an incidence of 1:3630 in Caucasians, but is rarer in dark-skinned people.

Other types of emphysema

Bullous emphysema

In bullous emphysema foci are present measuring more than 10 mm in diameter; these are typically apical and subpleural. Bullae are prone to rupture causing spontaneous pneumothorax. Bullous emphysema is not classed as a separate category of emphysema.

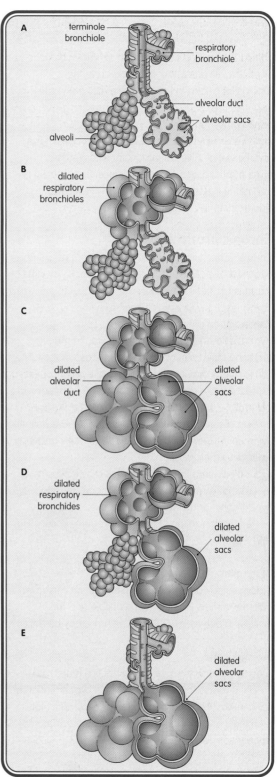

Fig. 11.8 Main types of emphysema. (A) Normal distal lung acinus; (B) centriacinar emphysema; (C) panacinar emphysema; (D) irregular emphysema; (E) paraseptal emphysema.

Interstitial emphysema

Interstitial emphysema is an inflation of the interstitium of the lung by air after laceration of lung substance (e.g. from a fractured rib). Air may spread to the mediastinum and to tissues at the root of the neck.

Senile emphysema

In senile emphysema, there is no destruction of the alveolar walls. Alveolar surface area decreases and alveolar ductal size increases. Senile emphysema is part of the ageing process and is of little clinical significance.

Chronic bronchitis

Chronic bronchitis is defined clinically as a persistent cough with sputum production for at least 3 months of the year for 2 consecutive years.

Pathology

Hyperplasia and hypertrophy occur to the mucus-secreting glands found in the submucosa of the large cartilaginous airways. Mucous gland hypertrophy is expressed as gland–wall ratio or by the Reid index (normally, <0.4). Hyperplasia of the intraepithelial goblet cells occurs at the expense of ciliated cells in the lining epithelium. Regions of epithelium may undergo squamous metaplasia.

Small airways become obstructed by intraluminal mucus plugs, mucosal oedema, smooth muscle hypertrophy, and peribronchial fibrosis. Secondary bacterial colonization of retained products occurs (Fig. 11.9).

Diagnosis

Diagnosis is made from the clinical history. In some patients, airflow limitation is reversible and the distinction between COPD and asthma may be difficult.

Investigations

Lung function tests show an obstructive pattern.

Chest radiography typically shows hyperinflation or flat hemidiaphragms, reduced peripheral vascular markings, and bullae. Alternatively, radiographs may appear normal.

Full blood counts may show secondary polycythaemia, but blood gas tests are often normal. α_1 antitrypsin levels should be measured.

Treatment

The most important step in treatment is to stop the patient smoking, thus reducing the rate of deterioration. Self-administration of inhaled drugs is the key to management of COPD: patients must be taught correct inhaler technique. Treatment options include:

- Bronchodilators—e.g. ipratropium bromide 40 μg four times a day may provide symptomatic relief.
- Corticosteroids—degree of reversibility can be assessed by prescribing 2 weeks of prednisolone 30 mg/day, with measurement of lung function. If there is improvement in FEV_1 of more than 15%, inhaled steroids should be prescribed. Corticosteroids prescribed after acute exacerbations may improve airway function considerably.
- Antibiotics—shortens exacerbations and should always be given in acute episodes.
- Vaccine—annual flu vaccine.
- Long-term domiciliary oxygen therapy—if necessary, administer for 19 hours per day at a flow rate of 1–3 L/min. Arterial oxygen saturation needs to be above 90%.

Prognosis

Prognosis is poor: 50% of patients with severe breathlessness die within 5 years.

Bronchial asthma

Bronchial asthma is a chronic inflammatory disorder of the lungs characterized by reversible spasmodic episodes of dyspnoea, coughing, and wheezing.

Prevalence

Five per cent of the population are receiving therapy for asthma at any one time. Prevalence of asthma in the Western world is rising, with a geographic distribution that is rare in the Far East and common in New Zealand.

Classification

Bronchial asthma may be categorized into two groups: extrinsic or intrinsic (Fig. 11.10). Precipitating factors are described in Fig. 11.11.

Occupational asthma is increasing; currently there are over 200 materials encountered at the workplace that are implicated.

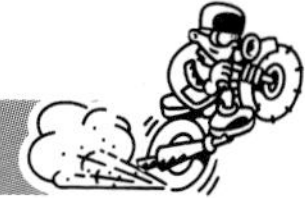

Pathogenesis of allergen-induced asthma

Pathogenesis of asthma is very complex. Usually one of two patterns of change in airway calibre can be observed with the inhalation of allergen by atopic asthmatics.

Immediate reaction

Maximal airway narrowing within 10–15 minutes of challenge with a return to baseline within 1–2 hours.

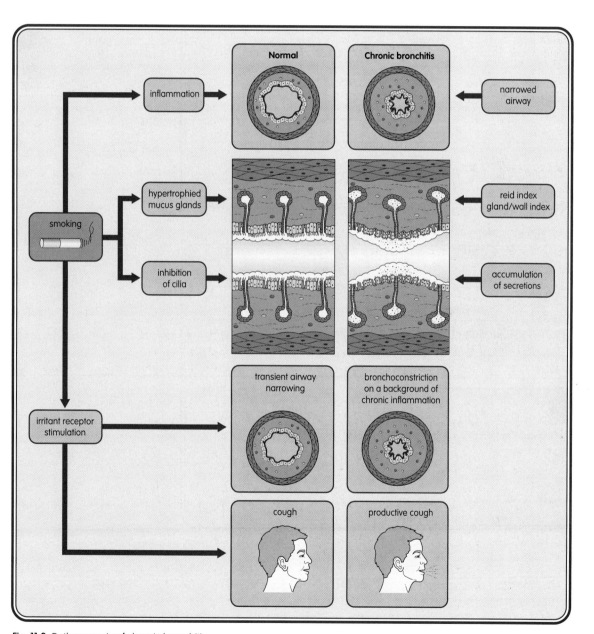

Fig. 11.9 Pathogenesis of chronic bronchitis.

Asthma		
	Extrinsic asthma	**Intrinsic asthma**
underlying abnormality	immune reaction (atopic)	abnormal autonomic regulation of airways
onset	childhood	adulthood
distribution	60%	40%
allergens	recognized	none identified
family history	present	absent
predisposition to form IgE antibodies	present	absent
association with chronic obstructive pulmonary disease	none	chronic bronchitis
natural progression	improves	worsens
eosinophilia	sputum and blood	sputum
drug hypersensitivity	absent	present

Fig. 11.10 Classification of asthma.

Precipitating factors for asthma					
Allergens	**Occupational sensitizers**	**Viral infections**	**Atmospheric factors**	**Drugs**	**Other factors**
house dust mite (*Dermato-phagoides pteronyssius*)	colophony fumes (from soldering)	para influenza	cigarette smoke	β-blockers	cold air
flour	isocyanates (from polyurethane varnishes)	respiratory syncytial virus	ozone	nonsteroidal anti-inflammatory drugs	emotion
animal danders	acid anhydrides (from industrial coatings)	rhinovirus	sulphur dioxide		fumes
grain					exercise

Fig. 11.11 Precipitating factors for asthma.

Late reaction

Airway narrowing begins after 3–4 hours and is maximal after 6–12 hours. This is much more difficult to reverse than immediate reaction asthma and there is an increase in level of airway hyperreactivity.

Inflammatory mediators play a vital role in the pathogenesis of asthma. Inflammatory stimuli activate cells within the airways, primary effector cells (mast cells, alveolar macrophages, and epithelial cells) causing the release of mediators that are chemotactic for cells derived from the circulation—secondary effector cells (eosinophils, neutrophils, and platelets).

Mediators that are thought to be involved in asthma include (Fig. 11.12):

- Preformed mediators—present in cytoplasmic granules ready for release. Associated with human lung mast cells and include histamine, neutral proteases, and chemotactic factors for neutrophils and eosinophils.
- Newly generated mediators—manufactured secondary to the initial triggering stimulus after release of preformed mediators. Many of these mediators are derived from the membrane phospholipid and are associated with the metabolism of arachidonic acid (e.g. prostaglandins and leukotrienes).

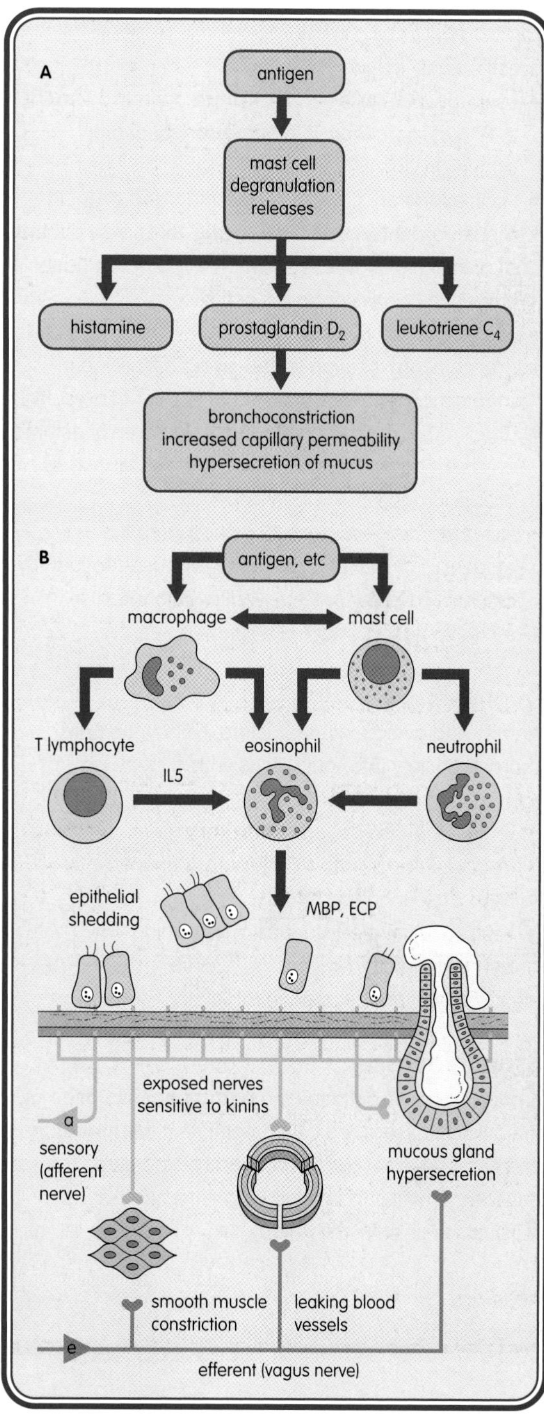

Fig. 11.12 Pathogenesis of asthma. (A) Preformed mediators; (B) newly generated mediators; IL5, interleukin 5; MBP, major basic protein; ECP, eosinophil cationic protein.

Macroscopically, a reddened, inflamed oedematous mucosa is seen. Microscopically, viscid mucus fills the bronchi, containing:

- Desquamated epithelial cells.
- Whorls of shed epithelium (Curshmann's whorls).
- Charcot Leyden crystal (eosinophil cell membranes).

Hyaline thickening of basement membrane, smooth muscle hypertrophy of the small bronchi and bronchioles, and an abundance of inflammatory cells are also seen.

Clinical features

Symptoms are often worse at night. Nocturnal coughing is a common presenting symptom, especially in children. Episodic wheezing and shortness of breath are almost universal.

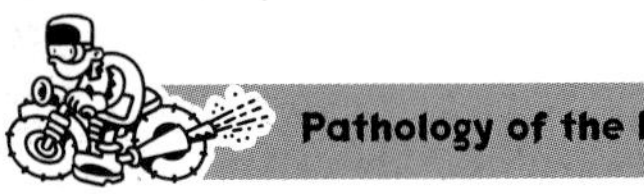

Investigations

Investigations include:

- Lung function tests—demonstrate an improvement in FEV_1 of more than 15% after bronchodilator administration.
- Peak expiratory flow rate—morning and evening measurements. Useful in the long-term assessment of asthma; a characteristic morning dipping pattern is seen in poorly controlled asthma.
- Exercise laboratory tests.
- Bronchial provocation tests—using histamine or methacholine to demonstrate bronchial hyperactivity.
- Chest radiography—no diagnostic features of asthma on chest radiograph; use to rule out a diagnosis of allergic bronchopulmonary aspergillosus.
- Skin prick tests—allergen injections into the epidermis of the forearm, which are used to identify extrinsic causes. Look for weal development in sensitive patients.

Treatment

Identify and avoid extrinsic factors. Follow the British Thoracic Society (BTS) guidelines with a stepwise approach to drug treatment:

- Occasional use of bronchodilators.
- Regular inhaled anti-inflammatory agents.
- High-dose inhaled steroids.
- High-dose inhaled steroids and regular bronchodilators.
- Addition of regular steroid tablets.

Bronchiectasis

Bronchiectasis is defined as a permanent dilatation of the bronchi associated with a persistent inflammatory process. The mucociliary transport mechanism is impaired and secondary bacterial infection occurs. Most cases arise in childhood.

Aetiology

Bronchiectasis is caused by infection (e.g. bronchopneumonia, measles, or whooping cough).

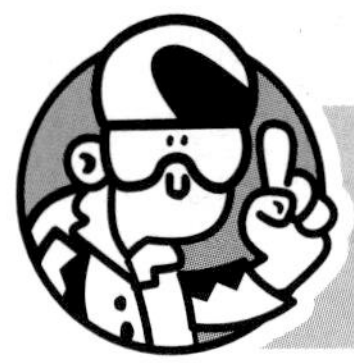

Examination questions on asthma are very common.

Inflammation can damage and weaken the bronchial wall, leading to dilatation. Bronchial obstruction followed by infection plays a key role.

Congenital abnormalities can lead to bronchiectasis.

Immunoglobulin deficiencies (e.g. IgA) may lead to recurrent infections and bronchiectasis.

Pathology

There are three pathological categories of bronchiectasis:

- Saccular, with large areas of bronchial dilatation and loss of bronchial subdivisions.
- Atelectatic.
- Follicular, which is the commonest variant—characterized by multiple lymphoid follicles.

Symptoms

Clinically mild cases present with a cough producing yellow or green sputum. Severe cases present with a chronic cough producing large quantities of foul-smelling sputum. Persistent halitosis, recurrent febrile episodes, and malaise also occur.

Haemoptysis may be present. Clubbing occurs and coarse crackles are heard on auscultation.

Complications

Complications of bronchiectasis include:

- Pneumonia.
- Pneumothorax.
- Empyema.
- Meningitis.
- Metastatic abscess (e.g. in brain).
- Amyloid formation (e.g. in kidney).

Investigations

Bronchiectasis can be investigated through:

- Radiology—chest radiograph may be normal or show bronchial wall thickening.
- High-resolution CT—the investigation of choice to detect bronchial wall thickening.
- Sputum tests—Gram stain, anaerobic and aerobic culture, and sensitivity testing are vital during an infective exacerbation. Major pathogens include *Staphylococcus aureus, Pseudomonas auerginosa, Haemophilus influenza* and anaerobes.
- Tests for cystic fibrosis where appropriate.
- Lung function spirometry.

Treatment

Treatment is by postural drainage for 10–20 minutes, three times a day. Patients are trained in the method by physiotherapists.

Antibiotics—bronchopulmonary infections should be eradicated if progression of the disease is to be halted. Treatment regimens depend on infecting organism (e.g. flucloxacillin 500 mg 6-hourly to treat *Staphylococcus aureus* infection). If there is no improvement with treatment, the patient is likely to be infected with *Pseudomonas aeruginosa*: treat with ceftazidine aerosol or parenterally.

Bronchodilators are useful if demonstrable airflow limitation exists.

Surgery is of limited value.

Congenital bronchiectasis

If associated with dextrocardia and sinusitis, this condition is termed Kartagener's syndrome. This is widespread, frequently cystic, and involves both lungs. Secondary infection appears in later life. Productive cough and purulent sputum are uncommon.

Acquired bronchiectasis

Bronchiectasis is often associated with bronchial obstruction (e.g. by a foreign body, tuberculous lymph nodes, or tumour). Destruction of the alveolar walls and fibrosis of lung parenchyma occur. The dependent portions of the lungs, usually the lower lobes, are affected most commonly. Infection is frequent because of poor drainage, and systemic symptoms may be present. Pulmonary haemodynamic changes can occur.

Cystic fibrosis

Cystic fibrosis is a disorder characterized by the production of abnormally viscid secretions by exocrine glands and mucus-secreting glands, such as those in the pancreas and respiratory tract.

Inheritance of cystic fibrosis

Cystic fibrosis is the commonest genetically transmitted disease in Caucasians. It is an autosomal recessive condition occurring in 1:2000 live births. The gene has been identified on the long arm of chromosome 7. Prevalence of heterozygous carriers is 4%.

Aetiology

The commonest mutation is a specific gene deletion in the codon for phenyalanine at position 508 in the amino-code sequence (ΔF508). This results in a defect in a transmembrane regulator protein known as the cystic fibrosis transmembrane conductive regulator (CFTR). Mutation causes a failure of opening of the chloride channels in response to elevated cAMP in epithelial cells, leading to:

- Decreased excretion of chloride into the airway lumen.
- Increased reabsorption of sodium into the epithelial cells.
- Increased viscosity of secretions.

Pathology

The thick secretions produced by the epithelial cells cause:

- Small airway obstruction, leading to recurrent infection and ultimately bronchiectasis.
- Pancreatic duct obstruction, causing pancreatic fibrosis and ultimately pancreatic insufficiency.

Clinical features

Presentation depends on age. Usually, the condition presents in infancy with gastrointestinal manifestations (Fig. 11.13)

Stools are bulky, greasy, and offensive in smell. Respiratory signs and symptoms are nonspecific:

- Lungs are normal at birth.
- Frequent infections with cough and wheeze as the child gets older.
- Clubbing and dyspnoea occur.

Cystic fibrosis	
Respiratory manifestations	**Gastrointestinal manifestations**
recurrent bronchopulmonary infection bronchiectasis	meconium ileus rectal prolapse diarrhoea failure to thrive malabsorption

Fig. 11.13 Manifestations of cystic fibrosis.

Investigations

Family history is sought (e.g. affected siblings). Genetic screening is available for couples with a family history.

Prenatal diagnosis is available by chorionic villous sampling or amniocentesis.

Tests include:

- Guthrie test.
- Immunoreactive trypsin test (IRT)—positive test shows low levels.
- Sweat test—raised levels of sodium and chloride in sweat.

The complications of cystic fibrosis are described in Fig. 11.14.

Treatment

Antibiotic treatment for respiratory disease is the same as for bronchiectasis. Multiple antibiotic resistance is common, and once *Pseudomonas aeruginosa* is established, it cannot be eradicated (Fig. 11.15).

Human DNase has been cloned, sequenced, and expressed by recombinant techniques:

- Capable of degrading DNA.
- Inhalation of this material has been shown to improve FEV_1.
- Expensive.

Heart–lung and liver transplantations are possible in severely affected patients.

Prognosis

Prognosis is improving: currently, mean survival is 29 years. Death is mainly caused by respiratory complications.

Complications of cystic fibrosis

Respiratory complications	Other complications
allergic aspergillosus bronchiectasis cor pulmonale haemoptysis lobar collapse nasal polyps pneumothorax sinusitis wheezing	abdominal pain biliary cirrhosis delayed puberty diabetes mellitus gall stones growth failure male infertility portal hypertension rectal prolapse

Fig. 11.14 Complications of cystic fibrosis.

Summary of treatment

Respiratory	Gastrointestinal
drain secretions, postural drainage	pancreatic enzyme supplements with all meals and snacks
prevent infection where possible	high-energy, high-protein diet
exercise encouraged	do not restrict fat in diet
regular sputum cultures	vitamin A, D, and E supplements
immunization against measles and influenza	

Fig. 11.15 Summary of treatment.

- **Describe the role of cigarette smoking in the development of COPD.**
- **What are the definitions of chronic bronchitis and emphysema?**
- **Describe the management of patients with chronic obstructive pulmonary disease?**
- **List the causative factors for asthma.**
- **Describe the management of a patient with bronchial asthma.**
- **What is the pathology of bronchiectasis?**
- **Explain the genetics of cystic fibrosis.**
- **List the complications of cystic fibrosis.**

INFECTIONS OF THE LUNG

Bacterial pneumonia

Bacterial pneumonia is defined as inflammation of the lung parenchyma in which the affected part of the lung is consolidated, the alveolar spaces being filled with blood cells and fibrin. Bacterial pneumonia is characterized by replacement of air in alveoli and alveolar ducts with a protein rich inflammatory exudate. On average, 4–8% of adults per year have lower respiratory tract infections, of which 4% are pneumonia.

Bacterial pneumonia is classified on the basis of aetiology or anatomy.

See Chapter 2 (Fig. 2.24) for a list of the defence mechanisms of the lung.

Aetiology

An aetiological factor can be found in up to 75% of cases. Precipitating factors are:

- Hospitalization.
- Alcohol excess.
- Cigarette smoking.
- Smoking-related diseases.
- Bronchiectasis.
- Bronchial obstruction.
- Immunosuppression.
- Drug abuse.

Two anatomical patterns exist: lobar pneumonia and bronchopneumonia.

Lobar pneumonia

Lobar pneumonia is an acute infection of the lung. Of these infections, 90% are caused by the Gram-positive diplococcus *Streptococcus pneumonia* (pneumococcus). The commonest sites for lobar pneumonia to occur are the lower lobes or right middle lobe, with consolidation sharply confined to the affected lung. Lobar pneumonia is prevalent in winter and early spring. Adults aged 20–50 years are affected, with a higher prevalence in men than in women.

Pathogenesis

In the untreated patient four stages of the disease are identified:

- Congestion.
- Red hepatization.
- Grey hepatization.
- Resolution.

The initial reactions in lobar peumonia are oedema and acute congestion, which last about 24 hours. Following an upper respiratory tract infection, there is an increase in nasopharyngeal secretions. Aspiration is facilitated by impaired defence barriers. Bacteria are carried by the secretions into the alveoli. Alveolar airspaces are filled with eosinophilic oedematous fluid containing neutrophil polymorphs. The oedema transports organisms through the pores of Kohn into the alveoli.

In days 2–4, a red hepatization occurs; there is accumulation in alveolar spaces of polymorphs, lymphocytes, and macrophages. The alveolar exudate contains a fine network of fibrin and large numbers of extravasated red cells. The lung is red, solid, and airless. Red hepatization corresponds to an area of oedema and haemorrhage.

In days 4–8, a grey hepatization occurs. Fibrinous pleurisy is present. Alveolar spaces are microscopically distended and filled by dense network of fibrin-containing neutrophil polymorphs. Grey hepatization represents a zone of advanced consolidation with destruction of red and white blood cells. The lung is grey or brown and solid.

Resolution occurs after 8–10 days in untreated cases. When bacteria have been eliminated, macrophages enter and replace granulocytes. The exudate is liquefied by fibrinolytic enzymes and coughed up or absorbed. There is preservation of the underlying alveolar wall architecture.

Clinical features

The clinical features (Fig. 11.16) of lobar pneumonia include abrupt onset of:

- High fever with rigors.
- Pleuritic chest pain on deep inspiration.
- Productive cough—sputum contains flecks of blood and is termed rusty.

Lower lobe involvement may cause referred pain to the shoulder because of diaphragmatic irritation. At extremes of age, presentation may be less typical and without typical respiratory signs.

Bronchopneumonia

Microorganisms colonize the bronchioles and extend into the surrounding alveoli, leading to numerous discrete foci of consolidation. Bronchopneumonia commonly occurs in old-age and infancy. It affects patients with concurrent disease (e.g. chronic renal failure and cardiac failure).

Typical clinical features of bacterial pneumonia	
Clinical feature	**Incidence (%)**
respiratory features	
cough	90
sputum	70
dyspnoea	70
chest pain	65
upper respiratory tract symptoms	33
haemoptysis	13
nonrespiratory features	
vomiting	20
confusion	15
diarrhoea	15
rash	5
abdominal pain	5
signs	
fever	80–90
tachypnoea	80–90
tachycardia	80–90
abnormal chest signs	80–90
hypotension	20
confusion	15
herpes labialis	10

Fig. 11.16 Typical clinical features of bacterial pneumonia.

Common pathogens in hospital and community infection	
Hospital-acquired infection	**Community-acquired infection**
Gram-negative bacteria (*Pseudomonas aeruginosa, Klebsiella pneumoniae, Escherichia coli,* and *Proteus*)	*Streptococcus pneumoniae*
	Mycoplasma pneumoniae
	influenzavirus A
	Haemophilus influenzae
Streptococcus pneumoniae	*Chylamidia*
Staphylococccus aureus	*Staphyloccocus aureus*
anaerobes	*Legionella pneumophilia*
fungi	*Coxiella burnetti*

Fig. 11.17 Table of common pathogens in hospital- and community-acquired infection.

Lobar pneumonia occurs when organisms widely colonize alveolar spaces, whereas bronchopneumonia occurs when organsims colonize bronchi and extend into alveoli.

Causative organisms tend to be of a low virulence: staphylococci, streptococci, *Haemophilus influenzae,* coliforms and fungi (Fig. 11.17).

Bronchopneumonia commonly affects the lower lobes and is bilateral. Patients become septicaemic.

Microscopically, there is an acute bronchiolitis: peribronchial alveoli are filled by an inflammatory exudate rich in neutrophil polymorphs; complete resolution is uncommon.

A variable amount of damage to the bronchiole walls with small areas of fibrosis occurs and bronchiectasis may develop if fibrosis is extensive.

Investigations

Several investigations are made:

- Sputum—culture and Gram stain.
- Blood—full blood count, blood culture (low sensitivity, high specificity).
- Chest radiography.
- Other specific tests—mycoplasma, legionella, and chlamydia antibodies; pneumococcal antigen testing by counter-immunoelectrophoresis (CIE) of the sputum, urine, and serum.

Treatment

Start treatment immediately, before microbiology results are available.

For mild cases use:

- Oral cefaclor 250 mg every 8 hours.
- Erythromycin 500 mg three times a day.

For severe cases, admit to hospital and use:

- Intravenous cefuroxime 1.5 g every 6 hours.
- Intravenous erythromycin 500 mg every 6 hours.
- Analgesia for pleuritic pain.
- Oxygen to correct hypoxia.

Treatment is modified on the basis of microbiological results.

Complications

Complications include pleural effusions, lung abscesses, and bacteraemia. Organization of exudate occurs as fibroblasts grow in from alveolar septa, leading to tissue fibrosis.

Prognosis

Overall mortality is 5%. Mortality is greater than 25% for bronchopneumonia caused by *Staphylococcus aureus.*

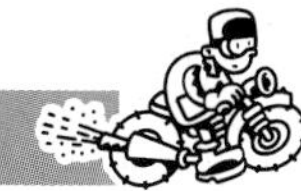

Community-acquired pneumonia is usually caused by Gram-positive bacteria, whereas hospital-acquired pneumonias are mainly caused by Gram-negative bacteria.

Primary atypical pneumonia: viruses and mycoplasma

Viral pneumonia

Viral pneumonia is uncommon in adults and is typically caused by influenza A virus (Fig. 11.18), a highly contagious virus.

Aetiology

Influenza virus is a spherical RNA virus covered by two antigens. Three forms exist (A, B, and C), with influenza A viruses more mutatable than B and C. Significant antigenic shifts in the surface antigens occur about every 10 years, leading to epidemics.

Complications of influenza occur most commonly in the elderly, in those with pre-existing cardiac and pulmonary disease, and late in pregnancy.

Primary influenza viral pneumonia

Primary influenza viral pneumonia is a serious disease with a high mortality rate; it develops 1–3 days after influenza onset. Patients present with high fever, dyspnoea, and cyanosis. On auscultation, signs of consolidation are absent. Chest radiography shows diffuse reticulonodular infiltrates more prominent in mid-lung fields.

Causative organisms of viral pneumonia	
Common	**Rare**
influenza virus	corona virus
measles virus (morbillivirus)	coxsackievirus
adenovirus	parainfluenza virus
varicellavirus	rhinovirus
cytomegalovirus	respiratory syncitial virus (pneumovirus)

Fig. 11.18 Causative organisms of viral pneumonia.

Respiratory failure and vascular collapse are common.

Pathology

Consolidation occurs because of hyperaemia; haemorrhagic oedema of the alveolar walls occurs. Infiltration by mononuclear cells and neutrophils is common.

There is thrombosis of alveolar capillaries and, in the most severely affected parts of the lung, there is focal necrosis of alveolar walls and hyaline membrane formation.

Capillary bleeding into alveolar spaces may occur.

Secondary bacterial pneumonia

This condition develops 3–6 days after influenza onset. Infection may be segmental or lobar, or as a patchy bronchopneumonia. Sputum contains neutrophils and bacteria.

Investigations

Isolate virus from sputum or throat washing.
Demonstrate a rise in antibody titre.

Prevention

Annual immunization with killed influenza vaccine is recommended in high-risk groups.

Treatment

Influenza viral pneumonia may require oxygen therapy. Appropriate antibiotics are necessary for secondary bacterial infections.

Mycoplasma pneumonia

Mycoplasma pneumonia is the second most common cause of community-acquired pneumonia.

Aetiology

Community outbreaks occur in 4–5-year cycles, with no seasonal prevalence. The condition affects patients in their teens and early twenties; asymptomatic infection is common. The incubation period is 3 weeks.

Clinical signs

Prominent headache is an early sign. A persistent, nonproductive cough becomes the dominant feature with time. Pharyngitis may be the only manifestation in some patients. Physical findings are often totally absent initially.

Diagnosis
Chest radiography shows:

- Patchy or confluent bronchopneumonia.
- In the lower lobe, unilateral marked infiltrate (more marked near hilus).

Leukocyte count is usually normal. Cold agglutinins occur in over 50% of patients. Diagnosis can be confirmed by rising antibody titre taken at presentation and 10 days later.

Treatment
Treatment is by erythromycin 500 mg four times a day for 7–10 days. Mortality is less than 0.1%

Lung abscess
Lung abscess is a localized inflammatory disease, with central necrosis surrounded by pneumonitis.

Aetiology
One causal factor is aspiration of infected material from the upper airway in an unconscious patient (e.g. an alcoholic).

Infection can occur by specific organisms (*Klebsiella pneumonias, Staphylococcus aureus,* and *Actinomyces bovis*) of the bronchiectactic or tuberculous cavities.

Beta-haemolytic streptococci and *Amoeba histolytica* can also cause abscesses.

Lung abscesses may form beyond bronchial obstructions (e.g. a foreign body or bronchial carcinoma). Lung abscess can be single (e.g. caused by aspiration) or multiple (e.g. caused by staphylococci).

A lung abscess can be a complication of pneumonia.

Clinical features
Onset may be acute or insidious. Acute symptoms include malaise, anorexia, fever, and a productive cough. Copious foul-smelling sputum is present, caused by the growth of anaerobic organisms.

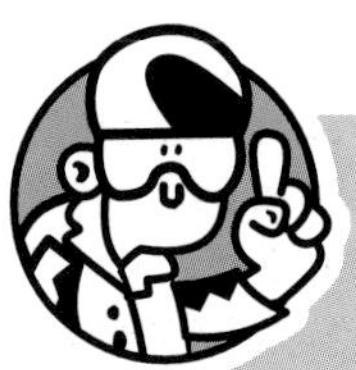

Questions on pneumonia are common in examinations.

A small area of dullness occurs over the area of pneumonitis. Pallor is common, caused by a moderate anaemia. Clubbing is a late sign.

Complications
Abscesses can heal completely leaving a small fibrous scar. Complications include empyema, bronchopleural fistula, pyopneumothorax, pneumatoceles, haemorrhage caused by erosion of a bronchial or pulmonary artery, meningitis, and cerebral abscess.

Investigations
Investigations must exclude necrosis in a malignant tumour or cavitation caused by tuberculosis.

Chest radiography shows a walled cavity with fluid level.

Sputum culture will identify a causative organism.

Blood culture and full blood count show that the patient is often anaemic with high erythrocyte sedimentation rate. Patients usually have mild to moderate leucocytosis.

Treatment
Follow disease carefully with regular chest radiographs and sputum collections. Resolution of disease is prompt after institution of appropriate antibiotics. Postural drainage should be used. Surgery is not usually indicated.

Pulmonary tuberculosis
The causative agent of pulmonary tuberculosis is *Mycobacterium tuberculosis.* Pulmonary tuberculosis is the world's leading cause of death from a single infectious disease. It is a notifiable disease and the prevalence is on the increase. In the UK, 7000 new cases occur per year, with the highest incidence among immigrants, who are 40 times more likely to develop the disease than the native Caucasian population. Their UK-born children are regarded as being at high risk and as such are immunised soon after birth.

Transmission and dissemination
Transmission is through the air or from direct contact. The pulmonary or bronchial focus ulcerates into an airway. A cough, sneeze, or exhalation then discharges droplets of viable *Mycobacterium tuberculosis.* The droplet nuclei are then inhaled by an uninfected person and can lodge anywhere in the lungs or airways.

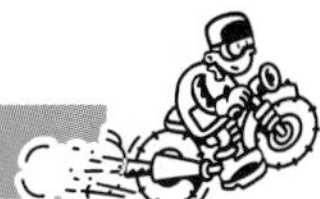

Primary tuberculosis

The initial lesion is usually solitary, 1–2 cm in diameter, and subpleural in the middle or upper zones. The focus of primary infection is called a Ghon complex. The primary infection has two components:

- The initial inflammatory reaction.
- Resultant inflammation in lymph nodes draining the area.

Within 3–8 weeks, the process becomes a tubercle, a granulomatous form of inflammation. The granulomatous lesion commonly undergoes necrosis in a process called caseation and is surrounded by mulitnucleated giant cells and epithelioid cells (both derived from macrophage). The caseous tissue may liquefy, empty into an airway, and be transmitted to other parts of the lung. Lymphatic spread of *Mycobacterium tuberculosis* occurs. The combination of tuberculous lymphadenitis and the Ghon complex is termed the primary complex.

In most cases, the primary foci will organize and form a fibrocalcific nodule in the lung with no clinical sequelae.

Secondary tuberculosis (postprimary tuberculosis)

Secondary tuberculosis results from reactivation of a primary infection or re-infection. Any form of immunocompromise may allow reactivation. The common sites are posterior or apical segments of the upper lobe or the superior segment of the lower lobe. Tubercle follicles develop and lesions enlarge by formation of new tubercles. Infection spreads by lymphatics and a delayed hypersensitivity reaction occurs.

In secondary tuberculosis, the lesions are often bilateral and usually cavitated. Most lesions are connected to fibrocalcific scars.

Progressive tuberculosis

Progressive tuberculosis may arise from a primary lesion or may be caused by reactivation of incompletely healed primary lesion or re-infection. Tuberculosis progresses to widespread cavitation, pneumonitis, and lung fibrosis. Early symptoms are seldom diagnostic.

Miliary tuberculosis

In miliary tuberculosis, an acute diffuse dissemination of tubercle bacilli occurs through the bloodstream. Numerous small granulomas form in many organs, with the highest numbers found in the lungs. These granulomas often contain numerous mycobacterium and are usually the result of a delay in diagnosis or commencement of treatment.

Miliary tuberculosis may be a consequence of either primary or secondary tuberculosis and is universally fatal without treatment.

Tuberculous bronchopneumonia

Tuberculous bronchopneumonia is an acute infection, usually bilateral. The lung tissue contains diffuse small pneumonic patches arranged around terminal bronchi. Tuberculous bronchopneumonia can develop from primary infection or reactivation.

The pathology of tuberculosis is shown in Fig. 11.19; complications are shown in Fig. 11.20.

Clinical features

Primary tuberculosis is usually asymptommatic. Gradual onset of symptoms occurs over weeks or months. Symptoms range from tiredness, anorexia, and malaise to bronchopneumonia with fever, cough, dyspnoea, and respiratory distress. Sputum is purulent, mucoid, or blood stained.

A pleural effusion or pneumonia may be the presenting complaint; an abnormal chest radiograph is often found, although the patient may be asymptomatic.

Diagnosis

Chest radiographs show upper zone shadows and fibrosis. Sequential sputum samples are taken:

- Stain with Ziehl–Neelson stain for acid-fast and alcohol-fast bacilli.
- Culture on Lowenstein–Jensen medium, which takes up to 8 weeks.

Bronchoscopy is useful if no sputum is available.

Biopsies from pleura, lymph nodes, and solid lesions within the lung may be necessary.

Prevention

BCG (bacille Calmette–Guérin) vaccination is a vaccine made from nonvirulent tubercle bacilli. The BCG vaccination is given to individuals who are tuberculin negative (Mantoux, Heaf, or tuberculin test). A positive test indicates prior infection. A 0.1 mL intradermal dose

primary

primary complex

3-8 weeks

post primary immunity

calcification

healing tuberculum test positive

reactivation or reinfection, usually years later, due to:

diabetes mellitus
malnutrition
immunosuppression:
drugs: cytotoxins
steroids
lymphoma
AIDS

erythema nodosum

small pleural effusion

6-9 months

collapse and bronchiectasis

adult pulmonary tuberculosis

miliary tuberculosis

TB meningitis

12 months

pleural effusion

pneumonia

within 3 years

tuberculosis affecting bones, joints, lymph nodes, kidneys, and gastrointestinal tract

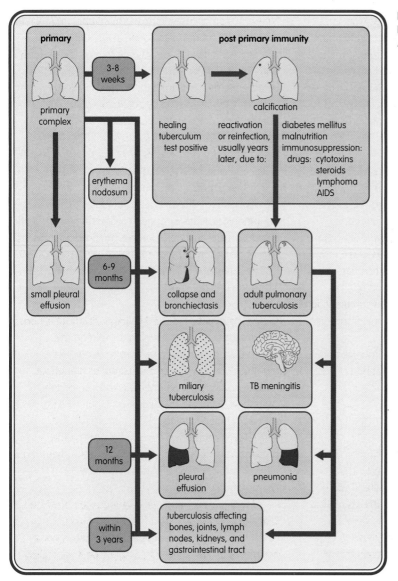

Fig. 11.19 Pathology of tuberculosis. From Kumar P, Clark M. *Clinical Medicine 3e*. Ballière Tindall; 1994.

Early and late complications of tuberculosis	
Early	**Late**
pneumonia	bronchiectasis
empyema	mycetomas in cavities
haemoptysis	colonization of fibrotic lung with a non-tuberculous mycobacterium
laryngitis	nonrespiratory disease
pneumothorax	

Fig. 11.20 Complications of tuberculosis.

(chosen dilution is usually 1:1000) is given to children and adults. BCG immunization occurs in newborns of high-risk groups (e.g. Asians). Immunization decreases the risk of developing tuberculosis by up to 70%. The BCG vaccination produces cellular immunity and a positive tuberculin test.

Treatment

Most patients are treated on an outpatient basis with combination therapy.

Treatment is provided in two phases:

- Initial phase lasting 2 months.
- Continuation phase lasting 3–6 months.

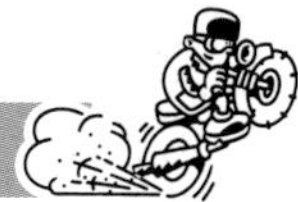

Rifampicin 600 mg is taken 30 mins before breakfast. Isoniazid 300 mg. Pyrazinamide 1.5–2.0 g daily for first 2 months.

Patients should be regularly followed up because lack of compliance is a major reason for treatment failure. Drug toxicity is a problem in a minority of cases.

Pneumonia in the immunocompromised

Pneumocystis carinii pneumonia

Pneumocystis carinii pneumonia (PCP) is a fungal infection that is largely confined to the lung. It is the commonest opportunistic infection in the immunocompromised.

PCP is an acute pulmonary infection which is often fatal. Infection occurs by inhalation of the organism. The patient presents with an insidious or abrupt onset of dry cough, fever, and dyspnoea.

Pleural effusions do not occur and there are no signs of consolidation.

Pathology

There is an interstitial infiltrate of mononuclear cells and alveolar airspaces filled with foamy eosinophilic material.

Diagnosis

Bilateral pneumonia in an immunocompromised patient should raise suspicion of PCP.

Diagnosed in 90% cases by staining using Giemsa, methanamine–silver, papanicocoau, or Gram–Weigert stains with monoclonal antibodies.

Chest radiography shows diffuse bilateral alveolar and interstitial shadowing, beginning in peripheral regions and spreading in a butterfly pattern.

Treatment

Oral trimethoprim sulphamethoxazole 120 mg/kg daily in divided dose.

Mortality of untreated patients is 100%; in treated patients, mortality is 20–50%.

Cytomegalovirus

Cytomegalovirus (CMV) is a DNA virus in the herpes group. Of patients with AIDS, 90% are infected with CMV. CMV also occurs in recipients of bone marrow and solid organ transplants. Only occasionally does CMV cause pneumonia.

Usual symptoms are a nonproductive cough, dyspnoea, and fever. Disseminated infection occurs, causing encephalitis, pneumonitis, retinitis, and diffuse involvement of the gastrointestinal tract.

Pathology

Features in the pathology of CMV infection include:

- Interstitial inflammatory infiltrate of mononuclear cells.
- Scattered alveolar hyaline membranes.
- Protein-rich fluid in alveoli.
- Intranuclear inclusion bodies found in alveolar epithelial cells.

Diagnosis

CMV infection can be diagnosed by the identification of characteristic intranuclear owl's eye inclusions in tissues and by direct immunofluorescence.

Treatment

Treatment is by ganaclovir 5 mg/kg daily for 14–21 days.

Aspergillus

Four pulmonary diseases are caused by the fungus *Aspergillus fumigatus*:

- Allergic aspergillosis.
- Mucoid impaction.
- Aspergilloma.
- Invasive aspergillosis.

Invasive aspergillosis

Invasive aspergillosis occurs in immunocompromised individuals with severe neutropenia or T-lymphocyte deficiency. It is confined to the lungs and may present as a necrotizing pneumonia, lung abscess, or solitary granuloma. Microabscesses contain the characteristic fungal filaments.

Recovery may occur after vigorous treatment with intravenous amphotericin. Prognosis is generally poor.

Cryptococcus

Cryptococcus is a budding, yeast-like fungus that may disseminate to all organs. Pulmonary lesions commonly involve the lower lobes, are nodular, and may simulate carcinoma. Other pulmonary manifestations include:

- Cavitation within lung nodules.
- Calcification.
- Pneumonitis.
- Pleural effusions.
- Intrathoracic lymph node enlargement.

Meningeal involvement is the commonest form of cryptococcosis.

Varicella zoster

Varicella zoster is an uncommon cause of pneumonia. The associated pustular rash confirms diagnosis. Treatment is with acyclovir.

Kaposi sarcoma

Kaposi sarcoma is a multifocal neoplastic condition typically seen in patients with AIDS. Lesions of the pleura, parenchyma, lymph nodes, and airways occur. Overall prognosis is poor.

- **Describe the differences between lobar pneumonia and bronchopneumonia.**
- **List the causes of hospital- and community-acquired pneumonia.**
- **Describe the management of a patient with pneumonia.**
- **What is the pathogenesis of tuberculosis?**
- **Describe primary and secondary tuberculosis.**
- **List the common causes of pneumonia in the immunocompromised patient.**

INTERSTITIAL DISEASE OF THE LUNG

Pulmonary fibrosis

Pulmonary fibrosis is the end result of many respiratory diseases (Fig. 11.21). The patient will have increased tissue within the lung causing decreased lung compliance.

The pathogenesis of pulmonary fibrosis is complex, involving many factors (Fig. 11.22). The main features are:

- A lesion affecting the alveolar capillary wall.
- Cellular infiltration, thickening, and fibrosis of the alveolar walls.
- Increased cells within the alveolar space, mainly macrophages and shed type II pneumocytes.

The end stage is characterized by a honeycomb lung, a nonspecific condition in which cystic spaces develop in fibrotic lungs with compensatory dilatation of unaffected neighbouring bronchioles.

Clinical features

Patients become progressively breathless and develop a dry, nonproductive cough. Irregular patchy infiltrative opacities are seen in the basal areas of chest radiographs. Lung function tests demonstrate a restrictive pattern along with a decreased transfer factor.

Pneumoconiosis

The pneumoconioses are a group of disorders caused by inhalation of mineral or biological dusts. The incidence is decreasing as working conditions continue to improve.

Four types of reaction occur:

- Inert (e.g. simple coal-worker's pneumoconiosis).
- Fibrous (e.g. asbestosis).
- Allergic (e.g. extrinsic allergic alveolitis).
- Neoplastic (e.g. mesothelioma).

Distribution of lung disease depends on the dust involved: particles measuring less than 2–3 μm in diameter reach the distal alveoli. Dust particles that are phagocytosed by alveolar macrophages drain into peribronchial lymphatics and hilar lymph nodes.

Radiological appearances are related to the degree of associated fibrosis and atomic number of dust particles involved.

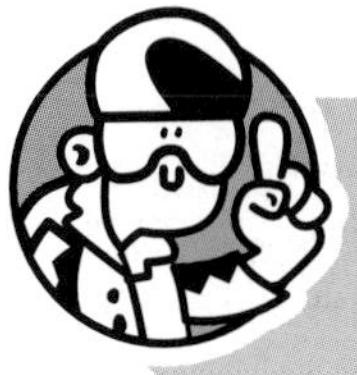

The end stage of chronic interstitial lung disease is termed honeycomb lung.

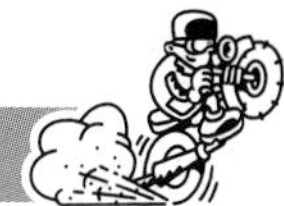

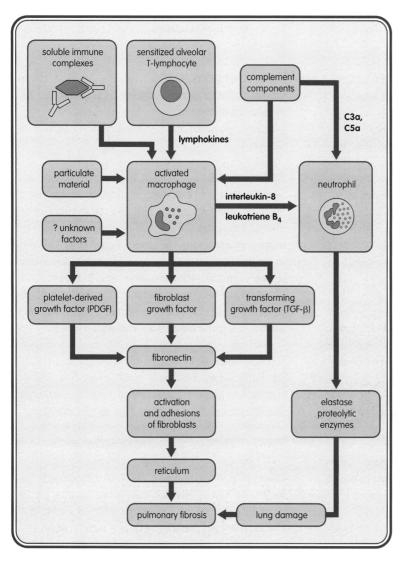

Causes of pulmonary fibrosis					
Dusts		Inhalants	Infection	Iatrogenic causes	Other causes
Mineral	Biological				
coal	avian protein	oxygen	postpneumonic infection	cytotoxic drugs	sarcoidosis
silica	*Actinomyces*	sulphur dioxide	acute respiratory disease	non-cytotoxics	connective-tissue disease
asbestos	—	nitrogen dioxide	—	toxins	—

Fig. 11.21 Causes of pulmonary fibrosis.

soluble immune complexes
sensitized alveolar T-lymphocyte
complement components
C3a, C5a
lymphokines
particulate material
? unknown factors
activated macrophage
interleukin-8
leukotriene B_4
neutrophil
platelet-derived growth factor (PDGF)
fibroblast growth factor
transforming growth factor (TGF-β)
fibronectin
activation and adhesions of fibroblasts
elastase proteolytic enzymes
reticulum
pulmonary fibrosis
lung damage

Fig. 11.22 Pathogenesis of pulmonary fibrosis. Macrophages can be activated by several factors (e.g. soluble immune complexes and sensitized T-lymphocytes), resulting in the release of various cytokines leading to fibrosis. From Kumar P, Clark M. *Clinical Medicine 3e.* Ballière Tindall; 1994.

Coal-worker's pneumoconiosis

The incidence of coal-worker's pneumoconiosis is related to total dust exposure: it is highest in men who work at the coal face. Two syndromes exist: simple pneumoconiosis and progressive massive fibrosis.

Simple pneumoconiosis

Simple pneumoconiosis is the commonest type of pneumoconiosis, reflecting coal dust deposition within the lung. It is asymptomatic. Two patterns exist:

- Macular coal-worker's pneumoconiosis—focal aggregates of dust laden macrophages. No significant scarring is present.
- Nodular coal-worker's pneumoconiosis—progression from the macular stage. Nodules are less than 10 mm in diameter. No significant scarring is present.

Simple pneumoconiosis is graded on radiographic appearance. Opacities on chest radiographs are mainly in the upper zone grades as follows:

1. A few small, round opacities are present.
2. Numerous small, round opacities are present. Normal lung markings are visible.
3. Very numerous small, round opacities are present. Normal lung markings are partially or totally obscured

Of patients with category 3 simple pneumoconiosis, 30% will develop progressive massive fibrosis.

Progressive massive fibrosis

In progressive massive fibrosis, large, round fibrotic nodules measuring more than 10 mm in diameter are seen, usually in the upper lobes. Scarring is present. Nodules may show central liquefaction and become infected by tuberculosis. The associated emphysema is always severe.

Symptoms include dyspnoea, cough, and sputum production (which may be black). Lung function tests show a mixed restrictive and obstructive pattern.

The disease may progress once exposure has ceased (unlike simple coal-worker's pneumoconiosis) and there is no specific treatment.

Asbestosis

Asbestos is a mixture of silicates of iron, nickel, magnesium, aluminium, and cadmium. It is mined in Southern Africa, the former Soviet Union, and Canada. Several types of asbestos exist: amphiboles are the fibres that cause pulmonary disease in man, of which crocidolite (blue asbestos) is the most important.

Blue asbestos exists in straight fibres measuring 50 μm in length and 1–2 μm in width; they are resistant to macrophage and neutrophil enzyme destruction.

Asbestos fibres may become coated in acid mucopolysaccharide and encrusted with haemosiderin to form the drumstick-shaped asbestos bodies. Histology shows features of pulmonary fibrosis and honeycomb lung, affecting the lower lobes more commonly. A considerable time lag exists between exposure and disease development. The first clinical symptoms are dyspnoea and a dry cough. Bilateral end inspiratory crackles indicate significant diffuse pulmonary fibrosis.

No treatment is available.

Caplan's syndrome

Caplan's syndrome is caused by a combination of coal-worker's pneumoconiosis and the disturbed immunity of rheumatoid arthritis.

Rounded lesions occur, measuring 0.5–5.0 cm in diameter.

Sarcoidosis

Sarcoidosis is a multisystem granulomatous disorder of unknown aetiology. Sarcoidosis is a common cause of interstitial lung disease, with only lymph nodes involved more commonly than the lungs. Women are more likely to develop the condition, which has a peak incidence in patients aged 20–40 years. Prevalence in the UK is 19:100 000. A geographical distribution shows that it is common in the USA and rare in Japan. The course of the disease is more severe in American blacks.

Clinical features

Sarcoidosis is asymptomatic in 30% of patients. The commonest presentation is with respiratory symptoms or radiographic abnormalities, notably bilateral hilar lymphadenopathy. Other symptoms include mild fever, malaise, arthralgia, and erythema nodosum.

Pulmonary infiltration leads to progressive fibrosis, causing dyspnoea, cor pulmonale, and eventually death.

Pulmonary infiltration

Pulmonary infiltration occurs as noncaseating granulomas distributed along the lymphatics and the walls of small airways and blood vessels. These

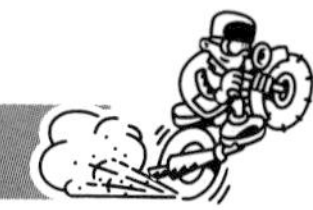

granulomas heal with minimal fibrosis. In progressive sarcoidosis, an interstitial fibrosis develops.

Extrapulmonary manifestations

Extrapulmonary manifestations are as follows:

- Skin sarcoidosis (e.g. erythema nodosum).
- Eye manifestations (e.g. anterior uveitis).
- Metabolic manifestations (e.g. hypercalcaemia).
- Central nervous system involvement (e.g. cranial nerve palsies).
- Bone and joint involvement (e.g. arthralgia).
- Hepatosplenomegaly.
- Cardiac involvement (e.g. cor pulmonale).

Sarcoidosis is diagnosed on histological evidence of widespread noncaseating epithelioid granulomas in more than one organ.

Investigations

Chest radiography can be useful:

- Bilateral hilar lymphadenopathy is characteristic feature.
- Reticular shadows typically appear in upper lobes after fibrosis starts.
- Although sarcoidosis is often asymptomatic, evidence from CT can indicate lung parenchymal involvement.

Full blood count can show mild normochromic normocytic anaemia and raised erythrocyte sedimentation rate. Serum biochemistry can reveal hypercalcaemia.

Lymph node transbronchial biopsy gives positive results in 90% of cases of pulmonary sarcoidosis.

In the past, the Kveim test has been used:

- Intradermal injections of splenic sarcoid tissue are undertaken.
- Granuloma formation occurs in affected patients.
- Transbronchial biopsy has superseded the Kveim test.

Serum ACE levels are two standard deviations above their normal mean value in 75% of patients. Serum ACE levels help to monitor response to treatment; the test is nonspecific, and is therefore of no diagnostic value.

Treatment

If the patient has hilar lymphadenopathy and no lung involvement, then no treatment is required.

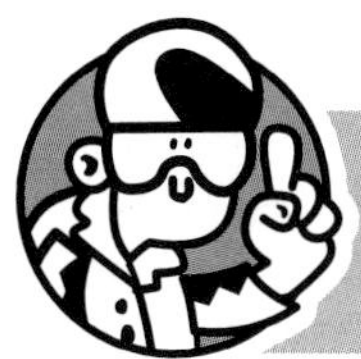

Sarcoidosis is a common topic for essays.

If infiltration has occurred for more than 6 weeks treat with corticosteroids (30 mg per day for 6 weeks then 15 mg on alternate days for 6–12 months).

Prognosis

Mortality is less than 5% in UK Caucasians and approximately 10% in Afro-Americans. If shadowing is present on chest radiographs for more than 2 years, the risk of fibrosis increases.

Idiopathic pulmonary fibrosis

Also known as fibrosing alveolitis or cryptogenic fibrosing alveolitis, idiopathic pulmonary fibrosis is a rare condition of progressive chronic pulmonary fibrosis of unknown aetiology. It has a peak incidence in patients aged 45–65 years.

Clinical features

Clinical features include progressive breathlessness and a dry cough. Fatigue and considerable weight loss can occur. There is progression to cyanosis, respiratory failure, pulmonary hypertension, and cor pulmonale over time.

Clubbing occurs in two-thirds of patients; bilateral, fine, end-inspiratory crackles are heard on auscultation.

Pathology

The alveoli walls are thickened because of fibrosis, predominantly in the subpleural regions of the lower lobes. An increased number of chronic inflammatory cells are in the alveoli and interstitium. This pattern is termed 'usual interstitial pneumonitis' and is a progressive condition.

Patterns of disease also include:

- Desquamative interstitial pneumonitis.
- Bronchiolitis obliterans.

Other patterns are observed and discussed elsewhere.

Idiopathic pulmonary fibrosis has been reported with a number of other conditions: connective-tissue disorders, coeliac disease, ulcerative colitis, and renal tubular acidosis.

Investigations

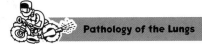

Several investigations are made:

- Transbronchial lung biopsy to confirm histological diagnosis.
- CT scan.
- Blood gases may show arterial hypoxaemia.
- Full blood count may show raised erythrocyte sedimentation rate.
- Lung function test shows a restrictive pattern.
- Bronchoalveolar lavage shows increased numbers of neutrophils.
- Autoantibody tests.
- Antinuclear factor is positive in one-third of patients. Rheumatoid factor is positive in one-half of patients.

Prognosis

Of patients with the condition, 50% die within 4–5 years.

Treatment

One-third of patients respond to immunosuppression:

- Prednisolone 30 mg daily—response may take 1–2 months.
- Azathioprine.
- Cyclophosphamide.

Single lung transplantation may be attempted where necessary.

Supportive treatment includes oxygen therapy.

Diffuse pulmonary haemorrhage syndromes

Goodpasture's syndrome

Goodpasture's syndrome usually occurs in patients older than 16 years. It usually begins with an upper respiratory tract infection. Goodpasture's syndrome is thought to be a type II hypersensitivity reaction.

Clinical features

Clinical features include haemoptysis, haematuria, and anaemia caused by massive bleeding.

Most patients have antiglomerular basement membrane antibody circulating in their blood, which causes glomerulonephritis and also acts on alveolar membranes, causing pulmonary haemorrhage. The coarse of the disease is variable: some patients resolve completely, others proceed to renal failure. There is an association with influenza virus A_2.

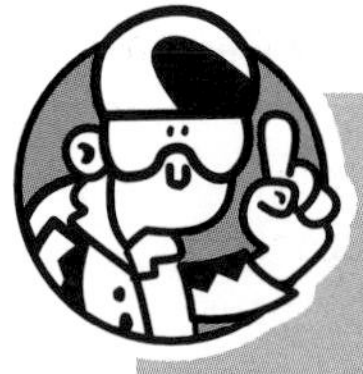

Goodpasture's syndrome is caused by autoantibodies to the alveolar basement membrane.

Treatment

Treatment is by corticosteroids or plasmapheresis to remove antibodies.

Idiopathic pulmonary haemosiderosis

Idiopathic pulmonary haemosiderosis is a rare condition, typically occurring in children aged under 7 years. An association with sensitivity to cow's milk has been suggested.

Clinical features

Patients present with haemoptysis because of recurrent episodes of intra-alveolar haemorrhage, cough, and dyspnoea.

Pathology

The more acute form of idiopathic pulmonary haemosiderosis shows evidence of diffuse alveolar damage and type II pneumocyte hyperplasia. Haemosiderin-containing macrophages are found in the sputum.

Treatment

Treatment is by corticosteroids and azathioprine. Prognosis is poor

Hypersensitivity pneumonitis

Hypersensitivity pneumonitis is also known as extrinsic allergic alveolitis. The condition is a widespread diffuse inflammatory reaction caused by a type III hypersensitivity reaction and results from the individual being already sensitized to the inhaled antigen. Antigens that can cause allergic lung disease include:

- Bird faeces (e.g. in bird fancier's lung).
- Cotton fibres (e.g. byssinosis).
- Sugar cane fibres (e.g. bagassosis).

Farmer's lung

In farmer's lung, a fungus present in mouldy hay is inhaled and a type III immune complex reaction follows if the individual is already sensitized. Initial

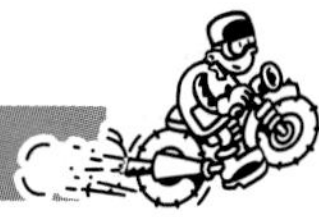

infiltration of small airways and alveolar walls with neutrophils occurs. Lymphocytes and macrophages then infiltrate, leading to the development of noncaseating granulomas, which may resolve or organize leading to pulmonary fibrosis.

Clinical features consist of fever, malaise, cough, and dyspnoea developing several hours after initial exposure to the antigen. Coarse end-inspiratory crackles are heard on auscultation.

Investigations include polymorphonuclear leucocyte count, precipitating antibodies (evidence of exposure not disease), lung function tests, and bronchoalveolar lavage.

Prevention is the aim of treatment. Corticosteroids help prevent onset of pulmonary fibrosis.

Pulmonary eosinophilia

The severity of these diseases can range from mild to fatal (Fig. 11.23).

Bronchiolitis obliterans

In bronchiolitis obliterans, characteristic histological appearance shows:

- Polypoid masses of organizing inflammatory exudate.
- Granulation tissue extending from alveoli to bronchioles.

Aetiology is unknown, although an association with a number of clinical conditions exists:

- Viral infections (e.g. respiratory syncitial virus).
- Aspiration.
- Inhalation of toxic fumes.
- Extrinsic allergic alveolitis.
- Pulmonary fibrosis.
- Collagen or vascular disorders.

Bronchiolitis obliterans is sensitive to corticosteroid treatment.

Collagen disorders and vascular disorders

Rheumatoid diseases

The respiratory system is affected in 10–15% of patients with rheumatoid disease; respiratory disease may occur before other systemic features. Patients characteristically have severe seropositive rheumatoid disease.

Diffuse pulmonary fibrosis can occur. Small-airway disease shows bronchiolitis obliterans or follicular bronchiolitis with lymphoid aggregates and germinal centres. Rheumatoid nodules are rare in the lung and when they do occur they usually cavitate. The pleura may show fibrosis and chronic unilateral pleural effusions are common.

Systemic lupus erythematosus (SLE)

In patients with systemic lupus erythematosus (SLE), pleurisy may develop, with or without an effusion. When present, effusions are small and bilateral.

Basal pneumonitis may be present and diffuse pulmonary fibrosis is rare.

Desquamative interstitial pneumonitis

Desquamative interstitial pneumonitis is found in

Pulmonary eosinophilia					
Disease	**Symptoms**	**Blood eosinophils (%)**	**Multisystem involvement**	**Duration**	**Outcome**
simple	mild	10	none	<1 month	good
prolonged	mild/moderate	<20	none	>1 month	good
asthmatic	moderate/severe	5–20	none	years	fair
tropical	moderate/severe	>20	none	years	fair
hyper-eosinophilic syndrome	severe	>20	always	months/years	poor
polyarteritis nodosa	severe	>20	always	months/years	poor/fair

Fig. 11.23 Table of causes of pulmonary eosinophilia.

Lung involvement is common in non-organ-specific autoimmune disease.

patients with fibrosing alveolitis. It is more diffuse than usual interstitial pneumonitis. A proliferation of macrophages in the alveolar airspaces occurs, along with interstitial thickening by mononuclear inflammatory cells. Lymphoid tissue and a small amount of collagen are sometimes present.

Desquamative interstitial pneumonitis has a distinctly uniform histological pattern. The alveolar walls show relatively little fibrosis.

Corticosteroids may be beneficial, and prognosis is good.

Alveolar proteinosis

Alveolar proteinosis is a rare condition, also known as alveolar lipoproteinosis. The aetiology is unknown in the majority of cases and pathogenesis is uncertain. It has been hypothesized that there is increased destruction or decreased clearance of type II cells and accumulation of eosinophilic material within the alveoli. Alveolar proteinosis is associated with a high incidence of concomitant fungal infections and may complicate other interstitial disease (e.g. desquamative interstitial pneumonitis.

The main symptoms of alveolar proteinosis are dyspnoea and cough. Chest pain and haemoptysis are rare.

The course of the disease is variable, but the majority of patients enjoy spontaneous remission.

- **What is the pathogenesis of pulmonary fibrosis?**
- **Describe the different forms of pneumoconioses.**
- **List the extrapulmonary manifestations of sarcoidosis.**
- **List the diseases which cause pulmonary eosinophilia.**
- **Describe pulmonary manifestations of vascular and collagen disorders.**

DISEASES OF IATROGENIC ORIGIN

Drug-induced lung disease

Pulmonary disease caused by medication is a growing problem. The mechanisms of drug-induced lung damage are either immunological or cytotoxic and the type of adverse reaction can be either:

- Predictable if caused by a dose-related effect.
- Unpredictable if caused by the development of hypersensitivity reactions.

There are no specific clinical, functional, or radiological findings in drug-induced pulmonary disease. The commonest symptoms include dyspnoea and cough (Fig. 11.24).

Examples of drug-induced lung diseases include:

- Bleomycin—the development of bleomycin-induced pulmonary disease is dose dependent. Bleomycin causes oxygen-radical-induced lung damage. Incidence is approximately 3%, with a mortality rate of 1–2%.
- Amiodarone—a class III antiarhythmic drug, which can cause fatal interstitial pneumonitis. Lung damage has its onset several months after commencement of amiodarone treatment. Incidence of toxicity is 1–2%. The condition responds well to corticosteroid treatment.

Pulmonary manifestations of adverse drug reactions	
Adverse reaction	**Examples**
diffuse alveolar damage	bleomycin, methotrexate, amiodarone, radiotherapy
interstitial pneumonitis	methotrexate, busulphan, amiodarone, gold
eosinophilic pneumonia	bleomycin, naproxzen, sulphasalazine
bronchiolitis obliterans	methotrexate, gold, mitomycin
pulmonary haemorrhage	amphotericin B, anticoagulants, hydralazine
pulmonary oedema	codeine, methadone, naloxone, salicylates
pleural effusions and fibrosis	amiodarone, hydralazine, bleomycin, bromocriptine

Fig. 11.24 Summary of pulmonary manifestations of adverse drug reactions.

- β blockers—β blockers are contraindicated in patients with asthma as they also block airway β receptors, thus precipitating bronchoconstriction.
- Aspirin—may induce asthma, either through decreased prostaglandin production or by increased leukotriene production. Recovery is usual on discontinuation of the drug.

Complications of radiotherapy

The lungs are very sensitive to radiation. Clinical effects depend on the dose given, volume of lung irradiated, and length of treatment. Pulmonary response to radiation is characterized by:

- Acute phase of radiation pneumonitis.
- Chronic phase of healing or fibrosis.

Acute radiation pneumonitis

Acute radiation pneumonitis is defined as an acute infiltrate precisely confined to the radiation area and occurring within 3 months of radiotherapy. Acute radiation pneumonitis rarely produces symptoms within the first month after therapy. Symptoms have an insidious onset and include nonproductive cough, shortness of breath on exertion, and low-grade fever.

Diffuse alveolar damage occurs, consisting of a proteinaceous exudate of material in the alveolar air spaces associated with hyaline membranes, especially in alveolar ducts. Endothelial damage, loss of normal respiratory epithelium, and hyperplasia of type II pneumocytes also occur.

Radiation pneumonitis results in a restrictive lung defect and corticosteroids should be given in the acute phase.

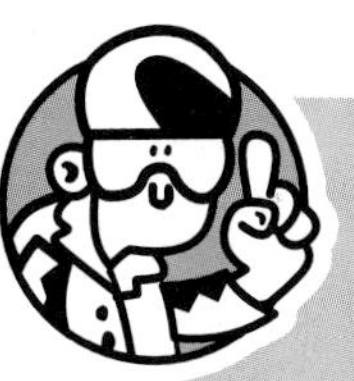

Do not give nonsteroidal anti-inflammatory drugs (NSAID) to asthmatics.

Chronic fibrosis

Acute radiation pneumonitis can resolve spontaneously or progress to pulmonary fibrosis. The chronic fibrosing state is usually asymptommatic. Proliferation and fragmentation of elastic fibres occurs and bronchiolitis obliterans and bronchial fibrosis may be present.

Chronic fibrosis is not precisely confined to irradiated areas.

Lung transplantation

Single lung transplantation is preferred to double transplantation because of donor availability. Bilateral lung transplantation is required in infective conditions to prevent bacterial spill-over from a diseased lung to a single lung transplant.

Patients must have end-stage lung or pulmonary vascular disease with no other treatment options (Fig. 11.25).

Complications

The complications of lung transplantation are described in Fig. 11.26.

Strategies for avoiding rejection

Lung transplantation does not require any significant degree of matching based on tissue type. The main criteria are compatibility of blood group and size match between organ and recipient.

Suppression of the immune system

All transplant patients require immunsuppression for life. This begins immediately before transplantation; drugs used include:

- Prednisolone.
- Azathioprine.
- Cyclosporin.

Large doses are given in the initial postoperative period. Lower maintenance doses are achieved after a few months. Rejection episodes are treated with high-dose intravenous corticosteroids.

Prognosis

One-year survival rates are 60–70%.

Lung transplantation	
Indications	**Diseases treated by transplantation**
age <60 years	pulmonary fibrosis
life expectancy <18 months without transplantation	primary pulmonary hypertension
no underlying cancer	bronchiectasis and cystic fibrosis
no serious systemic disease	emphysema including α_1-antitrypsin deficiency

Fig. 11.25 Indications and diseases treated by lung transplantation.

- Give examples of the pulmonary manifestations of adverse drug reactions.
- Describe the pulmonary effects of radiation.
- What is the rationale of lung transplantation?

NEOPLASTIC DISEASE OF THE LUNG

Bronchogenic carcinoma

Bronchial carcinoma accounts for 95% of all primary tumours of the lung and is the commonest malignant tumour in the Western world. It is the second most common cause of death in women after breast cancer; the mortality rate is rising in women but has stabilized in men. Bronchogenic carcinoma affects men more than women (M:F ratio, 3.5:1) and has an overall 5-year survival rate of 4–7%. Typically patients are aged 40–70 years at presentation; 2–3% occur in younger patients.

Complications of lung transplantation	
Complication	**Time**
hyperacute rejection	seconds/minutes
pulmonary oedema	12–72 hours
bacterial lower respiratory tract infection:	
donor-acquired	hours/days
recipient-acquired	days/years
acute rejection	day 5/years
airway complications	week 1/months
opportunistic infection	week 4/years
chronic rejection (e.g. bronchiolitis obliterans)	week 6/years

Fig. 11.26 Summary of the complications of lung transplantation.

Aetiology

Cigarette smoking is the largest contributory factor:

- It is related to the amount smoked, duration, and tar content.
- The rise in incidence of lung cancer correlates closely to the increase in smoking over the past century.
- In nonsmokers, the incidence is 3–5 cases per 100 000. In the UK, there are 100 deaths per 100 000 smokers per year.
- The risk in those who give up smoking decreases with time.

Environmental factors include:

- Radon released from granite rock.
- Passive smoking (increases risk by factor of 1.5).

Chronic inflammation predisposes to alveolar cell carcinoma.

There is a risk associated with occupational exposure to carcinogens (e.g. inhalation of asbestosis). Pulmonary fibrosis predisposes to adenocarcinoma.

Cell types

There are four main histological types of bronchogenic carcinoma:

- Non-small-cell carcinomas (70%):
  - Squamous cell carcinoma (52%).
  - Adenocarcinoma (13%).
  - Large-cell carcinoma (5%).
- Small-cell carcinomas (30%).

Tumours may occur as discrete or mixed histological patterns; the development from the initial malignant change to presentation is variable:

- Squamous cell carcinoma: 8 years.
- Adenocarcinoma: 15 years.
- Small-cell carcinoma: 3 years.

Squamous cell carcinoma

Squamous cell carcinoma arises from bronchial epithelium in the large bronchi. A strong association between cigarette smoking and squamous cell carcinoma exists. Males are affected most commonly, with a mean age at diagnosis of 57 years.

Squamous cell carcinomas arise from squamous metaplasia and are histologically well differentiated. Major mass of the tumour may occur outside the bronchial cartilage and encircle the bronchial lumen,

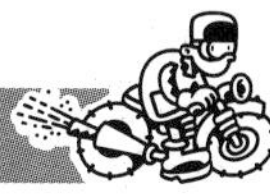

producing obstructive phenomena. The tumours are almost always hilar and are prone to massive necrosis and cavitation, with upper lobe lesions more likely to cavitate. Of squamous cell carcinomas, 13% show cavitation on chest radiographs. Peripheral lesions tend to be larger than those seen in adenocarcinomas.

If squamous carcinoma occurs in the apical portion of the lung, it may produce Pancoast's syndrome.

Symptoms include cough and sputum production. Haemoptysis, chest pain, pneumonia, and dyspnoea develop later.

Diagnosis

Diagnosis is by bronchoscopy (with biopsy and bronchial washings) and by sputum cytology.

In two-thirds of cases, exfoliated malignant cells can be identified in sputum. Squamous cell carcinoma tends to metastasize locally to hilar lymph nodes; distant metastases are a later feature. The condition should be treated surgically whenever possible. The tumour is radiosensitive.

Untreated, squamous cell carcinoma has the longest patient survival of any of the bronchogenic carcinomas.

Pancoast's syndrome

Pancoast's syndrome can be caused by all types of bronchogenic carcinoma, although two-thirds originate from squamous cells. As the tumour grows outward from the pulmonary parenchymal apex, it encroaches on anatomical structures, including:

- Chest wall.
- Subpleural lymphatics.
- Sympathetic chain.

Tumour extension can result in loss of sympathetic tone and an ipsilateral Horner's syndrome. Intractable shoulder pain occurs when the upper rib is involved. The subclavian artery and vein may become compressed. Destruction of the inferior trunk of the brachial plexus leads to pain in the ulnar nerve distribution and may lead to small-muscle wasting of the hand.

Pancoast's tumour is diagnosed by percutaneous needle aspiration of the tumour.

Rarely is the condition caused by nonbronchogenic tumours (e.g. metastatic lesions and tuberculosis).

Squamous cell carcinoma is the commonest cause of bronchogenic carcinoma.

Adenocarcinoma

Adenocarcinomas are most common in:

- Nonsmoking elderly women.
- The Far East.

Adenocarcinomas are associated with diffuse pulmonary fibrosis and honeycomb lung. Bronchogenic tumours associated with occupational factors are mainly adenocarcinomas. Ninety per cent of adenocarcinomas occur between 40–69 years of age, with the mean age for diagnosis being 53.3 years. Two-thirds of adenocarcinomas are found peripherally. Usually, tumours measure more than 4 cm in diameter.

Adenocarcinoma arises from glandular cells such as mucous goblet cells, type II pneumocytes, and clara cells. Histologically, they are differentiated from other bronchogenic tumours by their glandular configuration and mucin production. The gland structure may be acina or papillary.

Adenocarcinomas are classified according to four groups:

- Acinar.
- Papillary.
- Solid.
- Bronchoalveolar.

In practice, pathologists distinguish bronchioalveolar tumours, but treat the other three groups as similar. Two growth patterns are seen:

- Discrete nodule in the periphery with pleural tethering.
- Multifocal and bilateral diffuse tumour (so-called bronchioalveolar cell carcinoma).

Obstructive symptoms are rare, so the tumour tends to be clinically silent. Symptoms include coughing, haemoptysis, chest pain, and weight loss. Malignant cells are detected in the sputum in 50% of patients, and the commonest radiological presentation is a solitary peripheral pulmonary nodule, close to the pleural surface.

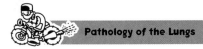

Resection is possible in a small proportion of cases; 5-year survival rate is less than 10%. Invasion of the pleura and mediastinal lymph nodes is common, as too is metastasis to the brain and bones.

Metastasis in the gastrointestinal tract, pancreas, or ovaries must be excluded after having made a diagnosis.

Large-cell anaplastic tumour

Large-cell anaplastic tumours are diagnosed by a process of elimination. No clear-cut pattern of clinical or radiological presentation distinguishes them from other malignant lung tumours. Under light microscopy, findings include:

- Pleomorphic cells with a large, darkly staining nuclei.
- Prominent nucleoli, abundant cytoplasm, and well-defined cell borders.
- Abundant mitoses.

Large-cell anaplastic tumours are variable in location, but are usually centrally located. Peripherally located lesions are larger than adenocarcinomas. The point of origin of the carcinoma influences symptomatic presentation of the disease: central lesions present earlier than peripheral lesions.

The tumour causes coughing, sputum production, and haemoptysis. When a tumour occurs in a major airway, obstructive pneumonia can occur. Sputum cytology and bronchoscopy with bronchial biopsy make the diagnosis.

On electron microscopy, these tumours turn out to be poorly differentiated variants of squamous cell carcinoma and adenocarcinoma; they are extremely aggressive and destructive lesions. Early invasion of blood vessels and lymphatics occurs, and treatment is by surgical resection whenever possible.

Small-cell carcinoma

Small-cell carcinomas arise from endocrine cells—Kulchitsky cells, members of the amine precursor uptake decarboxylase (APUD) system.

The incidence of this carcinoma is directly related to cigarette consumption and it is considered to be a systemic disease. Small-cell carcinomas are the most aggressive malignancy of all the bronchogenic tumours.

Most small-cell anaplastic tumours originate in the large bronchi and obstructive pneumonitis is frequently seen. Several histological subgroups of this carcinoma exist and all have:

- Cell size: 6–8 μm.
- High nucleus:cytoplasm ratio.
- Hyperchromatism of the nuclei.

When almost no cytoplasm is present, and the cells are compressed into an ovoid form, the neoplasm is called an oat-cell carcinoma. On radiography, the oat-cell carcinoma does not cavitate.

There is a high occurrence of paraneoplastic syndromes associated with this type of tumour, so presentation may be varied. The most frequent presenting complaint is coughing. Spread is rapid, and metastatic lesions may be the presenting sign. Small-cell carcinomas metastasize through the lymphatic route.

Chest radiography may help in diagnosis, although the diagnosis must be confirmed by histological or cytological means.

Prognosis is very poor, with a mean survival time for untreated patients with small-cell carcinoma of 7 weeks after diagnosis. Death is generally caused by metastatic disease.

Small-cell carcinoma is the only bronchial carcinoma that responds to chemotherapy.

Fig. 11.27 lists the paraneoplastic disorders associated with lung cancer.

Mixed tumours

A number of mixed tumour types exist that are commonly seen in resection material at autopsy.

Many pathologists base their diagnosis on the prominent cell type present because the predominant cell type predicts prognosis of the condition.

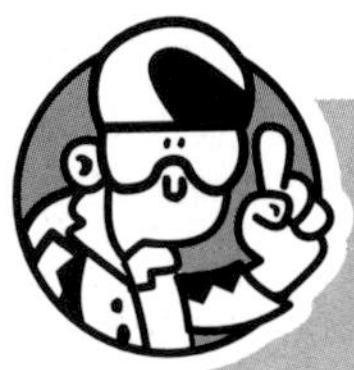

Adenocarcinoma of the lung is usually a peripheral tumour.

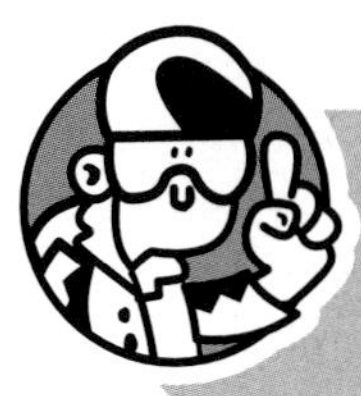

Large-cell anaplastic carcinomas lack features of differentiation.

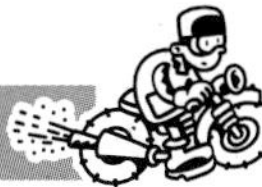

Common presenting symptoms

There are no specific signs of bronchogenic carcinoma. Diagnosis always needs to be excluded in cigarette smokers who present with recurrent respiratory symptoms:

- Persistent nonproductive coughing: 80%.
- Haemoptysis: 70%.
- Dyspnoea: 60%.
- Chest pain, often pleuritic caused by obstructive changes: 40%.
- Wheezing: 15%.

Unexplained weight loss is also a common presenting complaint.

Complications

Local

Ulceration of bronchus

Ulceration occurs in up to 50% of patients and produces haemoptysis in varying degrees.

Bronchial obstruction. The lumen of the bronchus becomes occluded; distal collapse and retention of secretions subsequently occur. This clinically causes dyspnoea, secondary infection, and lung abscesses.

Central necrosis. Carcinomas can outgrow their blood supply leading to central necrosis. The main complication is then the development of a lung abscess.

See Fig. 11.28 for an explanation of the effects and symptoms of local spread.

Metastatic

Local metastases to lymph nodes, bone, liver, and adrenal glands occurs.

Metastases to the brain present as:

- Change in personality.
- Epilepsy.
- Focal neurological lesion.

Investigations

Need to confirm diagnosis, assess tumour histology and spread.

Chest radiography

Good posteroanterior and lateral views are required. 70% of bronchial carcinomas arise centrally and chest radiography demonstrates over 90% carcinomas. The mass needs to be between 1–2 cm in size to be recognized reliably. Lobar collapse and pleural effusions may be present.

CT

CT scan gives good visualization of the mediastinum and is good at identifying small lesions. Valuable to assess extent of tumour and the operability of the mass. Lymph nodes >1.5 cm are pathological.

Scan should include brain, liver, and adrenals to identify distant metastases.

Fibreoptic bronchoscopy

Confirms central lesion, assesses operability, and allows accurate cell type to be determined. Used to obtain cytological specimens. Mucus secretions plus sputum examined for presence of malignant cells.

If carcinoma involves the first 2 cm of either main bronchus the tumour is inoperable.

Paraneoplastic disorders associated with lung cancer

Disorder	Incidence (%)
unexplained weight loss >6.4 kg	31
finger clubbing	29
fever	21
endocrine disorders	12
anaemia	8
neuromyopathy	1.4

Fig. 11.27 Paraneoplastic disorders associated with lung cancer. From McGee J, Isaacson P, Wright N. *Oxford textbook of pathology.* Oxford: Oxford University Press; 1992.

Effects of local spread

Site of spread	Symptoms
pleura/ribs	pain on respiration/pathological fractures
brachial plexus	shoulder pain and small muscle wasting of the hand
sympathetic ganglia	ipsilateral Horner's syndrome
recurrent laryngeal nerve	hoarse voice and bovine cough
superior vena cava	facial congestion; distended neck veins

Fig. 11.28 Effects and symptoms of local spread.

Transthoracic fine-needle aspiration biopsy

In transthoracic fine-needle aspiration biopsy, the needle is guided by X-ray or CT. Direct aspiration through chest wall of peripheral lung lesion; 25% of patients suffer pneumothorax due to the procedure.

Implantation metastases do not occur.

Treatment

Only treatment of any value in non-small-cell carcinoma is surgery; however, only 15% of cases are operable at diagnosis. A normal CT scan indicates no mediastinal spread and favours curative resection.

Lung function test must be performed as COPD has common aetiology and you need to assess fitness of the patient.

Radiation therapy

Treatment of choice if tumour is inoperable. Good for slowly growing squamous carcinoma.

Radiation pneumonitis develops in 10–15% and radiation fibrosis occurs to some degree in all cases.

Chemotherapy

Only effective treatment for small-cell carcinoma. Good results have been achieved with combination of mitomycin, ifosfamide, cisplatin.

Terminal care

Endoscopic therapy and transbronchial stenting are used to provide symptomatic relief in patients with terminal disease. Daily prednisolone (maximum dose: 15 mg) may improve appetite. Opioid analgesia is given to control pain and laxatives should be prescribed to counteract the opioid side effects. Candidiasis is a common treatable problem.

Both patient and relatives require counselling.

Prognosis

Poor prognosis: 20% patients are alive 1 year after diagnosis.

The different types of tumour are summarized in Fig. 11.29

Bronchoalveolar cell carcinoma

A distinctive type of adenocarcinoma occurring in the distal portions of the pulmonary parenchyma accounting for 3% of all primary neoplasm of lung. The carcinoma affects males and females equally and the incidence is not related to cigarette consumption.

Unifocal point of origin within the lung with the major bulk of the tumour seen in the alveoli rather than the bronchi. The lesion grows very slowly and spreads by the bronchial route to implant on other portions of the respiratory epithelium. The lesion may be stable for 5–10 years.

Tumour types

	Non-small-cell tumours			Small cell
	Squamous cell tumour	Adeno-carcinoma	Large cell	
incidence (%)	52	13	5	30
male/female incidence	M>F	F>M	M>F	M>F
location	hilar	peripheral	peripheral/ central	hilar
relationship to smoking	high	low	high	high
growth rate	slow	medium	rapid	very rapid
metastasis	late	intermediate	early	very early
treatment	surgery			chemotherapy
prognosis	2-year survival = 50%			3 months if untreated; 1 year if treated

Fig. 11.29 Summary of tumour types.

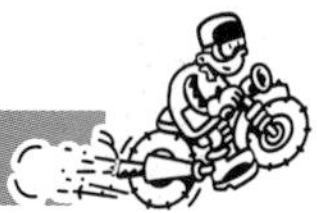

Associated with profuse mucoid sputum production.

In the early stage, radiography may show a nonspecific peripheral coin lesion. Diagnosis of the disease is based on histological examination of tissue obtained by transbronchial or open lung biopsy.

Surgical resection may be curative although surgical intervention is useless once dissemination has occurred.

Neuroendocrine tumours

Bronchial carcinomas may produce endocrine manifestations.

Corticotrophin

Oat cell carcinoma of the lung most commonly causes ACTH secretion. The adrenal glands subsequently secrete excessive quantities of:

- 17 hydroxysteroids.
- 17 ketosteroids.

Oat cell carcinoma induced ACTH secretion produces an atypical type of Cushing's syndrome. Hyperglycaemia, hypertension, and increased pigmentation are common and electrolyte disturbances are prominent.

The typical patient is a middle-aged male with muscular weakness, facial oedema, and severe hypokalemic alkalosis. There is seldom any suppression of hormonal activity following administration of dexamethasone.

ADH

Oat cell carcinoma is the most common cause of inappropriate ADH secretion.

Minimal criteria to make the diagnoses:

- Hyponatraemia.
- Decreased plasma osmolality.
- High urine sodium count.
- No renal, adrenal or cardiac disease sufficient to account for the defect.

Clinically the patient complains of headache, irritability, nausea, and vomiting. Mental confusion and muscle weakness are also features. Symptomatic treatment is restriction of water intake.

Parathormone

Caused by squamous cell carcinoma. The patient's symptoms depend on serum calcium levels; some patients may be asymptomatic with only slight calcium rises. Moderate hypercalcaemia causes:

- Lethargy.
- Polyuria.
- Polydipsia.
- Constipation.
- Abdominal pain.

Very high serum calcium levels causes:

- Comatose

May regress when the tumour mass is surgically removed.

Gonadotrophins

Squamous cell carcinoma, oat-cell carcinoma, and adenocarcinoma of the lung have all been implicated.

Clinical features are:

- Gynaecomastia.
- Testicular atrophy.

Hamartomas and miscellaneous mesenchymal tumours

Primary tumours other than carcinomas are rare.

Benign tumours

Adenomas

Arise from bronchial mucous glands. They present as polypoid or sessile lesions and symptoms are related to obstruction.

Benign mesenchymal tumours

Arise anywhere that mesenchyme occurs. The lesion is probably a hamartoma, it is a well circumscribed round lesion 1–2 cm composed of cartilage and found in the periphery of the lung. Rarely arises from a major bronchus and presents as an isolated coin lesion on radiographs.

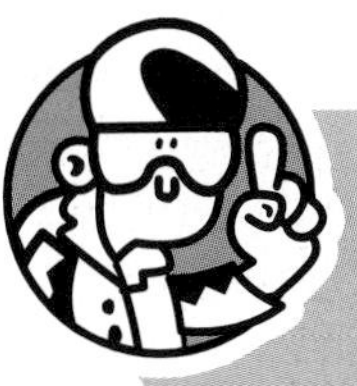

The majority of endocrine disturbances are caused by small-cell carcinomas.

Malignant tumours

Bronchial carcinoid

Low grade malignant tumour accounting for 1% of tumours found in the lungs. It affects males and females equally and presents < 40 yrs.

Bronchial carcinoids are locally invasive, highly vascular tumours that cause recurrent haemoptysis. The tumour grows slowly, eventually blocking a bronchus.

Rarely gives rise to the carcinoid syndrome and the 5yr survival > 80%.

Malignant mesenchymal tumours (sarcomas) are extremely rare.

Primary pulmonary lymphomas

Rare tumours composed of small B lymphocytes arising from the bronchus and bronchiole associated lymphoid tissue. Monotypic immunoglobulin may be secreted into the blood.

Metastatic malignancy to the lung

Metastases to the lung is a common clinical and radiological finding. Metastases are more likely to be multiple than solitary. Most haematogenous metastases are sharply circumscribed with smooth edges, and the appearance of multiple smoothly circumscribed nodules is highly suggestive of metastatic disease. Cavitation is unusual in metastatic lesions.

Solitary pulmonary metastases do occur as sarcomas of soft tissue or bone, carcinoma of the breast, colon, and kidney

Multinodular lung metastases may be of varying sizes (Fig. 11.30):

- Very large dimensions—cannonball pattern.
- Many small nodules—snowstorm pattern.

Calcification in metastatic malignancy is unusual. If it occurs it indicates chondrosarcoma or osteosarcoma. Carcinoma of the stomach, pancreas, and breast can involve the mediastinal glands and spread along lymphatics of both lungs—lymphangitis carcinomatosa.

Metastatic malignancy of lung and the resulting radiological appearance

Multinodular patterns		Solitary nodule
Cannonball	**Snowstorm**	
salivary gland	breast	breast
kidney	kidney	kidney
bowel	bladder	bowel
uterus/ovarian	thyroid	
testis	prostate	

Fig. 11.30 Metastatic malignancy of lung and the resulting radiological appearance.

- **What is the relationship between cigarette smoking and bronchogenic carcinomas?**
- **Classify bronchogenic carcinomas in terms of histology.**
- **List the bronchial carcinomas that are central and those that are peripherally located.**
- **Describe the differences between small-cell and non-small-cell carcinomas.**
- **List the common sites of metastases.**
- **Describe the care of the terminally ill patient with a bronchogenic carcinoma.**
- **Describe the endocrine manifestations of bronchogenic carcinomas.**
- **List the common malignancies that metastasize to the lung.**

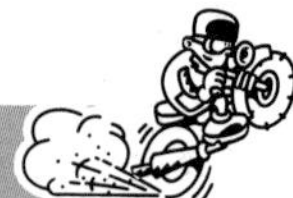

DISEASES OF THE PLEURA

Inflammatory pleural effusions

A pleural effusion is the presence of fluid between the visceral and parietal pleura (Fig. 11.31).

Transudative pleural effusions occur as a result of an imbalance between hydrostatic and osmotic forces. Exudative pleural effusions occur when local factors influencing pleural fluid formation and reabsorption are altered specifically through injury or inflammation (Fig. 11.32).

Inflammatory exudates are classified as:

- Serofibrinous.
- Suppurative (empyema).
- Haemorrhagic.

Suppurative

Also known as a pyothorax or empyema, this is a collection of pus within the pleural cavity caused by:

- Complication of thoracic surgery.

Pleural effusions			
Transudate		**Exudate**	
protein	<30 g/L	protein	>30 g/L
lactate dehydrogenase	<200 IU/L	lactate dehydrogenase	>200 IU/L
usually bilateral		unilateral in focal disease; bilateral in systemic disease	

Fig. 11.31 Classification of pleural effusions.

Causes of transudates and exudates	
Transudate	**Exudate**
left heart failure	bacterial pneumonia
hypoproteinaemia	carcinoma bronchus
constrictive pericarditis	pulmonary infarction
hypothyroidism	tuberculosis
cirrhosis	connective-tissue disease

Fig. 11.32 Causes of transudates and exudates.

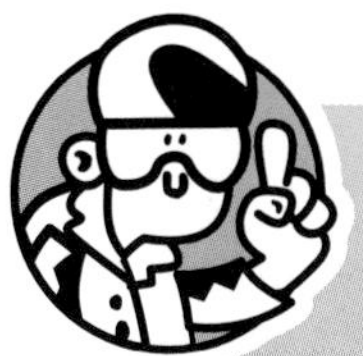

Questions on the cause of exudative and transudative pleural effusions are common in clinical examinations.

- Following rupture of lung abscess into the pleural space.
- Perforation of oesophagus.
- Mediastinitis.
- Bacterial spread of pneumonia.

Empyema cavity can become infected by anaerobes. The patients are pyrexial and ill. Empyemas require tube thoractomy and appropriate antibiotic treatment should be initiated immediately.

Haemorrhagic

If a haemorrhagic effusion exists neoplastic infiltration, pulmonary infarction, and TB need to be excluded. Leading malignancies that have associated pleural effusions are breast carcinoma, bronchial carcinoma, and lymphomas/leukaemia.

Clinical features of pleural effusions present only when >500 mL of fluid is present. Dyspnoea dependent on size of effusions develops.

Signs on examination see Chapter 8 (page 136).

Investigations

On a chest radiograph, it can be seen when >300 mL of fluid is present.

Pleural aspiration for microbiological examination.

Pleural biopsy.

Treatment

Treat the underlying disease. If the patient is symptomatic drain the effusion. Drain fluid slowly.

Malignant effusions—chemical pleurodesis can provide temporary relief. Use bleomycin/tetracycline.

Noninflammatory pleural effusions

Hydrothorax

A pleural effusion of transudated fluid of low protein

content. Hydrothorax is a common feature of congestive cardiac failure. High system venous pressure occurs causing:

- Increased transudation of fluid from pleural capillaries.
- Impaired drainage from the lymphatics and thoracic duct.

If large a hydrothorax may contribute to the dyspnoea of heart failure.

Hydrothoraces are commonly bilateral, if unilateral more likely to be right sided. The pleural fluid is a clear/light yellow colour.

A radiological finding specific to hydrothorax associated with congestive heart failure is the phantom tumour, in which fluid tends to localize in an interlobular pleural fissure.

Haemothorax

Blood in the pleural cavity. Common in both penetrating and nonpenetrating injuries of the chest and may cause hypovolaemic shock and reduce vital capacity through compression. Due to the defribinating action that occurs with motions of respiration and the presence of an anticoagulant enzyme the clot may be defribinated and leave fluid radiologically indistinguishable from effusions of another cause.

Blood may originate from lung, internal mammary artery, thoracicoacromial artery, lateral thoracic artery, mediastinal great vessels, heart, or abdominal structures via diaphragm. See Fig. 11.33 for the management of haemothorax.

Chylothorax

Accumulation of lymph in the pleural space. Commonest causes are rupture or obstruction of the thoracic duct due to surgical trauma or neoplasm, e.g. lymphoma. A latent period between injury and onset of 2–10 days occurs. The pleural fluid is high in lipid content and is characteristically milky in appearance. The prognosis is generally good.

Haemothorax	
Degree	**Management**
minimal (<350 mL)	blood usually reabsorbs spontaneously with conservative treatment
moderate (300–1500 mL)	thoracentesis and tube drainage with underwater seal drainage
massive (>1500 mL)	two drainage tubes inserted; immediate or early thoracotomy may be necessary to arrest bleeding

Fig. 11.33 Management of haemothorax.

Chylous effusion

Caused by the escape of chyle into the pleural space from obstruction or laceration of the thoracic duct.

Chyliform effusion

Results from degeneration of malignant and other cells in pleural fluid.

Pneumothorax

Accumulation of air in the pleural space. May occur spontaneously or following trauma.

Spontaneous

Results from rupture of a pleural bleb, the pleural bleb being a congenital defect of the alveolar wall connective tissue. Patients are typically tall, thin, young males. M:F ratio 6:1. Spontaneous pneumothoracies are usually apical affecting both lungs with equal frequency.

Secondary causes of spontaneous pneumothorax occur in patients with underlying disease such as, COPD, TB, pneumonia, bronchial carcinoma, sarcoidosis, and cystic fibrosis.

Patients present with sudden onset of unilateral pleuritic pain and increasing breathlessness.

Main aim of treatment is to get the patient back to active life as soon as possible.

Investigations

Chest radiography may show an area devoid of lung markings. May be more clearly seen on the expiratory film.

Management

Small pneumothorax: no treatment, but review in 7–10 days. Moderate pneumothorax: admit for simple aspiration.

Tension pneumothorax

Medical emergency.

Commonest causes:

- Positive pressure ventilation.
- Stab wound or rib fracture.

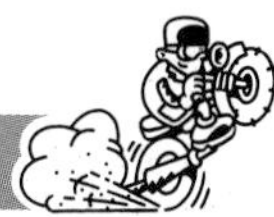

Air escapes into pleural space and the rise above atmospheric pressure causes the lung to collapse. At each inspiration intrapleural pressure increases as the pleural tear acts as a ball valve that permits air to enter but not leave the pleural space. Venous return to the heart is impaired as pressure rises and patient's experience dyspnoea and chest pain. They may also be cyanotic.

Clinically:

- Mediastinum pushed over into contralateral hemithorax. Tracheal deviation.
- Hyper resonance, absence of breath sounds.
- Intercostal spaces widened on ipsilateral side.

On ECG there is a rightward shift in mean frontal QRS complex, diminution in QRS amplitude, and inversion of precordial T waves.

Diagnosed on needle insertion.

Treatment immediate thoracostomy with underwater seal drainage, before requesting chest radiographs. See Fig. 11.34 for a radiograph of a tension pneumothorax. Fig. 11.35 gives a summary of noninflammatory pleural effusions.

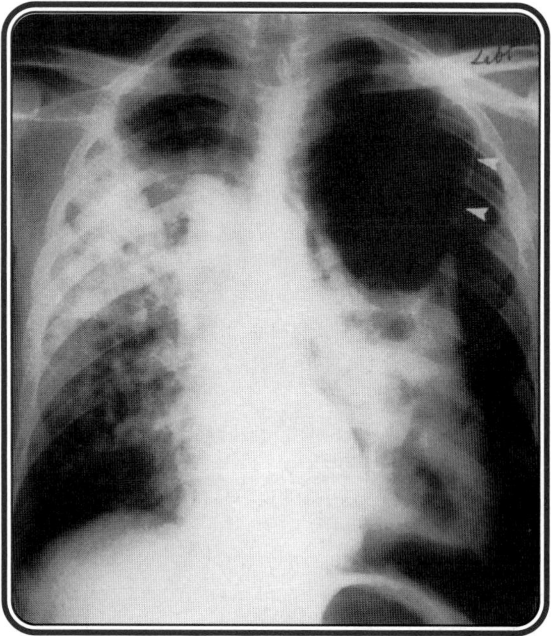

Fig. 11.34 Radiograph of a tension pneumothorax. Tension pneumothorax displacing mediastum and depressing left hemidiaphragm. Extensive consolidation and cavitation in both lungs is due to tuberculosis. A pleural adhesion (arrowheads) is visible. Courtesy of Dr D Sutton and Dr J W R Young.

Noninflammatory pleural effusions		
Disorder	**Collection**	**Cause**
haemothorax	blood	chest trauma; rupture of aortic aneurysm
hydrothorax	proteinaceous fluid	congestive cardiac failure
chylothorax	lymph	neoplastic infiltration; trauma
pneumothorax	air	spontaneous; traumatic

Fig. 11.35 Summary of noninflammatory pleural effusions.

Neoplasms of the pleura

Pleural fibroma

Rare neoplasm of the pleura not related to asbestos exposure which consists of:

- Fibrous connective tissue.
- Mesothelial cells.

A solitary mass can grow to be very large and hypertrophic pulmonary osteoarthropathy is a frequent association. Affects females most commonly with the mean age at presentation 50yrs.

Aetiology unknown. Most patients are asymptomatic.

Tumours grow slowly and behave generally in a benign fashion although malignant tumours do exist.

Surgical excision usually results in complete cure.

Up to 80% of localized fibrous tumour arise in relation to the visceral pleura.

Mesothelioma

The chest wall is covered by a thin sheet of mesothelial cells. Mesothelioma affects visceral or parietal pleura. There is formation of a layer of tissue which obliterates the pleural cavity; the tumour begins as nodules in the pleura. Mesothelioma is strongly associated with occupational exposure to asbestos especially fibres which are <0.25 μm diameter, e.g. crocidolite and amiosite.

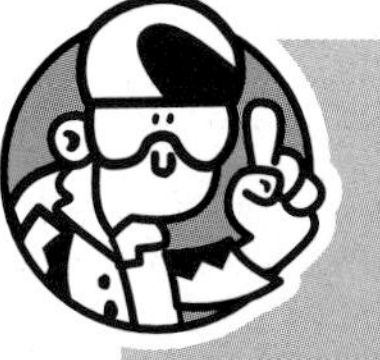

A tension pneumothorax should never be diagnosed by chest radiography. It is a clinical diagnosis which requires treatment before requesting a chest radiograph.

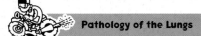

A latent period between exposure and development of illness can be up to 50 yrs.

Two histological varieties exist—50% of mesotheliomas have elements of both:

- Epithelial: Tubular structure.
- Fibrous: Solid structure with spindle-shaped cells.

Features of chest radiograph are:

- Pleural effusions commonest presentation.
- Unilateral pleural thickening.
- Nodular appearance.

Clinical features:

- Initial symptoms are very vague.
- Pain is the main complaint, often affecting sleep, along with dyspnoea.
- Pain results from infiltration of the tumour into the chest wall with involvement of intercostal nerves and ribs.

Open lung biopsy may be needed to confirm diagnosis.

No treatment is available and the condition is universally fatal. Pain responds poorly to therapy.

Metastases are common to hilar and abdominal lymph nodes with secondary deposits arising in lung, liver, thyroid, adrenals, bone, skeletal muscle, and brain. Death is due to infection, vascular compromise, and pulmonary embolus. The patient's symptoms become worse until death usually within 2yrs of diagnosis.

Patients eligible for industrial injuries benefit include those with mesothelioma, asbestosis, asbestos related carcinoma of bronchus, and coal-worker's pneumoconiosis.

Fig. 11.36 is a radiograph showing pleural thickening.

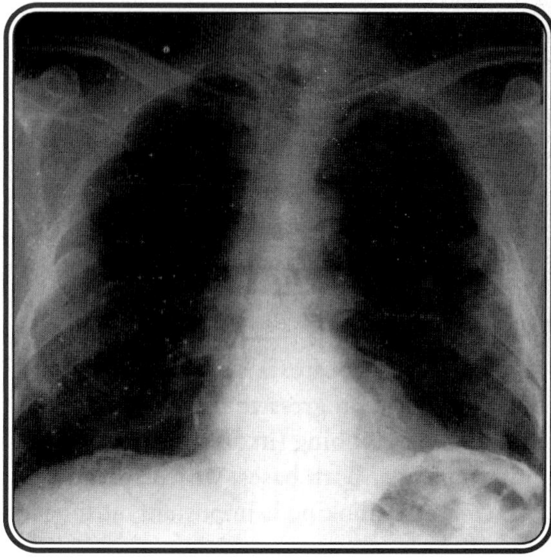

Fig. 11.36 Mesothelioma of the right pleura. The patient had a long history of asbestos exposure and has now developed a large pleural mass. Courtesy of Professor C D Forbes and Dr W F Jackson.

- **How do you differentiate between exudates and transudates in pleural effusions?**
- **Classify pleural effusions.**
- **Describe the different types of noninflammatory pleural effusions.**
- **Describe the clinical presentation of a tension pneumothorax and the subsequent management.**
- **Describe the relationship betwe en asbestos and pleural disease.**

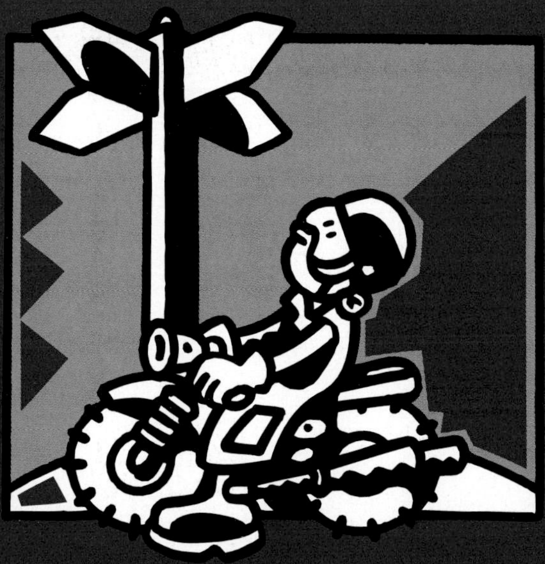

SELF-ASSESSMENT

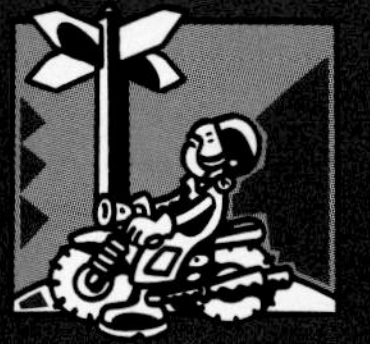

Multiple-choice Questions

Indicate whether each answer is true or false.

1. The following questions refer to adult haemoglobin (HbA):

(a) The concentration of HbA is higher in females than males, usually 13.5–17.5 g/L.
(b) Oxygen binds to iron in the ferric state.
(c) Haemoglobin is a good buffer because of its 38 histidine residues.
(d) Haemoglobin is capable of combining with both carbon dioxide and oxygen.
(e) It has a lower affinity for oxygen than fetal haemoglobin because of its α polypeptide chains.

2. Concerning sickle-cell anaemia:

(a) The disorder is autosomal dominant.
(b) The defective haemoglobin is caused by a substitution of valine for glutamate in position 6 of the β polypeptide chain.
(c) It is most prevalent in Caucasians.
(d) Crisis is more likely to occur at high-altitude.
(e) Crisis may lead to interpulmonary shunting and bone pain.

3. In asthma:

(a) Peak expiratory flow rate during an acute attack is usually decreased.
(b) The disease results from the destruction of lung parenchyma caused by smoking.
(c) An acute attack is characterized by bronchoconstriction which is not usually reversible.
(d) Acute asthma can be treated by using iprotropium bromide.
(e) Sodium cromoglycate inhibits phosphodiesterase therfore increasing cAMP which leads to bronchodilatation.

4. Concerning type I respiratory failure:

(a) PO_2 <8 kPa.
(b) Tolerance to high arterial oxygen tension develops.
(c) It must be treated effectively with low-dose oxygen.
(d) It differs from type II because it is of pulmonary vascular origin.
(e) It may be caused by spontaneous pneumothorax.

5. Bronchioles:

(a) Contain no smooth muscle in their walls therefore significantly reduce airway resistance.
(b) Differ from bronchi which contain cartilage in their walls.
(c) Contain clara cells which secrete highly proteinaceous fluid.
(d) Contribute to more than 50% of resistance to flow in the lower respiratory tract.
(e) Are a major site of gas exchange.

6. Peripheral chemoreceptors:

(a) Are located in the aortic bodies and carotid sinuses.
(b) Are sensitive to hypoxaemia.
(c) Have a relatively low blood flow enabling them to measure small changes in arterial blood gas tensions.
(d) Parasympathetic nerves cause vasoconstriction and reduce blood flow to these receptors.
(e) Are not sensitive to changes in arterial pH.

7. The following questions refer to the oxyhaemoglobin dissociation curve:

(a) Is shifted to the right with increased temperature.
(b) Is shifted to the left with decreased 2,3-DPG.
(c) Is identical for adult and fetal haemoglobin.
(d) The shape of the curve is unaffected by anaemia but the magnitude of the O_2 content is.
(e) Describes the variation of saturation of Hb with change in arterial PO_2

8. In fetal circulation:

(a) Ductus venosus carries oxygenated blood from the umbilical arteries to the inferior vena cava.
(b) Approximately 50% of the blood returning to the right side of the heart passes through the pulmonary circulation and back into the left atrium.
(c) The ductus arteriosus closes within the 1st 24 hours after birth in response to oxygenated blood.
(d) A patency usually exists between the left and right ventricles covered by the flap like septum secundum called the foramen ovale.
(e) The umbilical arteries carry oxygenated blood.

9. Mucosal associated lymphoid tissue in the respiratory tract:

(a) Is capsulated lymphoid tissue within the walls of the airways.
(b) It is a major site of lymphocytic activation in the airways.
(c) Activated lymphocytes will specifically home back to respiratory mucosa.
(d) Within the upper respiratory tract makes up Waldeyer's ring.
(e) Consists mainly of a distribution of T cells within the lamina propria covered by antigen tartgeting and transporting cells (M cells).

10. In quiet breathing:

(a) Ventilation is brought about by expansion of the chest mainly by the intercostal muscles.
(b) The abdominal muscles relax during inspiration.
(c) The elastic recoil forces of the lung parenchyma are responsible for expiration.
(d) Intrapleural pressure is more negative in expiration than inspiration.
(e) The diaphragm is responsible for approximately 75% of the work of ventilation.

11. Airway resistance:

(a) Increases with increasing air flow rate.
(b) Under laminar flow conditions is directly proportional to radius of the airway to the fourth power.
(c) Under laminar flow conditions is described by Poiseuille's law.
(d) Increases with increasing lung volume.
(e) Can be actively altered.

12. Central chemoreceptors:

(a) Can be found on the ventral surface of the medulla.
(b) Respond to hypoxaemia by increasing ventilation.
(c) Are sensitive to rapid changes in pH.
(d) Have a rapid response to PCO_2.
(e) Are responsible for about 10% of the control of ventialtion due to short term changes in PO_2.

13. Pulmonary vascular resistance:

(a) Is much lower than systemic vascular resistance.
(b) Can be further reduced by extension and recruitment of pulmonary capillaries.
(c) Is increased during exercise.
(d) Is lower than systemic vascular resistance since pulmonary vessels are easily distended.
(e) Is higher at the apex of the lung therefore reducing blood flow to the apex.

14. In emphysema:

(a) The distance for diffusion of O_2 is decreased due to destruction of the lung parenchyma.
(b) Over 10% of cases have α_1 antitrypsin deficiency.
(c) The overall surface area for gas exchange is decreased despite the increase in alveolar size.
(d) Patients develop stiff fibrotic lungs.
(e) Radial traction is increased therefore reducing airway resistance.

15. The following are true of V_A/Q:

(a) Ventilation increases towards the apex of the lung.
(b) Perfusion increases towards the base of the lung.
(c) V_A/Q is dependent on lung volume and posture.
(d) V_A/Q is uniform throughout the lung in the healthy patient.
(e) Perfusion is increased to those areas of lung which are under ventilated.

16. The following statements on the nasal cavities and air sinuses are true:

(a) The maxillary sinus and frontal nasal duct open into the middle meatus.
(b) Consist of three conchae and two air passages opening posteriorly into the choana.
(c) The sphenoethmoidal recess opens between the ethmoid sinus and the middle meatus.
(d) The nasolacrimal duct opens into the inferior meatus.
(e) The upper 2/3 of the nasal cavity is lined by olfactory mucosa.

17. Patent ductus arteriosus:

(a) Is a cyanotic heart disease.
(b) Gives a murmur of machinery quality.
(c) Results in blood flowing from the pulmonary artery to the aorta after birth.
(d) May lead to Eisenmenger's syndrome.
(e) Causes delay between radial and femoral pulses.

18. Metabolism in the lungs:

(a) The endothelium of the lungs is a major site of production of angiotensin converting enzyme (ACE).
(b) Administration of an ACE inhibitor such as captopril increases the breakdown of bradykinin.
(c) The lungs are involved in the removal of serotonin, prostaglandins, and leukotrienes.
(d) Type I pneumocytes produce surfactant.
(e) $PGF_{2\alpha}$ is removed by the lungs.

19. Mucociliary clearance:

(a) Cilia within the respiratory bronchioles waft mucus and debris up to the trachea.
(b) Is inhibited in smoking.
(c) Is reduced in Kartagener's syndrome due to highly viscous mucus secretion.
(d) Allows foreign material to be trapped in a sticky mucus film within the bronchi and bronchioles and then transported to the trachea and larynx.
(e) Forms part of the cough reflex.

20. The following statements about lung volumes are true:

(a) Functional residual capacity is that amount of air left within the lung following a maximal expiration.
(b) Vital capacity is usually about 4800 mL in the upright 70 kg male subject.
(c) Tidal volume can be measured by spirometry.
(d) Total lung volume is normally increased in fibrosing alveolitis.
(e) The ratio of FEV_1 / FVC is usually greater than 80% in asthmatics.

21. The following questions refer to gas diffusion from the lungs to the blood:

(a) Henry's law describes the solubility of a gas in a liquid.
(b) Carbon monoxide transfer is diffusion limited.
(c) The rate of diffusion of CO_2 is 15 times that of O_2.
(d) Diffusing capacity is an insensitive test of minor impediments to diffusion.
(e) The diffusion of oxygen from alveolar gas to the blood is dependent on the concentration difference between oxygen in the alveolar gas and oxygen in the blood.

22. The following statements relate to diffusion within the lungs:

(a) The rate of diffusion through a membrane is approximated by Fick's law.
(b) A reduced rate of diffusion may due to oedema of the alveola capillary wall.
(c) May be decreased due to a reduced overall area of the alveolar capillary membrane.
(d) O_2 therapy increases the rate of diffusion by increasing the partial pressure of oxygen in the blood.
(e) The transfer of N_2O across the alveolar capillary membrane is said to be diffusion limited.

23. The following questions relate to acid–base disturbance:

(a) Uncomplicated respiratory acidosis results from an increase in PCO_2.
(b) Renal compensation returns the blood gases and pH to normal in respiratory acidosis.
(c) Metabolic acidosis may cause respiratory compensation, increasing ventilation and therefore increasing PCO_2.
(d) The bicarbonate buffer system is important in the acid base balance because its pK is very close to physiological pH.
(e) Normal physiological pH range is 7.4–7.45.

24. During exercise:

(a) Moderate exercise causes an increased P_aCO_2 which drives the ventilatory increase.
(b) Oscillations in PCO_2 are similar in amplitude to those at rest due to the fine control achieved by the respiratory system.
(c) The build up of aerobic metabolites in severe exercise leads to an oxygen debt.
(d) In moderate exercise ventilation is excessive for metabolic demands and the subject hyperventilates.
(e) Exercise may be an important aetiological factor in some asthma.

25. Referring to α_1 antitrypsin:

(a) Deficiency results in increased breakdown of lung parenchyma due to the action of proteolytic enzymes.
(b) Is inhibited by aspirin.
(c) Deficiency accounts for approximately 2% of cases of emphysema.
(d) Deficiency is caused by smoking.
(e) Is important in the metabolism of angiotensin II to inactive peptides.

26. In asthma:

(a) The peak expiratory flow rate is increased.
(b) There is constriction of smooth muscle in bronchioles.
(c) There is mucosal oedema in the airways.
(d) Mucus secretion is decreased.
(e) House dust may be an allergen.

27. Ipatropium bromide:

(a) Is an antimuscarinic agent.
(b) May cuase urinary retention.
(c) Increases sputum viscosity.
(d) Causes bronchodilation.
(e) May affect intraocular pressure.

28. The following drugs are respiratory depressants:

(a) Barbiturates.
(b) Benzodiazepines.
(c) Alcohol.
(d) Doxapram.
(e) Aminophylline.

29. The following drugs used in the treatment of asthma have an anti-inflammatory action:

(a) Glucocorticoids.
(b) Salmeterol.
(c) Theobromine.
(d) Sodium chormoglycate.
(e) Terfernadine.

30. Pulmonary embolism:

(a) Is usually accompanied by lung infarction.
(b) Usually arises from the deep veins of the legs and pelvis.
(c) May cause sudden death.
(d) Is treated with anticoagulants.
(e) Is one of the most frequent causes of postoperative death.

31. Chronic bronchitis:

(a) Is associated with hypoplasia of bronchial mucus glands.
(b) Is defined as a productive cough for at least 3 months in 2 consecutive years.
(c) Is associated with *Haemophilus influenzae* infection.
(d) Usually coexists with emphysema.
(e) Is associated with cigarette smoking.

32. Coal worker's pneumoconiosis:

(a) Is caused by asbestos fibres.
(b) May cause respiratory failure.
(c) Is accompanied by focal emphysema.
(d) Has positive association with mesothelioma.
(e) May be caused by very low exposure to coal dust.

33. Salbutamol:

(a) Is an α agonist.
(b) May produce a tremor.
(c) Is usually administered sublingually.
(d) May cause hyperkalaemia with high doses.
(e) May cause peripheral vasoconstriction.

34. Small-cell carcinoma of the lung:

(a) Is usually treated by surgical resection.
(b) Shows keratin production on histological examination.
(c) Rarely metastasizes.
(d) Has a positive association with asbestos exposure.
(e) Usually arises in the periphery of the lung.

35. Malignant mesothelioma:

(a) Has a positive association asbestos exposure.
(b) Has usually metastasized by the time of presentation.
(c) May cause death by respiratory failure.
(d) May cause cardiac tamponade.
(e) Is an epithelial tumour.

36. Squamous cell carcinoma of the lung:

(a) Is associated with cigarette smoking.
(b) Shows mucin production on histological examination.
(c) May be treated by surgical resection.
(d) May produce ectopic hormones.
(e) May respond to radiotherapy.

37. Emphysema:

(a) Is associated with α_1 antitrypsin deficiency.
(b) Is defined as enlargement of airspaces distal to the terminal bronchiole with destruction of the alveolar walls.
(c) Causes decreased alveolar surface area.
(d) May cause respiratory failure.
(e) Is always associated with chronic bronchitis.

38. The following definitions are correct:

(a) Haemothorax—collection of blood in the pleural cavity.
(b) Pyothorax—collection of lymph in the pleural cavity.
(c) Pneumothorax—collection of air in the pleural cavity.
(d) Chylothorax—collection of pus in the pleural cavity.
(e) Hydrothorax—collection of fluid in the pleural cavity.

39. The following factors have a positive association with the development of lung carcinoma:

(a) Coal mining.
(b) Haematite mining.
(c) Asbestos exposure.
(d) Diffuse pulmonary fibrosis.
(e) Woodworking with hardwoods.

40. Sarcoidosis:

(a) May be diagnosed using the Shick test.
(b) Is characterized histologically by caseous granulomas.
(c) Affects the terminal ileum most frequently.
(d) May cause interstitial lung fibrosis.
(e) May cause hilar lymphadenopathy.

41. Adult respiratory distress syndrome (ARDS):

(a) Is associated with inhalation of sulphur dioxide.
(b) Is characterized by proliferation of type I pneumocytes.
(c) Is characterized by formation of hyaline membranes in the alveoli.
(d) Is rarely fatal.
(e) Is associated with endotoxic shock.

42. Cystic fibrosis:

(a) Is an autosomal dominant genetic condition.
(b) Is associated with meconium ileus in infants.
(c) May be confirmed by measuring sodium concentration in sweat.
(d) Is associated with bronchiectasis.
(e) Is associated with infertility in females.

43. Lobar pneumonia:

(a) Is most commonly due to *Klebsiella.*
(b) Is characterized by focal inflammation centred on airways.
(c) Affects females more commonly than males.
(d) Rarely produces pleural exudate.
(e) Produces grey hepatization before red hepatization.

44. Carcinoma of the larynx:

(a) Is usually of adenocarcinomatous differentiation.
(b) Usually affects subjects below 40 years of age.
(c) Affects females more commonly than males.
(d) Is associated with cigarette smoking.
(e) May produce dysphagia.

45. Wegener's granulomatosis:

(a) Is a necrotizing vasculitis.
(b) Affects mainly elastic arteries.
(c) Is caused by an anti-glomerular basement membrane antibody.
(d) Causes a necrotizing glomerulonephritis.
(e) Causes lung necrosis.

46. Bronchiectasis:

(a) Is associated with Kartagener's syndrome.
(b) Usually affects the upper lobes most prominently.
(c) May be complicated by amyloid formation.
(d) Is characterized by bronchial constriction.
(e) May be complicated by metastatic cerebral abscesses.

47. Doxapram:

(a) Is a respiratory depressant.
(b) May be given orally.
(c) May cause hypertension.
(d) Is contraindicated in coronary artery disease.
(e) Is used to treat asthma.

48. Fibrosing alveolitis:

(a) Usually occurs in young people.
(b) Is usually caused by inhaled dust.
(c) May result in 'honeycomb' lung.
(d) Gives an obstructive pattern of deficit on pulmonary function tests.
(e) Histologically shows proliferation of type II pneumocytes.

49. Atopic asthma:

(a) Is mediated by a type III hypersensitivity reaction.
(b) Is associated with hay fever.
(c) Is associated with eczema.
(d) Is associated with hypoplasia of bronchial wall smooth muscle.
(e) May be treated with β_2 agonists.

50. Aminophylline:

(a) Is a methylxanthine.
(b) Is given as a sustained-release oral preparation.
(c) May cause drowsiness.
(d) May cause a tachycardia.
(e) May be used with β_2 agonists to treat asthma.

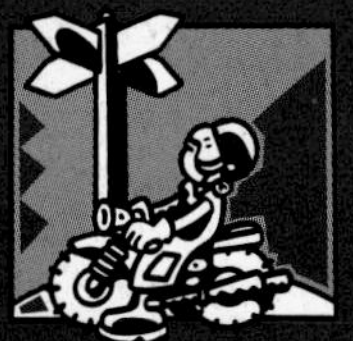

Short-answer Questions

1. What is surfactant? Describe its functions within the lung.
2. Define lung compliance and what factors change its value. What is meant by hysteresis of the pressure–volume curve?
3. Give the normal values for haemoglobin concentration in the blood. Draw the oxyhaemoglobin dissociation curve, giving arterial and venous PO_2.
4. Define the term venous admixture. If a patient presents with a pulmonary embolus how may their blood gases show a low PO_2 but a normal or lowered PCO_2?
5. Define airway resistance. How is calibre of the airway related to airway resistance under laminar flow conditions and what factors influence smooth muscle tone of the airways?
6. List three causes of hypoventilation. How does arterial PCO_2 relate to ventilation?
7. Define respiratory failure. What is the significance of type I and type II respiratory failure?
8. Define functional residual capacity and residual volume, giving normal values. How may these lung volumes be measured?
9. How does fetal haemoglobin differ from adult haemoglobin and what is meant by the double Bohr shift?
10. Define anatomical and physiological deadspace. Outline the Bohr method for measuring physiological deadspace.
11. Write short notes on lung carcinoma.
12. Write short notes on salbutamol.
13. Write short notes on pulmonary embolism.
14. Write short notes on pulmonary tuberculosis.
15. Write short notes on bronchial asthma.
16. Write short notes on bronchiectasis.
17. Write short notes on adult respiratory distress syndrome.
18. Write short notes on pneumonia in the immunocompromised.
19. Write short notes on malignant mesothelioma.
20. Write short notes on cystic fibrosis.

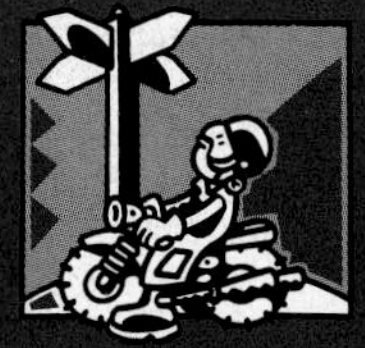

Essay Questions

1. Define airway resistance. What factors affect its magnitude?

2. What are peripheral and central chemoreceptors? Discuss the central control of breathing.

3. With the aid of a diagram, outline the fetal circulation. Discuss the changes at birth and give one example of a congenital defect resulting from failure of these changes to occur.

4. Discuss the changes that occur to the respiratory system in response to high altitude.

5. Write short notes on three of the following:
    - Carbon monoxide poisoning.
    - Sickle-cell anaemia.
    - Intrapleural pressure changes during breathing.
    - Dynamic compression of airways.
    - Regional variation of ventilation and perfusion in the upright lung.

6. Write an account of the pathologies which may be caused by asbestos in the lungs and chest.

7. Write an account of the respiratory diseases that have a proved association with cigarette smoking and the possible mechanisms for these associations.

8. Describe the pathologies of industrial lung disease.

9. Describe the different types of drugs which may be used in the treatment of asthma and their mechanisms of action.

10. Describe the different types of pulmonary function tests available in an average modern hospital and describe the abnormalities which may be seen in these: asthma; chronic obstructive pulmonary disease; and diffuse pulmonary disease.

1. a) F, b) F, c) T, d) T, e) F

2. a) F, b) T, c) F, d) T, e) T

3. a) T, b) F, c) F, d) T, e) F

4. a) T, b) F, c) F, d) F, e) T

5. a) F, b) T, c) T, d) F, e) F

6. a) F, b) T, c) F, d) F, e) F

7. a) T, b) T, c) F, d) T, e) T

8. a) F, b) F, c) T, d) F, e) F

9. a) F, b) T, c) T, d) T, e) F

10. a) F, b) T, c) T, d) F, e) T

11. a) T, b) F, c) T, d) F, e) T

12. a) T, b) F, c) F, d) T, e) F

13. a) T, b) F, c) F, d) T, e) T

14. a) T, b) F, c) T, d) F, e) F

15. a) F, b) T, c) T, d) F, e) F

16. a) T, b) F, c) F, d) T, e) F

17. a) F, b) T, c) F, d) T, e) F

18. a) T, b) F, c) T, d) F, e) T

19. a) F, b) T, c) F, d) T, e) F

20. a) F, b) T, c) T, d) F, e) F

21. a) T, b) T, c) F, d) F, e) F

22. a) T, b) T, c) T, d) F, e) F

23. a) T, b) F, c) F, d) F, e) F

24. a) F, b) F, c) F, d) F, e) T

25. a) T, b) T, c) T, d) F, e) F

26. a) F, b) T, c) T, d) F, e) T

27. a) T, b) T, c) F, d) T, e) T

28. a) T, b) T, c) T, d) F, e) F

29. a) T, b) F, c) F, d) T, e) T

30. a) F, b) T, c) T, d) T, e) T

31. a) F, b) T, c) T, d) T, e) T

32. a) F, b) T, c) T, d) F, e) F

33. a) F, b) T, c) F, d) F, e) F

34. a) F, b) F, c) F, d) T, e) F

35. a) T, b) F, c) T, d) T, e) F

36. a) T, b) F, c) T, d) T, e) T

37. a) T, b) T, c) T, d) T, e) F

38. a) T, b) F, c) T, d) F, e) T

39. a) F, b) T, c) T, d) T, e) F

40. a) F, b) F, c) F, d) T, e) T

41. a) T, b) F, c) T, d) F, e) T

42. a) F, b) T, c) T, d) T, e) F

43. a) F, b) F, c) F, d) F, e) F

44. a) F, b) F, c) F, d) T, e) T

45. a) T, b) F, c) F, d) T, e) T

46. a) T, b) F, c) T, d) F, e) T

47. a) F, b) F, c) T, d) T, e) F

48. a) F, b) F, c) T, d) F, e) T

49. a) F, b) T, c) T, d) F, e) T

50. a) T, b) T, c) F, d) T, e) T

1. Surfactant

Surfactant is a substance secreted by type II pneumocytes in the alveolus and contains phospholipid (dipalmitoyl phosphotidylcholine, DPC) which reduces the surface tension of the alveolar lining fluid. It therefore increases lung compliance. Surface tension of surfactant shows hysteresis, i.e. its surface tension is greater on expansion than on compression.

The function of surfactant in the lung:

- Reduce the work of breathing ($P \alpha T$—Laplace's law).
- Maintain alveolar stability ($P \alpha 1/R$—Laplace's law).

Alveoli vary in size, but because of surfactant the ST of the fluid that lines them is proportional to the surface area and so the $T:R$ ratio remains constant. Thus all the alveoli can be inflated by the same pressure. This prevents collapse of small alveoli and overinflation of large ones.

- Prevent transudation of fluid into the alveoli.

Surfactant reduces the hydrostatic pressure gradient across the capillary wall (by making tissue pressure less negative), so decreasing the ultrafiltration forces.

2. Lung compliance.

Lung compliance (C) is the ease of stretch of the lungs. It is the reciprocal of elastance (E).

C = 1/E

In the lungs this refers to the change in lung volume due to change of inflation pressure.

Compliance (C) = $\Delta V/\Delta P$

Factors affecting lung compliance.

- Disease, e.g.
  - Emphysema increases lung compliance.
  - Fibrotic lung desease decreases lung compliance.
- Lung volume.
- Surface tension forces within the lung.
- Production of surfactant.

Hysteresis:

If the pressure of inflation and deflation is plotted against lung volume this relationship forms a loop. This phenomenon is known as hysteresis of the pressure volume curve.

The reason for this hysteresis is due to a property of surfactant. The surface tension of surfactant is greater on expansion than on compression.

3. Normal values for Hb concentration:

Male: 13.5–18.0 g/dl
Female: 11.5–16.0 g/dl

Fig. 4.21A Oxyhaemoglobin dissociation curve.
Arterial PO_2 = 100 mmHg (13.3 kPa)
Venous PO_2 = 40 mmHg (5.3 kPa)

4. Venous admixture.

The venous admixture is that blood entering the systemic circulation that has bypassed gas exchange in the lungs. It will not have taken up oxygen or released its carbon dioxide, therefore its levels of PO_2 and PCO_2 are venous levels and for this reason it is termed venous admixture.

In a patient presenting with a pulmonary embolus, some of the pulmonary capillaries of the patient's lung will not be perfused with blood. The blood will not undergo gas exhange. This can be considered as a right-to-left shunt.

This initially causes a rise in arterial PCO_2 and a fall in PO_2. The rise in PCO_2 causes an increase in ventilation.

This allows those areas of lung that are well perfused and ventilated to lower the PCO_2 since a significant proportion (approximately 10%) of CO_2 is dissolved in the blood and is released in the alveoli.

Due to the shape of the oxyhaemoglobin dissociation curve any increase in ventilation doesn't increase O_2 carriage significantly and increases the dissolved O_2 by only a small amount (due to the low solubility of oxygen in the blood).

This non shunted blood returning to the systemic circulation has a higher PO_2 and a small amount of additional O_2 carriage (in dissolved form) but on mixing with shunted blood this additional dissolved O_2 quickly combines with the unsaturated Hb of the shunted blood and the PO_2 is lowered.

Fig. 10.4

Thus overventilating those areas which are well perfused allows the PCO_2 of arterial blood to be normal or lowered but arterial PO_2 cannot be increased to normal.

5. Airway resistance.

The resistance to flow of a gas within the airways of the lung, i.e. the resistance presented by the airways themselves, represented by the equation below:

$$\text{Airway resistance} = \frac{\text{mouth pressure} - \text{alveolar pressure}}{\text{air flow rate}}$$

$$\sim 0.5 - 1.5\ \text{cmH}_2\text{O}$$

In laminar flow, the flow of a fluid is in streamlines or laminae (parallel to the walls of the tube). The layer closest to the tube wall is believed to be stationary and therefore the resistance to flow is independent of roughness of the tube.

The resistance to flow is dependent on the viscosity of the fluid and the dimensions of the tube.

Poiseuille's law describes the resistance to flow under laminar flow conditions.

Resistance = $8\eta l/\pi r^4$

l = length of tube, r = radius of tube, η = viscosity of fluid.

Thus the resistance to flow is inversely proportional to the radius tube to the fourth power.

Factors affecting smooth muscle tone of the airways.

- Nervous factors

Parasympathetic (vagus) ==> bronchoconstriction. Acetyl choline (Ach) acting on muscurinic receptors. Major importance in control of bronchomotor tone

Sympathetic ==> bronchodilation. Noradrenaline acts via β_2 receptors. Not of major importance in controlling smooth muscle tone in man, but important in the treatment of asthma.

NANC (vagus) ==> bronchodilation. It is believed that vasoactive intestinal peptide (VIP) is the neurotransmitter responsible. Only effective neural bronchodilator pathway in man.

- Chemical factors

Constriction caused by: Histamine via H_1 receptors
Prostaglandins
Leukotrienes
Bradykinin
5-HT via 5-HT_2 receptors
Irritants
Cold air
Increased PCO_2 via central chemorecptors
Decreased PO_2 via peripheral chemoreceptors
Dilation caused by:
Adrenaline via β_2 receptors
NO
Fig. 3.30

6. Hypoventilation.

Causes:

- Obstruction—Asthma
  —Chronic obstructive airways disease (COAD).
  —Foreign body (e.g. peanut)
- Brainstem lesion.
- Pneumothorax.
- Trauma, e.g. fractured rib.
- Drugs, notably opiates which depress central chemoreceptors.
- Hypoventilation also occurs in alkalosis
  $pH = pK + \log [HCO_3^-]$
  P_aCO_2

The relationship between P_aCO_2 and ventilation is given by the equation

$P_aCO_2 = (VCO_2 / V_A) \times K$
K= constant, V_A = alveolar ventilation
VCO_2 = Amount of CO_2 expired
P_aCO_2 = Partial pressure of CO_2 in the alveolus

Under steady state conditions P_aCO_2 is in equilibrium with P_aCO_2. P_aCO_2 will therefore decrease with increased alveolar ventilation. This assumes the metabolic prodution of CO_2 is constant, e.g. under resting conditions.

7. Respiratory failure.

Respiratory failure is a clinical diagnosis made on the result of an arterial blood gas. If the P_aO_2 <8 kPa then the patient is in respiratory failure.

Type I respiratory failure is defined as a P_aCO_2 <6.5 kPa. This is a ventilation/perfusion mismatch.

Type II respiratory failure is defined as a P_aCO_2 >6.5 kPa. This is a situation of hypoventilation and the CO_2 in the blood cannot be blown off in the lungs.

The significance of type II failure is that tolerance to high levels of PCO_2 may have built up. High PCO_2 leads to renal compensation where plasma $[HCO_3^-]$ increases. The pH therefore returns to normal (Henderson–Hasselbalch equation, above), so reducing the central chemoreceptor drive. Hypoxic drive (low PO_2) from the peripheral chemoreceptors then becomes vital. This is significant clinically because if these patients are given high levels of oxygen, this raises the PO_2 reducing the drive for ventilation. The patient may therefore stop breathing and die. In type II respiratory failure limit the oxygen concentration to 24% using a venturi device.

8. Functional residual capacity is: that volume of air remaining in the lung at the end of quiet expiration and is about 2200 mL in the normal healthy subject.

Residual volume is: the amount of air left within the lung after maximal expiration and is about 1200 mL in the normal healthy subject.

Functional residual capacity and residual volume can be measured by the helium dilution method. The subject gives a maximum exhalation and then inhales a mixture of helium and oxygen from a bag, for a few breathes rebreathing into the bag. A simple component balance is carried out on helium. Because the initial volume and concentration of helium is known the initial volume (residual volume) of the lung can be calculated knowing the final helium concentration. To calculate the FRC the subject starts the procedure at end of quiet expiration.

Fig. 3.5

9. Fetal haemoglobin

Fetal haemoglobin differs from normal adult haemoglobin HbA as it has two α and two γ polypeptide subunits rather than two α and two β subunits.

Fetal haemoglobin (HbF):

- Has higher affinity for O_2 as its γ chain can bind 2,3, DPG less avidly than the β chains of HbA.
- Is able to bind O_2 at lower partial pressures (i.e. maternal venous PO_2)

The double Bohr shift

- Release of CO_2 from fetal Hb causes a shift to the left of the fetal oxyhaemoglobin dissociation curve, thus increasing the affinity of HbF for O_2.
- This CO_2 binds to maternal haemoglobin causing a shift to the right of the maternal oxyhaemoglobin dissociation curve, reducing the affinity of maternal Hb for O_2.
- O_2 is therefore released by maternal Hb and bound by fetal Hb.

10. Anatomical deadspace.

Anatomical deadspace refers to those areas of the airways not involved in gas exchange but involved in the bulk flow of gas to the gas exchange surface. i.e. the volume of the conducting zone.

Normal volume is approximately 150 mL (2 mL/kg) at rest.

Physiological deadspace

Physiological deadspace is a functional measure and it is the sum of the anatomical deadspace (volume of the conducting zone) and the volume of any non-functioning areas of the respiratory zone (alveolar deadspace).

In the normal healthy lung the alveolar deadspace is very small (<5 mL).

Fig. 3.8 shows the Bohr method for measuring physiological deadspace.

11.

- Incidence—most common malignant tumour in Britain.
- Age distribution—middle to old age.
- Sex distribution—males > females at present but incidence increasing in females.
- Predisposing factors—cigarette smoking; asbestos exposure; haematite mining; radon and other radioactive gases; chemical exposure: nickel, chromates, mustard gas, arsenic, coal-tar distillates; diffuse pulmonary fibrosis.
- Macroscopic appearances—tumour, usually central (squamous cell, small cell and large cell undifferentiated), sometimes peripheral (mainly adenocarcinoma).
- Microscopic appearances—squamous cell, small cell, adenocarcinoma, large cell undifferentiated.
- Spread—direct to pleural, lymphatics to hilar lymph nodes includes subcarinal node, blood to anywhere in systemic circulation if erodes into a pulmonary vein, transcoelomic across pleural cavities.
- Prognosis—related to type (worse with small cell) and stage (some squamous cell and adenocarcinomas may be surgically resectable) but overall 5-year survival rate 4–7%.

12.

- β2 adrenoceptor agonist drug.
- Used in the treatment of asthma.
- Actions—bronchodilation.
- Mechanism—β2 adrenoceptor stimulation leading to increased levels of cAMP within cells.
- Routes of administration—aerosol, oral, intramuscular, intravenous.
- Side effects—tremor, nervous tension, headache, peripheral vasodilatation, tachycardia, hypokalaemia after high doses.
- Drug interactions—no point in giving when the patient is on a β-blocking drug, may potentiate other sympathomimetics.

13.

- Types of embolic material:

  Thrombo-embolism—commonest by far, originate from deep veins of legs and pelvis

  Fat—from fractures of large bones containing bone marrow or massive subcutaneous injury

  Air—pressurized intravenous infusions, coronary bypass surgery, decompression sickness

  Amniotic fluid—during labour

  Tumour—important in development of metastases, rarely have haemodynamic effects.
- Effects of pulmonary embolism.
- Sudden death (filling main pulmonary arteries).
- Severe chest pain and breathlessness.
- Distal lung infarction.
- Development of pulmonary hypertension.

14.

- Causative organism—*Mycobacterium tuberculosis, Mycobacterium avium intracellulare* in immunocompromised host.
- Predisposing factors—alcoholism, diabetes mellitus, AIDS, other causes of immunosuppression.
- Primary tuberculosis—inhalation of mycobacteria leads to primary focus of infection in lung with accompanying lymph node enlargement (Ghon focus), focus becomes scarred and walled off from rest of lung but viable organisms may persist for years.
- Secondary tuberculosis—reactivation of primary focus, affects lung apices, progression if host immunity is reduced.
- Miliary tuberculosis—wide dissemination by blood in immunocompromised host.
- Immunization—BCG.

• Drug therapy—problems with resistance therefore more than one agent e.g. isoniazid, rifampicin, and pyrazinamide.

15.

• Definition—reversible airways obstruction due to increased irritability of bronchial tree
• Types—atopic, non-atopic, aspirin-induced, occupation, allergic bronchopulmonary aspergillosis
• Mechanisms—type I, type II, type III, or mixture of both hypersensitivity reactions. Release of histamine, slow-reacting substance of anaphylaxis (SRS-A), platelet activating factor, 5-hydroxytryptamine.
• Consequences—bronchial obstruction with distal overinflation, mucus plugging of bronchi, mucous gland hypertrophy, bronchial wall smooth muscle hypertrophy, inflammation extending into bronchioles, possible centrilobular emphysema.
• Treatment—β2 adrenoceptor agonists, sodium chromoglycate, aminophylline, corticosteroids.

16.

• Definition—permanent dilatation of bronchi and bronchioles.
• Causes—bronchial obstruction and severe inflammation e.g. measles, cystic fibrosis, chronic bronchitis, immotile cilia syndromes.
• Features—dilatation of bronchi and bronchioles, destruction of alveolar walls, pulmonary fibrosis.
• Complications—pneumonia, empyema, septicaemia, meningitis, metastatic abscesses, amyloid formation.
• Treatment—symptomatically, treat active infections, surgical resection of localized areas of bronchiectasis.

17.

• Definition—diffuse alveolar damage with hyaline membrane formation.
• Causes—shock (haemorrhagic, cardiogenic, septic, anaphylactic, endotoxic), trauma (direct lung trauma, multisystem trauma), viral or bacterial pneumonia, gas inhalation (nitrogen dioxide, sulphur dioxide, chlorine), narcotic abuse, ionizing radiation, gastric aspiration, disseminated intravascular coagulation, oxygen toxicity.
• Pathogenesis—diffuse alveolar damage +/- oxygen toxicity.
• Histological appearances—hyaline membranes, oedema, red cells, proliferation type II pneumocytes.
• Prognosis—50% mortality rate.

18.

• Causes of immunosuppression—human immunodefiency virus–acquired immune deficiency syndrome (AIDS), severe combined immunodeficiency (SCID), intensive chemotherapy and/or radiotherapy for disseminated malignancy.
• *Pneumocystis carinii* pneumonia—common in AIDS, protozoan, diffuse radiographic shadowing.
• Cytomegalovirus—common in AIDS, reactivation of dormant infection or acquisition through blood products, owl's eye nuclei.
• Aspergillus—any immunodeficiency state, fungus, diagnosis from bronchial washings.
• Cryptococcus—fungus, diagnosis by serology or direct examination of bronchial washings.
• Varicella zoster virus.
• Lymphoma—neoplastic but can give a pneumonic pattern on radiography.
• Kaposi's sarcoma—neoplastic but can give a pneumonic pattern on radiography.

19.

• Definition—malignant tumour derived from mesothelial cells.
• Site—usually pleural, sometimes peritoneal.
• Causes—asbestos especially blue asbestos, long latent period (20–30 years).
• Macroscopic appearances—malignant tumour, often spindle-celled, distinguished from diffuse adenocarcinoma.
• Spread—locally through pleural cavities, distant spread less common.
• Prognosis—poor, may remain localised for years but universally fatal.

20.

• Definition—autosomal recessive genetic condition affecting production of exocrine secretions.
• Pathogenesis—deletion in cystic fibrosis transmembrane conductance regulator leading to unresponsiveness to cAMP control and defective transport of chloride ions and water across epithelial cell membranes.
• Diagnosis—genetic or weat test (increased sodium concentration).
• Features—meconium ileus in infants, failure to thrive, recurrent lung infections, bronchiectasis, chronic pancreatitis, malabsorption, male infertility.

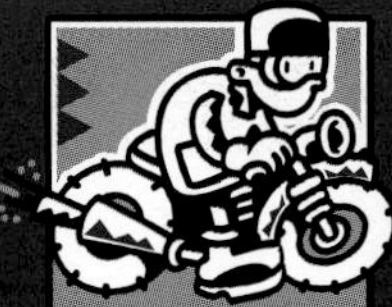

Index

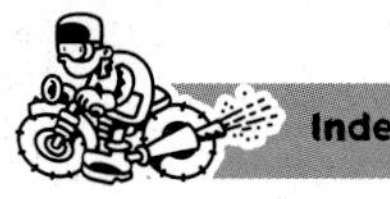

B

C

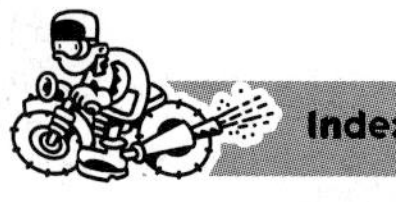

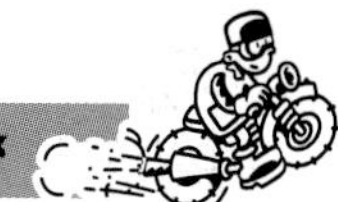

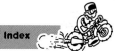

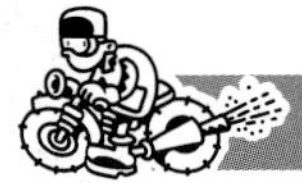

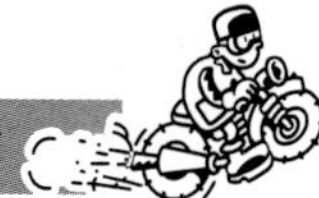

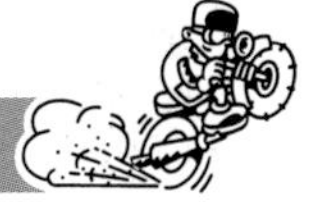

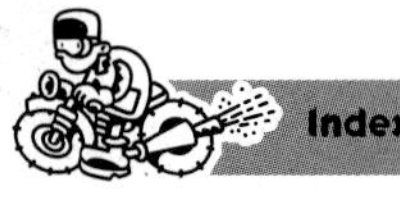

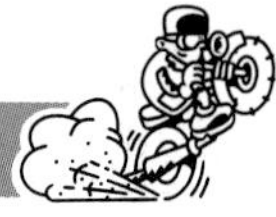

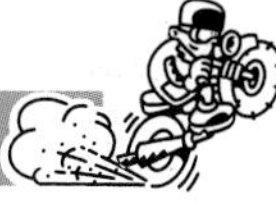

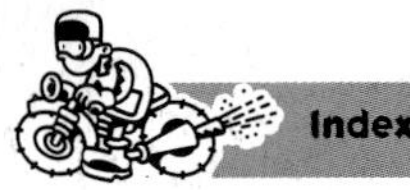